Developing Clinical Judgment

for Practical/Vocational Nursing and the Next-Generation **NCLEX-PN**® Examination

Developing Clinical Judgment

for Practical/Vocational Nursing and the Next-Generation **NCLEX-PN®** Examination

DONNA D. IGNATAVICIUS, MS, RN, CNE, CNEcl, ANEF
Speaker and Curriculum Consultant;
Founder, Boot Camp for Nurse Educators;
President, DI Associates, Inc.
Littleton, Colorado

ELSEVIER

Elsevier
3251 Riverport Lane
St. Louis, Missouri 63043

DEVELOPING CLINICAL JUDGMENT FOR PRACTICAL/VOCATIONAL NURSING AND THE NEXT-GENERATION NCLEX-PN® EXAMINATION ISBN: 978-0-323-76197-0

Library of Congress Control Number: 2021933784

Executive Content Strategist: Lee Henderson
Director, Content Development: Laurie Gower
Senior Content Development Specialists: Melissa Rawe; Laura Goodrich
Publishing Services Manager: Julie Eddy
Senior Project Manager: Jodi Willard
Design Direction: Amy Buxton

Printed in India

Last digit is the print number: 9 8 7 6 5 4 3 2 1

Contributor/Reviewers

CONTRIBUTOR

Tami Little, DNP, RN
Corporate Director of Nursing
Vista College
Richardson, Texas

REVIEWERS

Gayle Bassett, MSN, RN, CNE
Instructor of Nursing
Vista College
Las Cruces, New Mexico

Tami Little, DNP, RN
Corporate Director of Nursing
Vista College
Richardson, Texas

Preface

Purpose of This Workbook

As soon as 2023, the National Council of State Boards of Nursing (NCSBN) is expected to begin using the Next-Generation NCLEX® Examination (NGN) for nursing licensure based on its new model of clinical judgment. This one-of-a-kind workbook is designed to help students enrolled in prelicensure programs for licensed practical/vocational nursing (LPN/LVN) practice to:

- Develop clinical judgment skills for LPN/LVN practice to ensure patient safety and quality of care.
- Prepare for success on the NGN through practical thinking exercises in which students apply clinical reasoning (cognitive) skills to make appropriate clinical judgments.

This book is intended for students to use throughout their nursing program. Thinking exercises are available for all major areas of clinical specialty practice, with a heavy emphasis on the care of older adults. Each exercise provides challenging client situations with multiple NGN-style test items. For many thinking exercises, the clinical situation evolves into continuing care, requiring the student to address changing client conditions.

Organization of This Workbook

This student-friendly workbook is organized by nursing concepts but is easy to use in any type of prelicensure LPN/LVN nursing program; it is divided into three distinct parts for a total of 23 chapters. Each health problem throughout the book consists of 7 or 8 thinking exercises for student practice, including at least one unfolding case study followed by one or more single-episode/stand-alone cases with NGN-style test items:

Part 1 (Chapters 1 and 2). Chapter 1 provides an introduction to clinical judgment as a primary skill needed by practicing nurses. Chapter 2 offers tips for answering the practical thinking exercises in the workbook.

Part 2 (Chapters 3 to 14). This section focuses on thinking exercises that address nursing care for clients experiencing commonly occurring medical-surgical and mental health problems across the life span.

Part 3 (Chapter 15 to 23). This section includes thinking exercises that focus on coordinating care for older adults. Although pharmacology is integrated throughout this book, Chapter 23 is dedicated the nurse's role in medication administration.

Answer Key. The last section of this workbook presents the answers, rationales, and clinical judgment cognitive skills for each thinking exercise. In addition, the student is provided with reference pages where they can read more about each health problem.

References. At the end of the book is the list of textbook citations that are used for reference for the thinking exercises.

In summary, *Developing Clinical Judgment for Practical/Vocational l Nursing and the Next-Generation NCLEX-PN®* Examination is the first learning resource focused exclusively on developing the clinical judgment skills needed for LPN/LVN student success on the NGN and in clinical practice.

Donna D. "Iggy" Ignatavicius

To all of the nursing educators who are passionate about teaching,
and to all of the nursing students who are passionate about learning
and thinking-in-action like a nurse!

About the Author

Donna D. Ignatavicius received her diploma in nursing from the Peninsula General School of Nursing in Salisbury, Maryland. After working as a charge nurse in medical-surgical nursing, she became an instructor in staff development at the University of Maryland Medical Center. She then received her BSN from the University of Maryland School of Nursing. For 5 years she taught in several schools of nursing while working toward her MS in Nursing, which she received in 1981. Donna then taught in the BSN program at the University of Maryland, after which she continued to pursue her interest in gerontology and accepted the position of Director of Nursing of a major skilled-nursing facility in her home state of Maryland. Since that time, she has served as an instructor in several associate degree and baccalaureate nursing programs. Through her consulting activities, faculty development workshops, and international nursing education conferences (such as Boot Camp for Nurse Educators®), Donna is nationally recognized as an expert in nursing education. She is currently the President of DI Associates, Inc. (http://www.diassociates.com/), a company dedicated to improving health care through education and consultation for faculty. In recognition of her contributions to the field, she was inducted as a charter Fellow of the prestigious Academy of Nursing Education (ANEF) in 2007, received her Certified Nurse Educator (CNE) credential in 2016, and earned her Certified Clinical Academic Nurse Educator (CNEcl) in 2020.

Acknowledgments

Publishing a textbook would not be possible without the combined efforts of many people. With that in mind, I would like to extend my deepest gratitude to the many people who were such an integral part of this journey.

My contributor, Dr. Tami Little, developed excellent chapters to ensure clinical relevancy within the scope of PN/VN practice for this publication. Gayle Bassett, an expert clinician and instructor in an LPN program, provided invaluable suggestions and encouragement throughout the development of this textbook.

The staff of Elsevier has, as always, provided meaningful guidance and support throughout every step of the planning, writing, revision, and production of this new title. Executive Content Strategist Lee Henderson worked closely with me from the early stages of this title to help me hone and focus the project from start to finish. Senior Content Development Specialists Melissa Rawe and Laura Goodrich then worked with me to from vision to publication.

My acknowledgments would not be complete without recognizing the dedicated team of Educational Solutions Consultants and other key members of the Sales and Marketing staff who helped to put this book into your hands.

Contents

Exemplars

Mental Health Nursing

Pediatric Nursing

Pharmacology

Introduction: Developing Clinical Judgment

PART 1

1 The Use of Clinical Judgment in Practical/Vocational Nursing Practice

Learning Outcomes

1. Explain why the National Council of State Boards of Nursing (NCSBN) is planning to add a focus on clinical judgment for the Next-Generation NCLEX® (NGN).
2. Identify the six cognitive (thinking) skills of the NCSBN Clinical Judgment Measurement Model (NCJMM).
3. Compare the steps of the clinical problem-solving process (nursing process), the stages of Tanner's Model of Clinical Judgment, and the six cognitive (thinking) skills of the NCJMM.

Key Terms

Clinical judgment The observed outcome of critical thinking and decision making. It is an iterative process that uses nursing knowledge to observe and access presenting situations, identify a prioritized client concern, and generate the best possible evidence-based solutions in order to deliver safe client care (NCSBN, 2019b).

Clinical problem-solving process (nursing process) A scientific approach to client care that includes data collection, planning, implementation, and evaluation (NCSBN, 2020).

Clinical reasoning The process of thinking about a client situation *in a specific context* while considering client and family concerns.

Critical thinking Purposeful, informed, outcome-focused thinking that results in evidence-based clinical judgment.

At this point in your nursing program, you have likely learned about the clinical problem-solving process that is used by practical/vocational nurses to provide safe, client-centered care in a variety of health care settings. Depending on the state or province where your program is located, you may refer to this process as the *nursing process*. This chapter will help you build on what you know about the clinical problem-solving process (nursing process) and explain why the nursing profession currently supports clinical judgment as the best standard for making clinical decisions. This workbook focuses on helping you learn how to use thinking skills to make sound clinical judgments in a variety of clinical situations to keep clients safe.

Review of the Clinical Problem-Solving Process (Nursing Process) and Critical Thinking

The clinical problem-solving process (nursing process) is a systematic method for problem solving that nurses use to make safe, client-centered care decisions. It has been used since the 1960s as the gold

Table 1.1 Comparison of the RN and LPN/LVN Role Using the Nursing Process

Step of the Nursing Process	RN Role	LPN/LVN Role
Assessment	Performs the comprehensive client assessment	Collects and organizes client data (NCSBN, 2020; Williams, 2018)
Analysis (Diagnosis)	Interprets assessment data to identify client problems	Primarily an RN function but may assist in the identification of health needs for clients across the life span
Planning	Develops a plan of care to meet expected client outcomes	Contributes to the plan of care to meet desired or expected outcomes
Implementation	Uses knowledge, skills, and abilities to meet the needs of clients requiring promotion, maintenance, and/or restoration of health	Performs competencies and skills needed to care for clients with commonly occurring health problems that have predictable outcomes (NCSBN, 2020)
Evaluation	Assesses the client's response to interventions to determine if expected outcomes are met and if changes are needed in the plan of care	In coordination with the RN, measures the progress toward the expected client outcomes

LPN/LVN, Licensed practical nurse/licensed vocational nurse; *RN,* registered nurse.

standard to guide nursing practice and has been measured on the nursing licensure examinations (NCLEX) for many years. State and provincial regulatory bodies, such as state boards of nursing, have since differentiated the role of the registered nurse (RN) and licensed practical nurse/licensed vocational nurse (LPN/LVN) related to the nursing process (NCSBN, 2019a). As shown in Table 1.1, the LPN/LVN uses all of the steps of the nursing process.

As you might expect, using a problem-solving approach for the nursing process requires thinking and reasoning. In the 1990s the concept of **critical thinking** was introduced in nursing practice and nursing education. Since that time, experts have agreed that nurses use many types of thinking to make the best evidence-based decisions for their clients.

Clinical reasoning is also an important concept needed for the nursing process. In their landmark nursing education study, Benner et al. (2010) stated that **clinical reasoning** is the process of thinking about a client situation *in a specific context* while considering client and family concerns. The National Council of State Boards of Nursing (NCSBN) combined these concepts and defined the **clinical problem-solving process (nursing process)** for the LPN/LVN as "a scientific approach to client care that includes data collection [assessment], planning, implementation and evaluation" (NCSBN, 2020, p. 5). This definition is currently an Integrated Process for the NCLEX-PN®, but it does not include the analysis step.

Expanding From the Nursing Process to Clinical Judgment

In 2006 Tanner presented findings from her classic meta-analysis research that examined how practicing nurses actually think and make clinical decisions. She noted that nurses use *clinical thinking* skills more than the nursing process, and become more competent in these skills with experience and confidence. Tanner found that making sound clinical judgments requires thinking skills such as clinical reasoning and critical thinking. These skills include:

- *Noticing* a situation or changes in a client situation triggers the nurse to collect more data for an accurate and thorough assessment. Noticing is affected by what the nurse brings to the situation, such as knowledge, ethical perspective, and expectations. These factors are part of professional relational practice (Doane & Varcoe, 2015).
- *Interpreting* requires clinical reasoning to analyze the data to determine the client's problem(s).

Table 1.2 Comparison of the Nursing Process With Tanner's Model of Clinical Judgment

Tanner's Model of Clinical Judgment	Nursing Process (AAPIE)
Noticing	Assessment
Interpreting	Analysis
Responding	Planning Implementation
Reflecting	Evaluation

- *Responding* is taking action or monitoring the client based on current evidence to prevent, detect early, or resolve client problem(s).
- *Reflecting* allows the nurse to determine the client's status and think about what he or she learned from the situation that can be used in another similar situation.

As you might expect, Tanner's Model of Clinical Judgment can be aligned with the steps of the nursing process (Table 1.2). However, in some ways, Tanner's components are distinctly different from the nursing process steps. For example, *Noticing* is the trigger that informs the nurse to perform the assessment. The *Interpreting* component involves identifying the client's problems and encourages the nurse to communicate effectively with appropriate health care team members. *Responding* may require implementing one or more specific actions or frequently monitoring a client's clinical situation. *Reflecting* not only includes evaluating the results of client care, but it also allows the nurse to examine his or her actions in addressing the clinical situation.

The National League for Nursing (NLN) included *nursing judgment* as one of its four new nursing graduate competencies for all types of nursing programs. The NLN states that nursing judgment encompasses three processes: critical thinking, clinical judgment, and integration of best evidence into practice. Nurses use these processes when they make sound decisions about client care. More specifically, the use of nursing judgment involves these specific skills (www.nln.org):

- Processing information
- Thinking critically
- Evaluating the evidence
- Applying relevant knowledge
- Using problem-solving skills
- Reflecting on the situation

The National Council of State Boards of Nursing (NCSBN) Clinical Judgment Measurement Model (CJMM)

The NCSBN is responsible for the design and content of the registered and practical nursing licensure examinations known as the NCLEX-RN® and NCLEX-PN®. Over the past few years, the NCSBN conducted a study to determine if the current nursing licensure examinations for entry into practice are adequate to ensure that new nurses are competent in clinical judgment skills to protect the public. Current NCLEX® test items do not measure all layers or cognitive (thinking) skills of clinical judgment, but rather focus more on the nursing process (Dickison et al., 2019). Multiple-choice and SATA (Select All That Apply) questions are not currently presented in a detailed clinical situation and tend to primarily measure content knowledge as right or wrong. The current test items measure only whether new graduates are *minimally safe* to practice, such as the examples in Box 1.1. The NCSBN study showed that although knowledge is essential, it is not enough to ensure appropriate clinical judgement. Put another way, having knowledge does not translate to having good clinical judgment skills. However, using good clinical judgment requires adequate content knowledge (Dickison et al., 2019).

Box 1.1 Examples of Current NCLEX-PN® Test Item Formats

Multiple-Choice Test Item

A client is admitted to the memory care unit with a diagnosis of Alzheimer disease. What action by the nurse is the most important when caring for the client?

A. Be sure that the client receives environmental stimulation.
B. Reorient the client every time the nurse enters the room.
C. Protect the client and keep him or her safe.
D. Use validation therapy when communicating with the client.

To answer this test item, the student or graduate only needs to know that ensuring safety is essential when caring for a client with dementia. Choice C is the best response. Having this knowledge does not guarantee clinical judgment ability.

Select All That Apply Item

A nurse is caring for a client who has congestive heart failure. Which signs and symptoms would the nurse expect when collecting and organizing data? **Select all that apply.**

A. Shortness of breath
B. Lower extremity edema
C. Bruising on the chest and abdomen
D. Increased respiratory rate
E. Bounding radial pulse

To answer this test item, the student or graduate only needs to know the common signs and symptoms of a client who has heart failure. Choices A, B, D, and E are the correct responses. Bruising (Choice C) is not common in clients who have heart disease but is often found in clients who have clotting problems. Having this knowledge does not guarantee clinical judgment ability.

As a result of the study, NCSBN is planning a major change in the nursing licensure examinations, called the Next-Generation NCLEX® (NGN), that will include *measuring* new graduates' competence in clinical judgment. In one of their first steps toward meeting that outcome and based on an extensive literature review, the NCSBN defines **clinical judgment** as the observed outcome of critical thinking and decision making. It is "an iterative [repeating] process that uses nursing knowledge to observe and access presenting situations, identify a prioritized client concern, and generate the best possible evidence-based solutions in order to deliver safe client care" (NCSBN, 2018, p. 12).

In the near future, the NCLEX-RN® and NCLEX-PN® are expected to measure the ability of new graduates to use clinical reasoning skills based on the NCSBN Clinical Judgment Measurement Model (NCJMM) (Dickison et al., 2019; NCSBN, 2019b). Using case scenarios that contain more client clinical information, the six cognitive (thinking) skills in the model that you will need to use to make sound clinical judgments include:

- **Recognize Cues (What matters most?)**
  Cues are elements of data that provide important information for the nurse as a basis for making client decisions. In a clinical situation, determine which data are *relevant* (directly related to client outcomes or the priority of care) versus *irrelevant* (unrelated to client outcomes or priority of care). Decide what data are the *most* important and of *immediate* concern to the nurse.
- **Analyze Cues (What could it mean?)**
  Consider the cues in the context of the client history and situation. Think about how the identified relevant cues relate to the client's condition or history. Identify cues that support a particular cue in the situation and determine why certain cues are more concerning to the nurse than others. Determine what could be going on in the situation and what client condition(s) is (are) suspected.
- **Prioritize Hypotheses (Where do I start?)**
  Consider all possibilities about what is occurring in the client situation. Consider their urgency and risk for the client. Determine which explanations are *most likely* and *most serious* and why to identify the priority for care.

Table 1.3 Comparison of the Nursing Process, Tanner's Model of Clinical Judgment, and the NCSBN Clinical Judgment Measurement Model Cognitive Skills

Nursing Process (AAPIE)	Tanner's Model of Clinical Judgment	NCJMM Cognitive Skills
Assessment	Noticing	Recognize Cues
Analysis	Interpreting	Analyze Cues
Analysis	Interpreting	Prioritize Hypotheses
Planning	Responding	Generate Solutions
Implementation	Responding	Take Action
Evaluation	Reflecting	Evaluate Outcomes

NCSBN, National Council of State Boards of Nursing.

- **Generate Solutions (What can I do?)**
  Identify expected client outcomes. Using the priority or priorities identified, plan specific actions that could achieve the desirable outcomes. Consider which actual or potential actions should be *avoided* or are *contraindicated* because they could be harmful for the client in the given situation.
- **Take Action (What will I do?)**
  Decide which nursing actions will address the highest priorities of care and determine in what priority these actions will be implemented. Actions can include, but are not limited to, collecting additional data, documentation, requesting primary health care provider orders, performing nursing skills, health teaching, additional client monitoring, and coordination with health care team members.
- **Evaluate Outcomes (Did it help?)**
  Evaluate the actual client outcomes in the situation and compare to desired or expected outcomes. Determine what client findings indicate an improvement or a decline in the client's condition. Decide if the selected nursing actions were effective or ineffective.

The NCJMM incorporates the nursing process and Tanner's Model of Clinical Judgment and reasoning. Table 1.3 shows the alignment between these three models or processes. Chapter 2 in this workbook presents examples of the thinking exercises used in this book and how to approach them to determine the best responses using the thinking skills of the NCJMM. When possible the thinking exercises are similar to proposed test item formats that may be used in the future on the NGN.

Thinking and Discussion Questions

1. Consider the information about the lack of clinical judgment skills of nursing graduates as discussed in this chapter. Why do you think that new nurses lack these essential skills? Consider all factors in your response.

2. Review all three models of clinical decision making as presented in Table 1.3. What are the advantages and disadvantages of each model? Which model do you think is most useful in nursing practice and why?

References

Asterisk (*) indicates a classic or definitive work on this subject.

*Benner, P., Sutphen, M., Leonard, V., & Day, L. (2010). *Educating nurses: A call for radical transformation.* San Francisco: Jossey-Bass.

Dickison, P., Haerling, K. A., & Lasater, K. (2019). Integrating the National Council of State Boards of Nursing Clinical Judgment Model into nursing educational frameworks. *Journal of Nursing Education, 58*(2), 72–78.

Doane, G. H., & Varcoe, C. (2015). *How to nurse: Relational inquiry with individuals and families in changing health and health care contexts.* Philadelphia: Wolters Kluwer.

National Council of State Boards of Nursing (NCSBN). (Winter, 2018). Measuring the right things: NCSBN's next generation NCLEX® endeavors to go beyond the leading edge. In *Focus.* Chicago: Author.

National Council of State Boards of Nursing (NCSBN). (2020). *NCLEX-PN® Examination: Test plan for the National Council Licensure Examination for Practical Nurses.* Chicago: Author.

National Council of State Boards of Nursing (NCSBN). (2019a). *NCLEX-RN® Examination: Test plan for the National Council Licensure Examination for Professional Nurses.* Chicago: Author.

National Council of State Boards of Nursing (NCSBN). (2019b). The clinical judgment model. *Next generation NCLEX News. (Winter).* 1-6.

*Tanner, C. A. (2006). Thinking like a nurse: A research-based model of clinical judgment. *Journal of Nursing Education, 45,* 204–211.

Williams, P. (2018). *deWit's Fundamental concepts and skills for nursing* (5th ed.). St. Louis: Elsevier.

How to Apply Clinical Judgment Thinking Skills to Ensure Client Safety

2

Learning Outcomes

1. Describe how to apply the six cognitive (thinking) skills to client situations to make sound clinical judgments.
2. Identify tips for success when using the six clinical judgment thinking skills to answer various types of case study exercises in this workbook.

All nurses need to make sound clinical judgments to provide safe client care. As introduced in Chapter 1, the National Council of State Boards of Nursing (NCSBN) developed a clinical judgment model similar to well-respected existing models. This new model was the basis for a major NCSBN study on how to measure the clinical judgment ability of new nursing graduates to protect the public. This chapter will help you learn how to apply clinical judgment and "think like a nurse" using a variety of sample thinking exercises. Tips for applying the clinical judgment skills model to correctly answer these thinking exercises will also be described.

Clinical judgment cognitive skills are mental (thinking) processes that are required for appropriate and sound clinical judgment. As introduced in Chapter 1, these skills include:

- Recognize Cues
- Analyze Cues
- Prioritize Hypotheses
- Generate Solutions
- Take Action
- Evaluate Outcomes

Applying the Clinical Judgment Cognitive Skills

Clinical judgment can be learned through thinking exercises to apply nursing knowledge to clinical practice using a variety of client situations. Consider the case study in Box 2.1 on the next page.

Based on the assessment findings in the case study example, determine which data are relevant or important to the nurse in the situation. To *Recognize Cues* as a cognitive skill of clinical judgment in this thinking exercise, you need knowledge of:

- Normal physiologic and psychosocial changes associated with aging
- Adult normal or usual range for vital signs
- Signs and symptoms of adequate peripheral circulation
- Normal ranges for lab values

Tip for Success

To help identify the cues that are of greatest concern to the nurse, determine which data are unusual or abnormal for the client or clinical situation.

Box 2.1 Case Study Example

An 82-year old female client was admitted with a right hip fracture as a result of a fall at home. According to her daughter, she has a history of osteoporosis, for which she takes a bisphosphonate, and controlled diabetes mellitus type 2, for which she takes an oral hypoglycemic agent. The client lives alone in a senior housing apartment and depends on her daughter for appointments, food shopping, and other errands. Prior to her fall, she was ADL independent and had no history of dementia. Yesterday afternoon she had a right open reduction, internal fixation (ORIF) of the hip. Initial nursing shift assessment findings this morning include:

- Is alert but does not respond verbally to questions
- Apical pulse = 92 beats/min and irregular
- Blood pressure = 166/90 mm Hg
- Breath sounds clear in all lung fields
- Hypoactive bowel sounds × 4
- Restless and "picking at" bedcovers
- Right hip surgical dressing dry and intact
- Yells when right leg is touched
- No palpable right pedal pulse; left pedal pulse present
- Right foot cooler and paler than left foot
- Oxygen saturation = 95% (on 2 L/min via nasal cannula [NC])
- Finger stick blood glucose (FSBG) = 288 mg/dL (16 mmol/L)

To apply that knowledge, you likely selected the following *relevant* cues from the case study example that are most concerning to the nurse. The italicized phrases explain why these data are the most important.

- Apical pulse = 92 beats/min and irregular *(tachycardia with irregular heart rhythm)*
- Blood pressure = 166/90 mm Hg *(increased above normal range)*
- Restless and "picking at" bedcovers *(may suggest an underlying problem)*
- Yells when right leg is touched *(not usual behavior when one is touched)*
- No palpable right pedal pulse; left pedal pulse present *(peripheral pulses are usually present and equal in both legs)*
- Right foot cooler, swollen, and paler than left foot *(temperature and color should be same in both legs; swelling is not a normal finding)*
- FSBG = 288 mg/dL (16 mmol/L) *(increased above normal range)*

The next thinking skill is *Analyze Cues.* Analyzing or interpreting the meaning of data in this case requires you to have knowledge of:

- Postoperative complications of hip ORIF
- Normal range for FSBG

Based on your interpretation, you then need to *Prioritize Hypotheses.* For this thinking skill, consider all possibilities about what is happening in the case and then determine the *most likely* explanations and priority needs. The cues in the case study reveal that the client is *most likely* experiencing a musculoskeletal surgical complication, which is possible decreased blood circulation in the right (surgical) leg as evidenced by the findings that the right foot is cooler and paler than the left foot and there is no pedal pulse that the nurse can feel in the right foot. The client's elevated vital signs and restlessness are most likely due to acute pain. In addition, her FSBG value is above the normal range because surgery and trauma are stressors, especially for a client who has diabetes. The priorities for this client's care would be to:

1. Improve the circulation in the surgical (right) leg.
2. Reduce the client's acute pain.
3. Manage the client's elevated blood glucose.

The fourth thinking skill is to *Generate Solutions* that will meet expected client outcomes. The desired outcomes in this situation are that the client will:

- Have adequate peripheral circulation in both lower extremities.
- Have adequate pain control (2–3/10).
- Have vital signs within usual parameters.
- Have an FSBG within normal limits.

Consider which actual or potential nursing actions will meet these outcomes. Consider which ones should be *avoided* or are *contraindicated.* Remember that some actions could be harmful for the client in the given situation. This thinking skill requires you to have knowledge of how to care for the client and with which members of the health care team you will need to coordinate that care.

Tip for Success

To effectively Generate Solutions, first determine what expected outcomes are essential for the client. Then plan solutions or actions that will meet these outcomes.

When considering possible solutions, recall that poor lower extremity circulation is an arterial problem. That means that elevating the client's left leg will *decrease* peripheral circulation and can potentially cause harm. Possible nursing actions based on best practice (and not in priority order) might include:

- Notify the surgeon regarding peripheral circulation changes.
- Check right pedal pulse with a Doppler ultrasound device.
- Administer an analgesic as prescribed to manage pain.
- Administer regular insulin as prescribed to lower her blood glucose.
- Avoid elevating the left leg.

The fifth clinical judgment thinking skill is to *Take Action.* Determine the priority order that you want to take action from the list of possible actions. Priorities are determined by factors such as urgency, difficulty, or complexity of the client's situation. To meet the client's identified needs, the priority approach to care would be to:

1. Improve the peripheral circulation in the surgical (right) leg.
2. Reduce the client's acute pain.
3. Manage the client's elevated blood glucose.

Based on these priorities, the nurse's actions would include:

1. Check right pedal pulse with a Doppler ultrasound device.
2. Avoid elevating the right leg.
3. Notify the surgeon regarding peripheral circulation.
4. Administer an analgesic as prescribed to manage pain.
5. Administer regular insulin as prescribed to lower blood glucose.

Tip for Success

When deciding on actions to take and in what order of priority, determine which client problems are potentially life- or limb-threatening and the urgency of each problem. Notifying the primary health care provider is not usually the most important action because there are always other actions that you can take first as a nurse.

The last thinking skill is to *Evaluate Outcomes* by reassessing the client after nursing actions have been implemented. Remember that the desired outcomes are that the client will:

- Have adequate peripheral circulation in both lower extremities.
- Have adequate pain control (2–3/10).
- Have vital signs within usual range for the client.
- Have an FSBG within normal range.

When reassessing the client, if she met these outcomes, the nursing actions would be *effective.* If the outcomes were not met, then the nursing actions would be *ineffective* or *not related.*

Applying the Cognitive Skills for Thinking Exercises in this Workbook

The clinical case exercises in this workbook will help you apply the six thinking skills of the NCSBN's Clinical Judgment Measurement Model (NCJMM) using a variety of formats. Examples of these formats are described in this section with the thinking skill being assessed. Although the following examples are focused on adult medical-surgical and mental health nursing, this workbook presents thinking exercises across the life span and across all specialties.

The answers and rationales for the correct responses to the thinking exercises are provided in the last section of this workbook. Please note that the reference pages provided for each thinking exercise do not necessarily contain the answers, but rather provide the knowledge that is needed as a basis for answering the exercises. The thinking skill needed to answer each exercise is also identified in that section.

The five types of thinking exercises in this workbook are *similar* to the new test item format categories on the Next-Generation NCLEX® (NGN) that will measure the cognitive skills of clinical judgment and include:

- Highlight
- Cloze
- Drag and Drop
- Multiple Response
- Matrix

Highlight Thinking Exercises

The case study presented earlier in this chapter can be used as a Highlight Thinking Exercise as shown in to the following example to measure the cognitive skill of *Recognize Cues*. Many of these exercises in this book will ask you to select the most important or relevant information in a client scenario.

Highlight Thinking Exercise Example 1

An 82-year old female client was admitted with a right hip fracture as a result of a fall. According to her daughter, she has a history of osteoporosis, for which she takes a bisphosphonate, and controlled diabetes mellitus type 2, for which she takes an oral hypoglycemic agent. The client lives alone in a senior housing apartment and depends on her daughter for appointments, food shopping, and other errands. Prior to her fall, she was ADL independent and had no history of dementia. Yesterday afternoon she had a right open reduction, internal fixation (ORIF) of the hip. Initial nursing shift assessment findings this morning include:

- Is alert but does not respond verbally to questions
- Apical pulse = 92 beats/min and irregular
- Blood pressure = 166/90 mm Hg
- Breath sounds clear in all lung fields
- Hypoactive bowel sounds × 4
- Restless and "picking at" bedcovers
- Right hip surgical dressing dry and intact
- Yells when right leg is touched
- No palpable right pedal pulse; left pedal pulse present
- Right foot cooler and paler than left foot
- Oxygen saturation = 95% (on 2 L/min via nasal cannula [NC])
- Finger stick blood glucose (FSBG) = 288 mg/dL (16 mmol/L)

Highlight the client findings that require immediate follow-up by the nurse.

Answers

- Is alert but does not respond verbally to questions
- Apical pulse = 92 beats/min and irregular

- Blood pressure = 166/90 mm Hg
- Breath sounds clear in all lung fields
- Hypoactive bowel sounds × 4
- Restless and "picking at" bedcovers
- Right hip surgical dressing dry and intact
- Yells when right leg is touched
- No palpable right pedal pulse; left pedal pulse present
- Right foot cooler and paler than left foot
- Oxygen saturation = 95% (on 2 L/min via nasal cannula [NC])
- Finger stick blood glucose (FSBG) = 288 mg/dL (16 mmol/L)

Rationales

The findings indicate that the right leg may have peripheral circulation problems as indicated by an absent pulse, pallor, and coolness. The elevated vital signs and restlessness could be caused by acute pain. The oxygen saturation is within normal limits and needs to be monitored rather than followed up as an immediate concern for the nurse at this time. The finger stick blood glucose (FSBG) value is above normal and needs to be improved. Therefore these findings should concern the nurse and indicate an urgent need to follow up.

CJ Cognitive Skill

Recognize Cues

Reference

Linton & Matteson, 2020, pp. 890–895

A few of the thinking exercises in this book present a client situation and ask you to select or highlight the information that indicates that the client is or is not progressing as expected. This variation of the Highlight Exercise measures your ability to *Evaluate Outcomes*. For example, consider the following thinking exercise about a postoperative young adult who had a laparoscopic cholecystectomy.

Highlight Thinking Exercise Example 2

Nurses' Notes

10/12/21 11:30 a.m. (1130) Alert and oriented. Returned from a laparoscopic cholecystectomy to PACU with report of 7/10 pain with nausea. Vomited × 2 small amount greenish liquid. Wound closures intact and abdomen soft. Apical pulse 100 and B/P 152/88. Placed in semi-Fowler position and taking small sips of ginger ale. -- *D. L. Jones, LPN*

Highlight the data in the Nurses' Notes above that would indicate that the client is *not* progressing as expected.

Answers

Nurses' Notes

10/12/21 11:30 a.m. (1130) Alert and oriented. Returned from a laparoscopic cholecystectomy to PACU with report of 7/10 pain with nausea. Vomited × 2 small amount greenish liquid. Wound closures intact and abdomen soft. Apical pulse 100 and B/P 152/88. Placed in semi-Fowler position and taking small sips of ginger ale. -- *D. L. Jones, LPN*

Rationales

In the Nurses' Notes, the client is alert and oriented but has more pain than expected and has nausea and vomiting most likely due to general anesthesia. Vital signs are elevated, which may be caused by acute pain and nausea and vomiting. The expected findings would be that the client's pain and nausea are under control and that the pulse and blood pressure return to the client's usual values.

CJ Cognitive Skill

Evaluate Outcomes

Reference

Linton & Matteson, 2020, pp. 284–296

Cloze Thinking Exercises

Cloze Thinking Exercises will ask you to complete statements about a presented client clinical situation. For each blank, you will have one or more lists of options from which to select. Consider the following example, which requires you to *Prioritize Hypotheses.*

Cloze Thinking Exercise Example

An 82-year-old female client is admitted with a left fractured hip. She is scheduled for an open reduction, internal fixation (ORIF) of the hip. Her history reveals a diagnosis of osteoporosis, for which she takes a bisphosphonate; diabetes mellitus type 2, for which she takes an oral hypoglycemic agent; and hypertension, for which she takes a diuretic. The client quit smoking 10 years ago but enjoys an occasional glass of wine to help her sleep. **Complete the following sentences by choosing the *most likely* options for the missing information from the lists of options provided.**

The nurse should recognize that after hip surgery the client will be at a high risk for ____1____ because of ____2____ and for ____3____ because of her ____4____. The overall ***priority*** for her postoperative care will be to prevent ____5____ and manage her ____6____.

Options for 1	Options for 2	Options for 3
Dementia Infection Stroke Dysreflexia Myocardial infarction Depression	History of smoking Alcoholism Osteoporosis Hypertension Diabetes mellitus Dehydration	Delirium Urinary incontinence Bowel obstruction Alcohol withdrawal Nausea and vomiting Persistent pain
Options for 4	**Options for 5**	**Options for 6**
History of smoking and drinking Advanced age and hip fracture Multiple medications Persistent pain High blood pressure Hypoxia	Fat embolism syndrome Diabetic ketoacidosis Skin breakdown from traction Immobility complications Lung congestion Vertebral compression fractures	Blood pressure Serum glucose levels Emotional behaviors Persistent pain Alcohol withdrawal Hypothermia

Answers

The nurse should recognize that after hip surgery the client will be at a high risk for <u>infection</u> because of <u>diabetes mellitus</u> and for <u>delirium</u> because of her <u>advanced age and hip fracture</u>. The overall ***priority*** for her postoperative care will be to prevent <u>immobility complications</u> and manage her <u>serum glucose levels</u>.

Rationales

Clients who have diabetes are always at risk for acquiring an infection after surgery. Even for clients who are alert and oriented, those of advanced age who experience a hip fracture are at a very high risk for delirium (acute confusion). A large number of clients who have a hip fracture die from complications of immobility, and therefore preventing those complications is a desired postoperative outcome. Surgery is a trauma to the body and affects the ability of most clients to have stable serum glucose levels. These clients are often placed on sliding scale insulin during their hospital stay.

CJ Cognitive Skill

Prioritize Hypotheses

Reference

Linton & Matteson, 2020, pp. 284–296

Drag and Drop Thinking Exercises

Drag and Drop Thinking Exercises are used in this workbook to help you learn to apply the cognitive skills of *Generate Solutions* or *Take Action.* If this type of item was presented electronically, you could "drag and drop" the actions on the left to the column on the right using a computer mouse. An example of this type of thinking exercise is presented below. In this exercise a list of nursing actions is provided from which you will choose to match with actual or potential client problems.

Drag and Drop Thinking Exercise Example

A 65-year-old male client was admitted to the orthopedic surgical unit following a right total knee arthroplasty (TKA) for severe osteoarthritis. The nurse is developing an individualized client plan of care that includes actions to help prevent or detect potential complications as early as possible during his hospital stay. **Indicate which nursing action listed in the far-left column is appropriate for each potential TKA complication. Note that not all actions will be used.**

Nursing Action	Potential TKA Complication	Appropriate Nursing Action for Each TKA Complication
1 Maintain sequential or pneumatic compression stockings or devices while client is in bed.	Surgical site infection	
2 Provide cold application to the surgical area.	Deep vein thrombosis (DVT)	
3 Monitor the surgical wound daily for increased redness or cellulitis.	Urinary tract infection (UTI)	
4 Assess the client's ability to void without discomfort.	Pressure injury	
5 Maintain client's right leg in a neutral position while in bed.	Decreased surgical knee range of motion	
6 Keep the client's heels off of the bed.		
7 Remind the client to perform knee and leg exercises as instructed by the physical therapist.		

Answers

Nursing Action	Potential TKA Complication	Appropriate Nursing Action for Each TKA Complication
1 Maintain sequential or pneumatic compression stockings or devices while client is in bed.	Surgical site infection	**3** Monitor the surgical wound daily for increased redness or cellulitis.
2 Provide cold application to the surgical area.	Deep vein thrombosis (DVT)	**1** Maintain sequential or pneumatic compression stockings/devices while client is in bed.
3 Monitor the surgical wound daily for increased redness or cellulitis.	Urinary tract infection (UTI)	**4** Assess the client's ability to void without discomfort.
4 Assess the client's ability to void without discomfort.	Pressure injury	**6** Keep the client's heels off of the bed.
5 Maintain client's right leg in a neutral position while in bed.	Decreased surgical knee range of motion	**7** Remind the client to perform knee and leg exercises as instructed by the physical therapist.
6 Keep the client's heels off of the bed.		
7 Remind the client to perform knee and leg exercises as instructed by the physical therapist.		

Rationales

To detect surgical infection early, the nurse would carefully monitor the client's surgical wound for redness, swelling, and inflammation (cellulitis) (Action 3). To help prevent DVT from venous stasis and decreased mobility, venous return from the lower extremities is assisted by use of sequential or pneumatic compression stockings or devices (Action 1). The client will be in bed immediately after surgery, so he is at a potential risk for heel breakdown (pressure injury). Therefore the nurse would position his heels such that they are not on the bed by using pillows or other devices (Action 6). The nurse would assess the client's urinary output and ability to void without discomfort to monitor for UTI (Action 4). The client would be assisted out of bed to a chair later in the day, and physical therapy would begin at the bedside. Therefore the client needs to practice knee and leg exercises to promote knee flexion and extension needed to ambulate and climb stairs (Action 7).

CJ Cognitive Skill

Generate Solutions

Reference

Linton & Matteson, 2020, pp. 861–863

Multiple Response Thinking Exercises

Multiple Response Thinking Exercises may be used to measure one of several cognitive skills. For this type of exercise you will need to select the correct responses from a list of choices to answer the question. You might recognize this type of question because it is used now for the NCLEX but with only 5 or 6 choices. The Multiple Response exercise usually has 5 to 10 choices. The following example assesses the thinking skill of *Take Action*.

Multiple Response Thinking Exercise Example

The nurse is assessing a 37-year-old female client who had a partial thyroidectomy this afternoon.

Vital Signs	
Temperature	98°F (36.7°C)
Heart rate	84 beats/min
Respirations	22 breaths/min
Blood pressure	108/68 mm Hg
Oxygen saturation	100% (on oxygen via nasal cannula 2 L/min)
Laboratory Test Results This Morning	
Hematocrit	37% (0.37)
Serum sodium	141 mEq/L (141 mmol/L)
Serum potassium	3.9 mEq/L (3.9 mmol/L)
Serum calcium	9.5 mg/dL (2.37 mmol/L)

Physical Assessment Findings

- Reports throat pain as a 7/10 on a 0 (no pain) to 10 (severe pain) pain scale
- Reports hoarseness at times
- Breath sounds clear in all lung fields
- No respiratory distress
- Bowel sounds active × 4
- Neck surgical dressing intact

Which of the following actions would the nurse take? **Select all that apply.**

_____ A. Administer an analgesic as soon as possible.

_____ B. Monitor the client for muscle twitching and tingling.

_____ C. Request an order for oral potassium.

_____ D. Check behind the client's neck for bleeding.

_____ E. Place the client in a flat position to increase blood pressure.

_____ F. Teach the client that hoarseness is usually temporary.

_____ G. Perform orthostatic blood pressure checks.

Answers

A, B, D, F

Rationales

Choice A is an appropriate action for the nurse to take because the client reports a pain level of 7, indicating uncontrolled surgical pain. The desired pain level for most clients is 2 to 3. The client's most current serum calcium level is within the normal range of 9 to 10.5 mg/dL (2.25 to 2.62 mmol/L), but the nurse would assess for signs of low calcium, including tetany (muscle twitching) and tingling, especially around the mouth, in case there was parathyroid injury during surgery (Choice B). The nurse would check for active bleeding by inspecting and feeling behind the client's neck (Choice D). Temporary hoarseness is not unusual for clients having thyroid removal because the laryngeal nerve can become injured or irritated (Choice F).

CJ Cognitive Skill

Take Action

Reference

Linton & Matteson, 2020, pp. 954–956

Matrix Thinking Exercises

In this workbook, Matrix Exercises may be used to practice one of several thinking skills. To measure *Generate Solutions,* you will be given a list of nursing actions and asked to determine if each action would be ***Anticipated*** or ***Indicated, Contraindicated,*** or ***Non-Essential*** for the client situation presented. The following Matrix Thinking Exercise is used to *Evaluate Outcomes* as to whether the implemented nurse's actions were ***Effective, Ineffective,*** or ***Unrelated.***

Matrix Thinking Exercise Example

The nurse is assessing a 75-year-old female client after implementing interventions to manage delirium. **For each assessment finding, use an X to indicate whether the implemented interventions were <u>Effective</u> (helped to meet expected outcomes), <u>Ineffective</u> (did not help to meet expected outcomes), or <u>Unrelated</u> (not related to the expected outcomes).**

Assessment Finding	Effective	Ineffective	Unrelated
Oriented to person and place			
Becomes combative when touched			
Recognizes her visiting daughter			
Uses her call light appropriately			
Awake all night but sleeps all day			
States she has no pain			

Answers

Assessment Finding	Effective	Ineffective	Unrelated
Oriented to person and place	X		
Becomes combative when touched		X	
Recognizes her visiting daughter	X		
Uses her call light appropriately	X		
Awake all night but sleeps all day		X	
States she has no pain			X

Rationales

Delirium is acute confusion that commonly occurs in older adults and clients who have substance use disorder. In addition to confusion, the client often has problems with his or her sleep-wake cycle and had behavioral or emotional manifestations, such as yelling, agitation, and aggression. Being oriented, recognizing her daughter, and using her call light appropriately indicate that her delirium is resolving as a result of appropriate nursing and interprofessional collaborative actions.

CJ Cognitive Skill

Evaluate Outcomes

Reference

Morrison-Valfre, 2017, pp. 192–193

Thinking and Discussion Questions

1. Which of the six cognitive skills in the NCJMM do you think will be the *least* difficult for you to apply in the thinking exercises and why? Which one(s) will be the *most* difficult to apply and why?

2. For the cognitive skills you think are *most* difficult, what strategies might you need to develop or what resources might you need to use to help improve your thinking?

Clinical Judgment for Clients Across the Life Span Experiencing Commonly Occurring Health Problems

PART 2

Perfusion

3

Exemplar 3A. Bradycardia/Pacemaker (Medical-Surgical Nursing: Older Adult)

Unfolding Case (3A-1 Through 3A-6)

Thinking Exercise 3A-1

An 82-year-old female client who lives in a senior living facility contacts the nurse after a fall. The client is alert and oriented when the nurse arrives to her room; the client reports, "I was sitting on the toilet and then I was on the floor. I'm not sure what happened but I wasn't feeling well so I used my alert button to call for help." The client's vital signs are: heart rate (HR), 55 beats/min; respirations, 18 breaths/min; blood pressure (BP), 136/48 mm Hg, oxygen saturation, 96% (on room air [RA]). After completing an initial assessment and ensuring the client is safe, the nurse reviews the client's medical record.

History and Physical	Nurses' Notes	Vital Signs	Laboratory Results

82-year-old female residing in an independent living senior center

Heart rate (HR), 55 beats/min

Medications:

- Acetaminophen 650 mg orally every 4–6 hours PRN
- Aspirin (ASA) 325 mg orally daily
- Atenolol 50 mg orally daily
- Calcium carbonate 1000 mg chewable tabs every 4–6 hours PRN
- Clopidogrel 75 mg orally daily
- Nifedipine ER 30 mg orally daily

Recent physical assessment (2 weeks ago):

- Alert and oriented × 3
- Lung fields clear throughout
- Denies chest pain or shortness of breath
- Bowel sounds present × 4
- Reports constipation, encouraged to drink more fluids
- Denies incontinence or difficulty voiding
- Right forearm skin tear, 2 mm × 4 mm, scant serous drainage

Highlight client data in the History and Physical Note above that may have contributed to the client's fall.

Thinking Exercise 3A-2

An 82-year-old female client who lives in a senior living facility contacts the nurse after a fall. The client is alert and oriented when the nurse arrives to her room; the client reports, "I was sitting on the toilet and then I was on the floor. I'm not sure what happened but I wasn't feeling well so I used my alert button to call for help." The client's vital signs are: heart rate (HR), 55 beats/min; respirations, 18 breaths/min; blood pressure (BP), 136/48 mm Hg; oxygen saturation, 96% (on room air [RA]). The client has a history of hypertension, coronary artery disease, and gastroesophageal reflux disease (GERD), for which she is prescribed aspirin, atenolol, nifedipine, clopidogrel, and chewable calcium carbonate tabs. Which questions would the nurse ask to determine the effect of the health history on her recent fall? **Select all that apply.**

_____ A. "What did you eat for breakfast?"

_____ B. "Do you get light-headed when you rise from a chair or bed?"

_____ C. "Are you experiencing burning when you urinate?"

_____ D. "Do you remember your heart rate prior to taking your medications this morning?"

_____ E. "Do you have to strain to move your bowels?"

_____ F. "Did you feel nauseated or sweaty prior to fainting?"

_____ G. "What is your name, today's date, and the place where we are currently?"

_____ H. "Did you start smoking cigarettes again?"

Thinking Exercise 3A-3

An 82-year-old female client who lives in a senior living facility contacts the nurse after a fall. The client is alert and oriented when the nurse arrives to her room; the client reports, "I was sitting on the toilet and then I was on the floor. I'm not sure what happened but I wasn't feeling well so I used my alert button to call for help." The client's vital signs are: heart rate (HR), 55 beats/min; respirations, 18 breaths/min; blood pressure (BP), 136/48 mm Hg; oxygen saturation, 96% (on room air [RA]). The client has a history of hypertension, coronary artery disease, and gastroesophageal reflux disease (GERD), for which she is prescribed aspirin, atenolol, nifedipine, clopidogrel, and chewable calcium carbonate tabs. **Complete the following sentences by choosing the *most likely* options for the missing information from the lists of options provided.**

This client is ***most likely*** experiencing _______1_______, which refers to a heart rate slower than 60 beats/min. The ***most likely*** explanation for this client's slow heart rate is _______2_______. If the heart rate is too slow, the brain and other organs may not get enough oxygen, causing symptoms of dizziness and fainting. Additional symptoms may include _______3_______, _______4_______, and _______5_______.

Options for 1 and 2	Options for 3, 4, 5
Antihypertensive drugs	Aortic murmur
Atrial fibrillation	Bounding pulses
Bradycardia	Chest pain
Hemorrhage	Confusion
Hypertension	Diaphoresis
Old age	Erythema
Pulse deficit	Fatigue
Tachycardia	Pulmonary edema

Thinking Exercise 3A-4

An 82-year-old female client who resides in a senior living facility contacts the nurse after a fall. The client is alert and oriented when the nurse arrives to her room; the client reports, "I was sitting on the toilet and then I was on the floor. I'm not sure what happened but I wasn't feeling well so I used my alert button to call for help." The client's vital signs are: heart rate (HR), 55 beats/min; respirations, 18 breaths/min; blood pressure (BP), 136/48 mm Hg; oxygen saturation, 96% (on room air [RA]). The client has a history of hypertension, coronary artery disease, and gastroesophageal reflux disease (GERD), for which she is prescribed aspirin, atenolol, nifedipine, clopidogrel, and chewable calcium carbonate tabs. **Use an X to show whether the nursing actions below are Indicated (appropriate or necessary) or Contraindicated (could be harmful) for the client's care at this time.**

Nursing Action	Indicated	Contraindicated
Administer oxygen via nasal cannula.		
Teach the client to rise slowly from lying or sitting positions.		
Hold the client's atenolol dose.		
Encourage the client to exercise daily.		
Assess orthostatic vital signs.		
Administer a laxative each morning.		

Thinking Exercise 3A-5

An 82-year-old female client who lives in a senior living facility experienced an episode of syncope 2 days ago and was admitted to a telemetry unit. Current medications are aspirin 325 mg orally daily, clopidogrel 75 mg orally daily, atenolol 25 mg orally daily, heparin 5000 units subcutaneously three times a day, and famotidine 20 mg orally twice a day. After dinner, the client's telemetry monitor alerts the nurse to an irregular cardiac rhythm. The nurse collects the following assessment data. Client findings include:

- Alert and oriented × 3
- Heart rate (HR) = 44 beats/min
- Reports chest pain and shortness of breath
- Chest rise symmetrical
- Respirations = 20 breaths/min
- Oxygen saturation = 92% (on room air [RA])
- Blood pressure (BP) = 118/48 mm Hg
- Electrocardiography indicates third-degree atrioventricular block

After implementing emergent interventions, the nurse prepares to transfer the client's care to a registered nurse. What essential information will the nurse include in a hand-off report to the registered nurse? **Select all that apply.**

_____ A. Activity level including ambulating in the hall independently this morning

_____ B. Administration of atropine as needed

_____ C. Current vital signs and any supplemental oxygen administered

_____ D. Immunization record including seasonal influenza and pneumococcal vaccines

_____ E. Client's level of consciousness and orientation status

_____ F. Family history of neurovascular events including ischemic and hemorrhagic strokes

_____ G. When the last schedule doses of clopidogrel and heparin were administered

_____ H. Any use of a temporary transcutaneous pacemaker and the settings

Thinking Exercise 3A-6

An 82-year-old female client participates in cardiac rehabilitation activities after several episodes of syncope and the insertion of a permanent pacemaker. The client has a history of hypertension, coronary artery disease, and gastroesophageal reflux disease (GERD). The pacemaker is set on a demand mode at 60 beats/min. A nurse evaluates the progress of the client's recovery. **For each client finding below, use an X to indicate whether the client is progressing as expected or is <u>not</u> progressing as expected.**

Client Finding	Is Progressing	Is Not Progressing
An ECG tracing presents pacemaker spikes.		
The client reports dyspnea and chest pain during physical therapy.		
A medical identification card describing the pacemaker is in the client's wallet.		
The client reports light-headedness when rising from a chair.		
Heart rate is 72 beats/min during occupational therapy.		
The client takes his pulse rate for a full minute each morning.		

Single-Episode Case (3A-7)

Thinking Exercise 3A-7

A nurse assesses a 77-year-old client who has a history of atrial fibrillation for which he is prescribed metoprolol, digoxin, and warfarin. The client's findings are as follows:

- Alert and oriented
- Reports light-headedness when standing
- Denies blurred vision or halos around bright lights
- Orthostatic vital signs
  - Lying
    - Heart rate: 54 beats/min
    - Blood pressure: 136/52 mm Hg
    - Oxygen saturation: 96% (on room air [RA])
  - Sitting
    - Heart rate: 60 beats/min
    - Blood pressure: 125/50 mm Hg
    - Oxygen saturation: 98% (on room air [RA])
  - Standing
    - Heart rate: 58 beats/min
    - Blood pressure: 115/44 mm Hg
    - Oxygen saturation: 95% (on room air [RA])

Which nursing actions are ***most appropriate*** at this time? **Select all that apply.**

_____ A. Position the client safely in a chair or back in bed.

_____ B. Remind the client to call for assistance when getting out of bed.

_____ C. Assess the client for signs of dehydration.

_____ D. Provide the client with a bedpan to defecate while in bed.

_____ E. Ensure that an informed consent form is signed for insertion of a permanent pacemaker.

_____ F. Contact the primary health care provider to adjust the client's digoxin dose.

_____ G. Send a urine sample to the laboratory to evaluate for a urinary tract infection.

Exemplar 3B. Heart Failure (Medical-Surgical Nursing: Older Adult)

Unfolding Case (3B-1 Through 3B-6)

Thinking Exercise 3B-1

A 74-year-old male client was recently admitted to a skilled nursing and rehabilitation facility after hospitalization for an episode of heart failure. The client's medical history includes atrial fibrillation and hyperlipidemia, for which he is prescribed aspirin, atorvastatin, digoxin, and warfarin. The nurse assesses the client after a physical therapy session. The nurse's assessment findings include:

- Oriented to person, place, and time
- Irregular heart rhythm
- Dyspnea when resting
- Auscultated crackles in basal lung fields
- Hemoglobin = 15 g/dL (150 g/L)
- Hematocrit = 50%
- Prothrombin time = 18 seconds
- International normalized ratio (INR) = 2.5

Highlight or place a check mark next to the assessment findings that require follow-up by the nurse.

Thinking Exercise 3B-2

A 74-year-old male client was recently admitted to a skilled nursing and rehabilitation facility after hospitalization for an episode of heart failure. The client's medical history includes atrial fibrillation and hyperlipidemia. The client is alert and oriented, has an irregular heart rhythm, experiences dyspnea when resting, and has auscultated crackles in basal lung fields. **For each client finding below, identify if the finding is associated with heart failure, atrial fibrillation, or hyperlipidemia. Each finding may be associated with more than one disease process.**

Client Finding	Heart Failure	Atrial Fibrillation	Hyperlipidemia
Ejection fraction <45%			
Dyspnea			
Palpitations			
Activity intolerance			
Low-density lipoprotein = 160 mg/dL (4.14 mmol/L)			

Thinking Exercise 3B-3

A 74-year-old male client was recently admitted to a skilled nursing and rehabilitation facility after hospitalization for an episode of heart failure. The client's medical history includes atrial fibrillation and hyperlipidemia, for which he is prescribed aspirin, atorvastatin, digoxin, and warfarin. The client is alert and oriented, has an irregular heart rhythm, experiences dyspnea when resting, and has auscultated crackles in basal lung fields. Current vital signs are: heart rate (HR), 110 beats/min; respirations, 28 breaths/min; blood pressure (BP), 140/68 mm Hg; and oxygen saturation, 88% (on room air [RA]). **Complete the following sentences by choosing the *most likely* options for the missing information from the lists of options provided.**

The client is ***most likely*** experiencing ______1______. Based on the client findings, he has hypoxemia, activity intolerance, and fluid overload. These symptoms are complications of ______2______ and decreased ______3______.

Options for 1	Options for 2	Options for 3
Aortic stenosis	Arterial occlusions	Afterload
Cor pulmonale	Infection	Blood pressure
Deep vein thrombosis	Medication therapy	Cardiac output
Left ventricular dysfunction	Pulmonary congestion	Heart rate
Pneumonia	Pulse pressure	Peristalsis

Thinking Exercise 3B-4

A 74-year-old male client was recently admitted to a skilled nursing and rehabilitation facility after hospitalization for an episode of heart failure. The client's medical history includes atrial fibrillation and hyperlipidemia, for which he is prescribed aspirin, atorvastatin, digoxin, and warfarin. The client is alert and oriented, has an irregular heart rhythm, experiences dyspnea when resting, and has auscultated crackles in basal lung fields. Current vital signs are: heart rate (HR), 110 beats/min; respirations, 28 breaths/min; blood pressure (BP), 140/68 mm Hg; and oxygen saturation, 88% (on room air [RA]). **Select the appropriate expected or desired outcome listed in the far-left column below for each identified client problem. Note that not all outcomes will be used.**

Expected Outcome	Client Problem	Appropriate Outcome for Each Client Problem
1 The client performs ADLs without fatigue.	Hypoxemia	
2 Intake and output are equal, and no peripheral edema is present.	Activity intolerance	
3 Respiratory rate and oxygen saturation are within normal limits.	Increased fluid volume	
4 The cllient denies dizziness, chest pain, and dyspnea.		
5 The client participates in physical therapy three times daily.		

Thinking Exercise 3B-5

A 74-year-old male client was recently admitted to a skilled nursing and rehabilitation facility after hospitalization for an episode of heart failure. The client's medical history includes atrial fibrillation and hyperlipidemia, for which he is prescribed aspirin, atorvastatin, digoxin, and warfarin. The client is alert and oriented, has an irregular heart rhythm, experiences dyspnea when resting, and has auscultated crackles in basal lung fields. Current vital signs are: heart rate (HR), 110 beats/min; respirations, 28 breaths/min; blood pressure (BP), 140/68 mm Hg; and oxygen saturation, 88% (on room air [RA]). Which interventions are ***most appropriate*** for the nurse to implement or delegate at this time? **Select all that apply.**

_____ A. Administer supplemental oxygen to keep oxygen saturation levels greater than 90%.

_____ B. Schedule activities with frequent periods of rest.

_____ C. Place the client in a private isolation room.

_____ D. Reposition the client every 2 hours while in bed.

_____ E. Explain interventions to the client to help reduce anxiety.

_____ F. Report nausea, anorexia, and visual disturbances to the primary health care provider.

_____ G. Weigh the client each morning at the same time on the same scale.

Thinking Exercise 3B-6

A 74-year-old male client participated in cardiac rehabilitation activities at a skilled nursing and rehabilitation facility after hospitalization for an episode of heart failure. The client's medical history includes atrial fibrillation and hyperlipidemia, for which he is prescribed aspirin, atorvastatin, digoxin, and warfarin. The nurse assesses the client and evaluates for potential discharge. **For each client finding below, use an X to indicate if nursing and collaborative interventions were Effective (helped to meet expectations) or Ineffective (did not help to meet expected outcomes).**

Client Finding	Effective	Ineffective
Chooses low-sodium food options for each meal		
Denies dyspnea when ambulating with physical therapy		
Had a bowel movement this morning		
Gained 3 lb (1.4 kg) of weight since yesterday		
Respirations = 15 breaths/min; oxygen saturation = 95% (on room air [RA])		

Single-Episode Cases (3B-7 Through 3B-9)

Thinking Exercise 3B-7

Pharmacology

A nurse cares for a 68-year-old female client who has chronic heart failure, hypertension, and aortic stenosis. While administering prescribed medications, the nurse reinforces health teaching associated with each medication. **Match the appropriate nurse's reinforced teaching statement listed in the far-left column with each medication. Note that not all teaching statements by the nurse will be used.**

Health Teaching	Prescribed Medications	Appropriate Teaching for Each Medication
1 "Eat foods high in potassium including bananas and orange juice."	Captopril	
2 "Perform good oral hygiene to prevent dry mouth."	Digoxin	
3 "Take your radial pulse for 1 minute at the same time each day."	Furosemide	
4 "Contact your primary health care provider if you experience a dry cough or dizziness."	Atenolol	
5 "Keep the drug in a dark container to avoid air and light exposure."		
6 "Do not abruptly discontinue this medication."		

Thinking Exercise 3B-8

Pharmacology

A 61-year-old male client is admitted to acute cardiac rehabilitation. The client has a history of chronic heart failure, hyperlipidemia, and atrial fibrillation. A nurse completes a medication reconciliation and identifies that some information is missing. **Choose the *most likely* options for the information missing from the drug table by selecting from the lists of options provided below the table.**

Medication	Dose, Frequency, Route	Drug Class	Indication
Aspirin	325 mg once a day orally	Salicylate	**1**
Atorvastatin	20 mg once a day orally	HMg-CoA reductase inhibitor	**2**
Digoxin	0.125 mg once a day orally	**3**	Increases myocardial contractile force and cardiac output
Warfarin	2.5 mg once a day orally	**4**	Reduces risk of embolic strokes

Options for 1 and 2	Options for 3 and 4
Treats angina	Angiotensin-converting enzyme inhibitor
Manages atrial fibrillation	Anticoagulant
Treats heart failure	Beta-adrenergic blocker
Decreases cholesterol	Cardiac glycoside
Reduces blood pressure	Corticosteroid
Decreases platelet aggregation	Selective serotonin reuptake inhibitor

Thinking Exercise 3B-9

A 81-year-old male client prepares to be discharged from an acute rehabilitation center after a myocardial infarction and exacerbation of heart failure. The client has a history of chronic kidney disease and coronary artery disease. Before reinforcing discharge teaching, the nurse assesses the client's understanding. Which statements by the client indicate that he correctly understood the teaching? **Select all that apply.**

_____ A. "I will avoid table salt and salty foods and read labels on all food items to ensure my diet is low in sodium."

_____ B. "I'll weigh myself each day at the same time on the same scale to monitor for fluid retention."

_____ C. "Activity can cause my heart failure to get worse, so I'll have my wife help me with activities of daily living."

_____ D. "I'll contact my primary health care provider if I gain 3 or more pounds in 1 week."

_____ E. "I will be sure to monitor my vital signs and skip a dose of metoprolol if my heart rate is less than 60 beats per minute."

_____ F. "I'll notify my primary health care provider if I experience shortness of breath or chest pain while resting."

_____ G. "I plan to drink a glass of red wine every evening with dinner to prevent further damage to my heart."

Clotting: Deep Vein Thrombosis *(Medical-Surgical Nursing: Middle-Age Adult)*

4

Unfolding Case (4-1 Through 4-6)

Thinking Exercise 4-1

A 45-year-old male client had a partial colectomy with descending colostomy secondary to colon cancer 3 days ago. The client has a history of colorectal polyps and ulcerative colitis and a body mass index (BMI) of 42. He is married and has three children, works as a computer programmer, and was independent prior to surgery. The shift report indicates that the client had a difficult recovery after surgery and has been on bedrest since admission. Which client statements require a follow-up assessment by the nurse? **Select all that apply.**

_____ A. "I have pain my left calf. It's tolerable but I would rate it as a 4 on a scale of 0 to 10."

_____ B. "My wife plans on bringing the kids to see me today. Hopefully they won't bother anyone."

_____ C. "I didn't sleep well last night. The tech turned on the lights at 4:00 a.m. to take my blood."

_____ D. "My right leg seems skinnier than my left leg, which is warm and swollen."

_____ E. "There is finally some stool in my colostomy bag. I think that's a good sign, right?"

_____ F. "The tech said that my vital signs are back to normal. I feel like I can get out of bed today."

_____ G. "The incision looks better, but the ostomy is red and appears a little moist."

Thinking Exercise 4-2

A 45-year-old male client had a partial colectomy with descending colostomy secondary to colon cancer 3 days ago. The client has a history of colorectal polyps and ulcerative colitis and a BMI of 42. The nurse is concerned that the client may have a blood clot and performs an assessment of the left lower extremity (LLE). **For each client finding below, identify if the finding is consistent with the presence of an arterial thrombus or deep vein thrombosis (DVT). Client findings may support one medical complication or both of them.**

Client Findings	Arterial Thrombus	DVT
Capillary refill = more than 3 seconds		
Dull ache or heaviness in the left calf		
Peripheral pulses difficult to palpate because of pitting edema		
Left extremity is pale when elevated on pillows		
Decreased mobility		

Thinking Exercise 4-3

A 45-year-old male client had a partial colectomy with descending colostomy secondary to colon cancer 3 days ago. The client has a history of colorectal polyps and ulcerative colitis and a BMI of 42. The shift report indicates that the client had a difficult recovery after surgery and has been on bedrest since admission. The nurse's focused assessment findings include:

- Left lower extremity is pink and warm with 2+ pitting edema
- Client reports left calf pain, which he rates 4/10 and describes as a dull ache

Choose the *most likely* options for the information missing from the statements below by selecting from the lists of options provided.

The client is ***most likely*** experiencing ________1________. The nurse would provide care to prevent ________2________, which is a potentially life-threatening complication. Together these two health problems are referred to as ________1________.

Options for 1	Options for 2
Arteriosclerosis	Acute coronary syndrome
Arterial embolism	Aortic aneurysm
Lymphedema	Gangrene
Raynaud disease	Pulmonary embolism
Deep vein thrombosis	Stroke
Venous thromboembolism	

Thinking Exercise 4-4

A 45-year-old male client had a partial colectomy with descending colostomy secondary to colon cancer 3 days ago. The client has a history of colorectal polyps and ulcerative colitis and a BMI of 42. The nurse's focused assessment findings are consistent with venous thromboembolism and include unilateral lower extremity pitting edema and pain. Venous duplex ultrasonography confirms the client has a left lower extremity deep vein thrombosis. **Use an X to show whether each nursing action below is Indicated (appropriate or necessary), Contraindicated (could be harmful), or Non-Essential (makes no difference or is not necessary) for the client's care at this time.**

Nursing Action	Indicated	Contraindicated	Non-Essential
Apply sequential compression device to unaffected lower extremity.			
Instruct the client to gradually increase activity and to stop any activity temporarily if pain occurs.			
Administer supplemental oxygen via a nonrebreather mask.			
Use ice packs to decrease leg swelling and pain.			
Administer prescribed anticoagulant therapy.			
Place client's legs in a dependent position when sitting in a chair.			

Thinking Exercise 4-5

A 45-year-old male client had a partial colectomy with descending colostomy secondary to colon cancer 3 days ago. The client has a history of colorectal polyps and ulcerative colitis and a BMI of 42. The client is diagnosed with a left deep vein thrombosis (DVT), and primary health care provider orders are implemented. Later in the day the nurse finds the client ambulating in the hallway with his wife. The client stops suddenly, grabs his chest, and states, "I can't breathe." The nurse helps the client to bed and completes an assessment. Client findings include:

- Sinus tachycardia (102 beats/min)
- Reports chest pain 9/10
- Respirations labored, using accessory muscles
- Chest rise symmetrical
- Respiratory rate = 28 breaths/min
- Oxygen saturation = 86% (on room air [RA])
- Crackles auscultated bilaterally

After implementing emergent interventions, the nurse prepares to transfer the client's care to a registered nurse. What essential information will the nurse include in a hand-off report to the registered nurse? **Select all that apply.**

_____ A. A list of scheduled morning medications that were administered

_____ B. Current oxygen saturation level and percentage of oxygen being administered

_____ C. The client's respiratory pattern and auscultated lung sounds

_____ D. Colostomy assessment and current intake and output balance

_____ E. Immunization history including influenza and pneumococcal vaccines

_____ F. Notification of the laboratory technician about orders for blood work

_____ G. Assessment of available intravenous access for heparin

Thinking Exercise 4-6

Pharmacology

A 45-year-old male client had a partial colectomy with descending colostomy secondary to colon cancer 3 days ago. The client has a history of colorectal polyps and ulcerative colitis and a BMI of 42. Three days after surgery, the client was diagnosed with a left deep vein thrombosis and pulmonary embolism, for which he was treated. The client is scheduled for discharge today and is prescribed warfarin for continuous anticoagulant therapy at home. After reinforcing discharge instructions, the nurse assesses the client's understanding. **For each client statement, use an X to indicate whether the nurse's reinforced teaching was <u>Effective</u> (helped the client understand the instructions), <u>Ineffective</u> (did not help the client understand the instructions), or <u>Unrelated</u> (not related to the instructions).**

Client Statement	Effective	Ineffective	Unrelated
"I will elevate my legs when sitting to improve circulation."			
"I will use a raised desk to stand at work instead of sitting."			
"I will eat a healthy diet with green leafy vegetables every other day."			
"I will contact my primary health care provider if I have chest pain or shortness of breath."			
"I will drink at least 50 ounces of water each day."			

Single-Episode Case (4-7)

Thinking Exercise 4-7

A 55-year-old male client is diagnosed with a right lower extremity deep vein thrombosis (DVT). The client has several questions about his diagnosis and care. **Indicate which nursing response listed in the far-left column is appropriate for the client's question. Note that not all actions will be used.**

Nurse's Response	Client Question	Appropriate Nurse's Response for Each Client Question
1 "When the clot in your leg dislodges and moves to your lung it is called a pulmonary embolism. Smoking increases the risk of this complication."	"The night nurse said I needed to stop smoking. What does smoking have to do with my swollen leg?"	
2 "Increasing your activity slowly may decease your fear. Let's start with getting out of bed and then a short walk later today."	"What can I do to decrease the swelling in my leg?"	
3 "Swelling will decrease when the clot is gone, and the medication you are on will dissolve the clot."	"I read on the Internet that the clot can go to my lungs if I move my leg. Is that true?"	
4 "You have many risk factors for a DVT, including smoking."		
5 "Nicotine causes your blood vessels to constrict or narrow, which makes it easier for blood clots to become stuck in the vein."		
6 "Wearing compression stockings as well as elevating your legs when in bed and the chair will help."		
7 "If you have pain when you flex your foot, you should stay in bed."		

Gas Exchange

5

Exemplar 5A. Asthma (Pediatric Nursing: School-Age Child)

Unfolding Case (5A-1 Through 5A-6)

Thinking Exercise 5A-1

An 8-year-old boy is brought to the local urgent care center after experiencing dyspnea while participating in the school's physical education course. His mother was called and plans to meet him there. Which data will the nurse initially collect? **Select all that apply.**

_____ A. Height and weight

_____ B. Temperature

_____ C. Heart rate

_____ D. Oxygen saturation

_____ E. Inspection of chest symmetry and movement

_____ F. Auscultation of lung sounds

_____ G. Palpation of abdomen

_____ H. Inspection of head and neck

Thinking Exercise 5A-2

An 8-year-old boy is brought to the local urgent care center after experiencing dyspnea while participating in the school's physical education course. The nurse's initial assessment findings include:

- Temperature = 98.6°F (37°C)
- Heart rate = 135 beats/min
- Respirations = 32 breaths/min
- Oxygen saturation = 88% (on room air [RA])
- Chest symmetrical and movements equal
- Reports dyspnea at rest
- Use of respiratory accessory muscles
- Audible expiratory wheezes without auscultation
- Productive cough with tenacious secretions

Complete the following sentences by choosing the *most likely* option for the missing information from the lists of options provided.

The nurse recognizes that the assessment findings could be caused by several medical disorders. _____1_____ is a hereditary disorder characterized by dysfunction of the exocrine glands. Common signs and symptoms are _____2_____, progressive dyspnea, activity intolerance, and weight loss. _____3_____ is a common respiratory infection that causes bronchiolitis in young children. Symptoms frequently include rhinitis, coughing, and wheezing. _____4_____ is a potentially reversible, chronic obstructive airway disorder characterized by bronchoconstriction and airway inflammation. Manifestations during an exacerbation usually include dyspnea, anxiety, and _____5_____.

Options for 1, 3, and 4	Options for 2 and 5
Asthma	Audible expiratory wheezes
Chronic bronchitis	Cor pulmonale
Cystic fibrosis	Hemoptysis
Emphysema	Tracheal obstruction
Pulmonary tuberculosis	Thick, tenacious mucous
Respiratory syncytial virus	Pulmonary hypertension

Thinking Exercise 5A-3

An 8-year-old boy is brought to the local urgent care center after experiencing dyspnea while participating in the school's physical education course. The nurse completes an initial assessment and suspects the client is having an exacerbation of asthma. Assessment findings are consistent with several health problems, and additional data are collected to assist the nurse in assessing and prioritizing the client's condition.

Initial Assessment Findings
- Temperature = 98.6°F (37°C)
- Heart rate = 135 beats/min
- Respirations = 32 breaths/min
- Oxygen saturation = 88% (on room air [RA])
- Chest symmetrical and movements equal
- Reports dyspnea at rest
- Use of respiratory accessory muscles
- Audible expiratory wheezes without auscultation
- Productive cough with tenacious secretions

Additional Client Findings
- Alert and oriented
- Sitting in chair with hands on knees
- States, "I can't breathe, I need help getting air."
- Peak expiratory flow rate = 160 L/min (personal best = 240 L/min)
- Confirmed history of asthma and prescription for a rescue inhaler

Use an X to show whether the potential health problems below are <u>Urgent</u> (intervention needed immediately), <u>Non-Urgent</u> (intervention needed but not immediately), or <u>Irrelevant</u> (not a current problem for this client).

Potential Health Problems	Urgent	Non-Urgent	Irrelevant
Inadequate oxygenation related to air trapping			
Airway obstruction related to bronchospasm			
Potential for injury related to infection			
Anxiety related to perceived threat of suffocation			
Inadequate nutrition related to dyspnea			

Thinking Exercise 5A-4

An 8-year-old boy is brought to the local urgent care center after experiencing dyspnea while participating in the school's physical education course. The nurse completes an initial assessment and determines the client is having an exacerbation of asthma. Assessment findings are:

- Heart rate = 135 beats/min
- Respirations = 32 breaths/min
- Oxygen saturation = 88% (on room air [RA])
- Reports dyspnea at rest

- Use of respiratory accessory muscles
- Audible expiratory wheezes without auscultation
- Productive cough with tenacious secretions
- Peak expiratory flow rate = 160 L/min (personal best = 240 L/min)

Which interventions would the nurse implement to achieve desirable outcomes for this client? **Select all that apply.**

_____ A. Administer supplemental oxygen.

_____ B. Perform a skin test to identify common allergens.

_____ C. Administer an inhaled leukotriene modifier.

_____ D. Monitor for signs of impending respiratory failure.

_____ E. Administer an inhaled short-acting $beta_2$-receptor agonist.

_____ F. Initiate an intravenous line for hydration.

_____ G. Compare current peak expiratory flow rate with the client's personal best value.

Thinking Exercise 5A-5

An 8-year-old boy who has a medical history of asthma experiences dyspnea while participating in a physical education course and is evaluated at the urgent care center. The nurse completes an initial assessment and determines the client is having an exacerbation of asthma. The nurse coordinates with a registered nurse to develop the plan of care, which includes:

- Positioning the client to improve the use of accessory muscles.
- Administering the client's short-acting $beta_2$-agonist bronchodilator.
- Providing supplemental oxygen to keep saturation greater than 92%.
- Evaluating peak expiratory flow rates to determine treatment effectiveness.

After obtaining consent from the child's mother, the nurse prepares to implement the plan of care. **Indicate how each intervention from the plan of care will be implemented by matching the appropriate nursing action listed in the far-left column with each intervention from the plan of care. Note that not all the nursing actions will be used.**

Specific Nursing Action	Planned Intervention	Appropriate Nursing Action for Each Planned Intervention
1 Supply oxygen at 3 L/min via a facemask.	Position the client to improve the use of accessory muscles.	
2 Perform chest physiotherapy.	Administer the client's short-acting $beta_2$-agonist bronchodilator.	
3 Place a continuous pulse oximetry probe on the client's finger.	Provide supplemental oxygen to keep saturation >92%.	
4 Support the client in a Fowler or tripod position.	Evaluate peak expiratory flow rates to determine treatment effectiveness.	
5 Ask the client to blow out as hard and as quickly as possible until all of the air is out of the lungs.		
6 Position the client in modified left lateral recumbent position.		
7 Ask the client to breathe in slowly and as deeply as possible, then hold the breath for a count of 10 if possible.		

Thinking Exercise 5A-6

An 8-year-old boy who has a medical history of asthma experiences dyspnea while participating in a physical education course and is evaluated at the urgent care center. The nurse determines the client is having an exacerbation of asthma and implements an appropriate plan of care, which includes:

- Positioning the client to improve the use of accessory muscles.
- Administering the client's short-acting $beta_2$-agonist bronchodilator.
- Providing supplemental oxygen to keep saturation greater than 92%.
- Evaluating peak expiratory flow rates to determine treatment effectiveness.

After interventions are implemented, the nurse evaluates the client's response to these interventions. The client's current findings include:

- Heart rate = 130 beats/min
- Respirations = 28 breaths/min
- Oxygen saturation = 98% (on supplemental oxygen)
- Reports breathing more easily, less shortness of breath
- Decreased use of respiratory accessory muscles
- Expiratory wheezes heard via auscultation only
- Productive cough with tenacious secretions
- Peak expiratory flow rate = 180 L/min (personal best = 240 L/min)

Highlight or place a check mark next to the assessment data that indicate the client's condition is improving.

Single-Episode Case (5A-7)

Thinking Exercise 5A-7

Pharmacology

A nurse reconciles the medication list of a 13-year-old female client who has a history of asthma. The home medication list is missing some information. **Choose the *most likely* options for the information missing from the drug table by selecting from the lists of options provided below the table.**

Medication	Dose, Frequency, Route	Drug Class	Indication
Albuterol	1–2 aerosol metered doses inhaled every 4–6 hr as needed	**1**	Relaxes smooth muscles in the bronchial tree to relieve bronchial constriction
Montelukast	5-mg chewable tablet orally once a day	Leukotriene inhibitor	**2**
Diphenhydramine	25-mg tablet orally every 6 hr as needed	**3**	Blocks histamine and dries respiratory secretions
Guaifenesin	1 teaspoon orally every 4 hr as needed	Expectorant	**4**

Options for 1 and 3	Options for 2 and 4
Antihistamine	Constricts blood vessels to reduce inflammation
Antipyretic	Prevents bronchospasms
Beta-adrenergic agonist	Stabilizes mast cells to reduce inflammation and edema
Corticosteroid	Suppresses cough reflex
Mucolytic	Thins respiratory secretions for easier expectoration

Exemplar 5B. Chronic Obstructive Pulmonary Disease (Medical-Surgical Nursing: Middle-Age Adult)

Unfolding Case (5B-1 Through 5B-6)

Thinking Exercise 5B-1

A 44-year-old male client who has a history of chronic obstructive pulmonary disease (COPD) was admitted to the hospital 2 days ago with shortness of breath and hypoxia. The client was treated with supplemental oxygen, positive airway pressure, and intravenous antibiotics. He is scheduled to be discharged tomorrow. Which client statements are of immediate concern to the nurse? **Select all that apply.**

_____ A. "I'd like to go outside to smoke."

_____ B. "I can't catch my breath even when sitting."

_____ C. "My chest feels really heavy."

_____ D. "I've had this cough for years."

_____ E. "I'm having trouble concentrating."

_____ F. "I lost 15 pounds in the past 6 months."

_____ G. "This is my third hospitalization this year."

Thinking Exercise 5B-2

A 44-year-old male client who has a history of chronic obstructive pulmonary disease (COPD) was admitted to the hospital 2 days ago with shortness of breath and hypoxia. He was treated with supplemental oxygen, positive airway pressure, and intravenous antibiotics. The client was scheduled to be discharged tomorrow but presents this morning with dyspnea at rest and heaviness in his chest. The nurse completes a focused assessment and documents the findings.

History and Physical	**Nurses' Notes**	Vital Signs	Laboratory Results

0900: Alert and oriented to person and place. Answers questions appropriately but reports having difficulty concentrating during the assessment. Respirations labored with use of intercostal and accessory muscles. Wheezes auscultated and productive cough present. Skin cool and pale with cyanotic lips. Pitting edema on bilateral lower extremities; jugular veins are distended. Vital signs: temperature = 98°F (36.7°C), pulse = 102 beats/min, respirations = 28 breaths/min, blood pressure = 144/56 mm Hg, oxygen saturation = 86% on 2 L/min O_2 via NC.--*P. Quinn, LPN*

For each client finding below, determine if the finding is consistent with a complication of COPD: inadequate oxygenation, cor pulmonale, or pulmonary infection. Each client finding may be associated with more than one complication.

Client Findings	Inadequate Oxygenation	Cor Pulmonale	Pulmonary Infection
Chest tightness/discomfort			
Difficulty concentrating			
Cyanotic lips			
Dyspnea			
Dependent edema			

Thinking Exercise 5B-3

A 44-year-old male client who has a history of chronic obstructive pulmonary disease (COPD) was admitted to the hospital 2 days ago with shortness of breath and hypoxia. He was treated with supplemental oxygen, positive airway pressure, and intravenous antibiotics. The client presents this morning with dyspnea at rest and heaviness in his chest. The nurse documents these assessment findings.

History and Physical	Nurses' Notes	Vital Signs	Laboratory Results

0900: Alert and oriented to person and place. Answers questions appropriately but reports having difficulty concentrating during the assessment. Respirations labored with use of intercostal and accessory muscles. Wheezes auscultated and productive cough present. Skin cool and pale with cyanotic lips. Pitting edema on bilateral lower extremities; jugular veins are distended. Vital signs: temperature = 98°F (36.7°C), pulse = 102 beats/min, respirations = 28 breaths/min, blood pressure = 144/56 mm Hg, oxygen saturation = 86% on 2 L/min O_2 via NC.--*P. Quinn, LPN*

Complete the following sentence by choosing from the lists of options.

The nurse recognizes that the client is experiencing an exacerbation of COPD with several complications. The ***priority*** client condition is ______1______. The nurse would intervene immediately to prevent hypoxia, ______2______, and ______3______.

Options for 1	Options for 2	Options for 3
Activity intolerance	Atelectasis	Anorexia
Cor pulmonale	Hypercapnia	Fluid imbalance
Impaired gas exchange	Muscle wasting	Hemorrhaging
Inadequate nutrition	Pneumonia	Hypertension
Pulmonary infection	Respiratory alkalosis	Respiratory acidosis

Thinking Exercise 5B-4

A 44-year-old male client who has a history of chronic obstructive pulmonary disease (COPD) was admitted to the hospital 2 days ago with shortness of breath and hypoxia. He was treated with supplemental oxygen, positive airway pressure, and intravenous antibiotics. The client presents this morning with dyspnea at rest and heaviness in his chest. The nurse documents these assessment findings.

History and Physical	Nurses' Notes	Vital Signs	Laboratory Results

0900: Alert and oriented to person and place. Answers questions appropriately but reports having difficulty concentrating during the assessment. Respirations labored with use of intercostal and accessory muscles. Wheezes auscultated and productive cough present. Skin cool and pale with cyanotic lips. Pitting edema on bilateral lower extremities; jugular veins are distended. Vital signs: temperature = 98°F (36.7°C), pulse = 102 beats/min, respirations = 28 breaths/min, blood pressure = 144/56 mm Hg, oxygen saturation = 86% on 2 L/min O_2 via NC.--*P. Quinn, LPN*

Use an X to show whether the nursing actions below are <u>Indicated</u> (appropriate or necessary), <u>Contraindicated</u> (could be harmful), or <u>Non-Essential</u> (makes no difference or is not necessary) for the client's care at this time.

Nursing Action	Indicated	Contraindicated	Non-Essential
Slowly increase the oxygen flow rate by 1 liter every 15 minutes until oxygen saturation reaches 90%.			
Teach the client that smoking caused his chronic lung disease and that he must quit or he will die.			
Type and cross-match for blood products.			
Help the client to a comfortable high-Fowler position in bed or supported at the bedside.			
Schedule treatments, meals, and physical activity so that the client has time to rest.			
Administer salmeterol 1 inhalation as needed 15 minutes prior to meals and physical activity.			
Place the client on a 1200-mL fluid restriction.			

Thinking Exercise 5B-5

A 44-year-old male client who has a history of chronic obstructive pulmonary disease (COPD) was admitted to the hospital 2 days ago with shortness of breath and hypoxia. He was treated with supplemental oxygen (2 L/min via nasal cannula), positive airway pressure, and intravenous antibiotics. The client presents this morning with dyspnea at rest and heaviness in his chest.

The nurse receives the following orders from the primary health care provider:

- Oxygen at 3 L/min; titrate to maintain blood oxygen saturation at 90% to 92%
- High-calorie, high-protein supplements with each meal
- Daily weights before breakfast using the same scale
- Fluticasone propionate 88 mcg oral inhalation twice daily 12 hours apart

Which actions will the nurse take to implement these orders? **Select all that apply.**

_____ A. Request a soft diet with frequent small meals instead of three large meals.

_____ B. Initiate continuous pulse oximetry.

_____ C. Consult a registered dietitian nutritionist.

_____ D. Recommend chest physiotherapy to mobilize tenacious secretions.

_____ E. Help the client to rinse his mouth after inhalant administration.

_____ F. Encourage a family member who has a calming influence to remain at the bedside.

_____ G. Remind assistive personnel to use the same scale before breakfast for weights.

Thinking Exercise 5B-6

A 44-year-old male client who has a history of chronic obstructive pulmonary disease (COPD) was admitted to the hospital 2 days ago with shortness of breath and hypoxia. The client presented this morning with dyspnea at rest and heaviness in his chest. The nurse implements the following orders from the primary health care provider:

- Oxygen at 3 L/min; titrate to maintain blood oxygen saturation at 90% to 92%
- High-calorie, high-protein supplements with each meal
- Daily weights
- Fluticasone propionate 88 mcg oral inhalation twice daily 12 hours apart

The nurse evaluates the client afterward. **For each assessment finding, indicate if the client's condition has improved, has not changed, or has declined.**

Client Finding	Improved	No Change	Declined
Respirations = 34 breaths/min			
Dependent pitting edema bilaterally			
Oxygen saturation = 91% (on room air [RA])			
Bilateral wheezes and crackles			
Oral mucosa and lips pinkish red			

Single-Episode Cases (5B-7 and 5B-8)

Thinking Exercise 5B-7

A nurse is caring for a 63-year-old female client who was admitted 4 days ago with an upper respiratory infection and an exacerbation of chronic obstructive pulmonary disease (COPD). The client has a history of cigarette smoking; she quit 5 years ago after smoking a half-pack a day for 32 years. The client has been admitted three times in the past 8 months for complications of COPD. The nurse reinforces teaching to assist the client to manage COPD symptoms and complications more effectively. Which statements would the nurse include as part of the client teaching? **Select all that apply.**

_____ A. "Let me help you to make a list of substances that irritate your airway so that we can determine how best to avoid them."

_____ B. "Take your quick-relief rescue inhaler when you have increased symptoms and repeat the dose every 15 minutes until symptoms are controlled."

_____ C. "Exercise is important to your health, so try to push through your symptoms and get a good workout in at least 5 days a week."

_____ D. "Influenza and pneumococcal vaccines are safe for clients with COPD and help protect against respiratory infections."

_____ E. "When using your metered dose inhaler, remember to take a slow, deep breath through your mouth and then hold your breath for 10 seconds."

_____ F. "Drinking plenty of fluids can help keep the mucus in your airway thin and easier for you to cough up.

_____ G. "Use several pillows or a recliner for sleeping to help you breathe better."

Thinking Exercise 5B-8

A 58-year-old client with severe chronic obstructive pulmonary disease (COPD) developed an increased cough and dyspnea over the past week. Current client findings include:

- Lethargic but responds appropriately to direct questions
- Vital signs: heart rate = 89 beats/min, respirations = 28 breaths/min, BP = 144/68 mm Hg, oxygen saturation = 85% (on room air [RA])
- Wheezes present throughout bilateral lung fields
- Arterial blood gas (ABG) results: pH = 7.34, $Paco_2$ = 55 mm Hg, Pao_2 = 68 mm Hg, HCO_3 = 30 mEq/L (30 mmol/L)

The nurse consults with the registered nurse and primary health care provider to develop a coordinated plan of care, which includes:

- Bi-level positive airway pressure (BiPAP) therapy
- Albuterol nebulizer
- Supplemental oxygen, 2 L/min

After implementing care, the nurse reassesses the client. **For each client finding, use an X to indicate if the client's condition has improved, has not changed, or has declined.**

Client Finding	Improved	Not Changed	Declined
Pao_2 = 75 mm Hg			
Stuporous			
Lung fields clear throughout			
$Paco_2$ = 65 mm Hg			
BP = 145/66 mm Hg			

6 Elimination

Exemplar 6A. Benign Prostatic Hyperplasia/Transurethral Resection of the Prostate (Medical-Surgical Nursing: Older Adult)

Unfolding Case (6A-1 Through 6A-6)

Thinking Exercise 6A-1

The nurse reviews a portion of the history and physical for a 76-year-old male client.

History and Physical | **Nurses' Notes** | **Vital Signs** | **Laboratory Results**

Reports new onset of urinary symptoms including frequency, weak urinary stream, and postvoid dribbling. He also states that he has nocturia 2–3 times and urgency. The client denies burning on urination. His previous history includes diabetes mellitus type 2, hypertension, hyperlipidemia, and early chronic obstructive pulmonary disease (COPD). His wife provides his medication list, which includes metformin, losartan, amlodipine, and simvastatin.

Indicate which client assessment findings below require immediate follow-up by the nurse at this time.

Assessment Finding	Assessment Finding That Requires Immediate Follow-Up
Urinary frequency	
Diabetes mellitus type 2	
Hypertension	
Weak urinary stream	
Nocturia 2–3 times	
Postvoid dribbling	
COPD	

Thinking Exercise 6A-2

A 76-year-old male client reports new onset of urinary symptoms including frequency, weak urinary stream, and postvoid dribbling. He also states that he has nocturia 2–3 times and urgency. The client denies burning on urination. His previous history includes diabetes mellitus type 2, hypertension, hyperlipidemia, and early chronic obstructive pulmonary disease (COPD). His wife provides his medication list, which includes metformin, losartan, amlodipine, and simvastatin. For which complication(s) does the nurse recognize that the client may be at risk related to his urinary symptoms? **Select all that apply.**

_____ A. Urinary retention

_____ B. Urolithiasis

_____ C. Urinary tract infection

_____ D. Chronic kidney disease

_____ E. Polycystic kidney

_____ F. Bladder cancer

_____ G. Urethral obstruction

_____ H. Atonic bladder

Thinking Exercise 6A-3

A 76-year-old male client reports new onset of urinary symptoms including frequency, weak urinary stream, and postvoid dribbling. He also states that he has nocturia 2–3 times and urgency. The client denies burning on urination. After physical and diagnostic examination, the primary health care provider prescribes a combination drug regimen of finasteride and tamsulosin. **Choose the *most likely* options for the information missing from the statements below by selecting from the lists of options provided.**

The nurse determines, based on the client's urinary symptoms and his prescribed drug regimen, that he ***most likely*** has _______________ 1 _______________. If drug therapy is not effective, the client may need to have a partial or total __________ 2 __________.

Options for 1	Options for 2
Polycystic kidney	Vasectomy
Acute kidney injury	Cystoscopy
Benign prostatic hyperplasia	Cystectomy
Hydronephrosis	Ureteroscopy
Hyperactive bladder syndrome	Prostatectomy

Thinking Exercise 6A-4

A 76-year-old male client reports new onset of urinary symptoms including frequency, weak urinary stream, and postvoid dribbling. He also states that he has nocturia 2–3 times and urgency. The client denies burning on urination. After physical and diagnostic examination, the primary health care provider prescribed a combination drug regimen of finasteride and tamsulosin. The nurse provides health teaching related to his health problem and drug therapy. **Use an X to show whether each health teaching listed below is Indicated (appropriate or necessary), Contraindicated (could be harmful), or Non-Essential (makes no difference or is not necessary) for the client's care at this time.**

Health Teaching	Indicated	Contraindicated	Non-Essential
"Increase your daily intake of caffeine to help prevent urinary retention."			
"Monitor your blood pressure frequently because one of your drugs may cause it to decrease."			
"Perform Kegel exercises every day to help manage incontinence."			
"Avoid alcoholic beverages to help prevent urgency and dribbling."			
"Strain your urine with every voiding to remove any stones."			
"Report burning when you void or cloudy urine to your primary health care provider."			

Thinking Exercise 6A-5

A 76-year-old male client reported new onset of urinary symptoms including frequency, weak urinary stream, and postvoid dribbling. He also stated that he has nocturia 2–3 times and urgency. The client denied burning on urination. After physical and diagnostic examination, the primary health care provider prescribed a combination drug regimen of finasteride and tamsulosin. After the client took these drugs for 6 months, his urinary symptoms did not resolve and he had transurethral resection of the prostate (TURP). What postoperative nursing actions will the nurse include in the client's plan of care? **Select all that apply.**

_____ A. Maintain the continuous bladder irrigation to clear the bladder of blood clots.

_____ B. Do not remove the tape that secures the three-way urinary catheter.

_____ C. Change the surgical dressing as needed and provide incisional care.

_____ D. Administer pain medication for postoperative bladder spasms that commonly occur.

_____ E. Monitor the client's urine for large, thick, bright red clots.

_____ F. Monitor the client's vital signs to detect infection or bleeding.

_____ G. Teach the client that his sexual function should not be impaired.

_____ H. Encourage oral fluids when able to tolerate.

_____ I. Irrigate the suprapubic urinary catheter every 8 hours and as needed.

Thinking Exercise 6A-6

A 76-year-old male client had a transurethral resection of the prostate (TURP) 4 weeks ago and is returning to the surgeon's office for a follow-up visit. Before being examined by the surgeon, the nurse performs a brief assessment and documents the findings. **Highlight the client findings in the** Nurses' Notes **below that demonstrate that the client is progressing well.**

Nurses' Notes

Client states that he is feeling much better and has only occasional bladder spasms. Is voiding less frequently in larger amounts, has no feeling of urgency, and typically has nocturia 2–3 times. Has not tried to have intercourse since surgery but is hoping to try after this visit. Vital signs include: temperature = 98°F (36.7°C), pulse = 78 beats/min, respirations = 18 breaths/min, blood pressure = 154/90 mm Hg. Oxygen saturation = 96%. No adventitious breath sounds. Bowel sounds present × 4. -- *J. L. Miller, LPN*

Single-Episode Cases (6A-7 and 6A-8)

Thinking Exercise 6A-7

A 68-year-old male client returned from the postanesthesia care unit (PACU) this morning after a transurethral resection of the prostate (TURP). The client has a three-way indwelling urinary catheter, and the nurse prepares to document his intake and output. The client's intake and output includes:

Intake	Output
5%D/0.45%NS solution = 125 mL × 8 hr Water = 2 cups (12 oz each) Apple juice = 4 oz Bladder irrigation solution = 110 mL × 8 hr	Drainage in bag = 1600 mL

Choose the correct options for the information missing from the statement below by selecting from the list of options provided.

The nurse calculates that the client's total fluid intake for the 8 hours since he was transferred from the PACU is __________ mL and his total urinary output for the 8-hour period is ___________ mL.

Options
720
960
1030
1250
1480

Thinking Exercise 6A-8

The nurse is reinforcing discharge teaching for a client who had a transurethral resection of the prostate (TURP) yesterday. Which statements would the nurse include? **Select all that apply.**

_____ A. "Report any changes in urinary color or amount to your surgeon."

_____ B. "Check with your surgeon if you need to take over-the-counter drugs."

_____ C. "Drink plenty of fluids, especially water, every day."

_____ D. "Avoid drinking lots of caffeine-containing beverages."

_____ E. "Be aware that retrograde ejaculation may occur when having sex."

_____ F. "Report increased or acute pain to your surgeon immediately."

_____ G. "Be aware that your prostate may enlarge again and need further treatment."

Exemplar 6B. Ulcerative Colitis/Colostomy (Medical-Surgical Nursing: Middle-Age Adult)

Unfolding Case (6B-1 Through 6B-6)

Thinking Exercise 6B-1

A 38-year-old female client visits her primary health care provider with report of anorexia, increasing diarrhea, moderate to severe abdominal cramping, and blood in her stool. She was diagnosed as having ulcerative colitis 2 years ago. Her current assessment findings include:

- Temperature = 99.8°F (37.7°C)
- Heart rate = 92 beats/min

- Respirations = 20 breaths/min
- BP = 110/58 mm Hg
- Oxygen saturation = 95% (on room air [RA])
- Pain = 6/10

Highlight the client findings that are of immediate concern of the nurse.

Thinking Exercise 6B-2

A 38-year-old female client visits her primary health care provider with report of anorexia, increasing diarrhea, moderate to severe abdominal cramping, and blood in her stool. She was diagnosed as having ulcerative colitis 2 years ago. Her current assessment findings include:

- Temperature = 99.8°F (37.7°C)
- Heart rate = 92 beats/min
- Respirations = 20 breaths/min
- BP = 110/58 mm Hg
- Oxygen saturation = 95% (on room air [RA])
- Pain = 6/10

Choose the *most likely* options for the information missing from the statement below by selecting from the list of options provided.

Based on the client data, the nurse recognizes that the client is currently at risk for complications of ulcerative colitis, especially ______________________ and ______________________.

Options
Nausea and vomiting
Crohn's disease
Fluid and electrolyte imbalance
Peptic ulcer disease
Inadequate nutrition

Thinking Exercise 6B-3

A 38-year-old female client visits her primary health care provider with report of anorexia, increasing diarrhea, moderate to severe abdominal cramping, and blood in her stool. She was diagnosed as having ulcerative colitis 2 years ago. Her current assessment findings include:

- Temperature = 99.8°F (37.7°C)
- Heart rate = 92 beats/min
- Respirations = 20 breaths/min
- BP = 110/58 mm Hg
- Oxygen saturation = 95% (on room air [RA])
- Pain = 6/10

Choose the *most likely* options for the information missing from the statement below by selecting from the list of options provided.

The nurse determines that the ***priority*** for care for this client is ______________________ and ensuring that she has adequate ______________________.

Options
Oxygenation
Pain management
Elimination
Fever management
Hydration

Thinking Exercise 6B-4

A 47-year-old female client had her first colonoscopy last week because she is at a high cancer risk due to ulcerative colitis for almost 11 years. She was referred to an oncologist for confirmed colorectal cancer and scheduled for a partial colectomy with colostomy. **Place an X to show whether the nursing actions below are <u>Indicated</u> (appropriate or necessary), <u>Contraindicated</u> (could be harmful), or <u>Non-Essential</u> (makes no difference or is not necessary) for the client's preoperative care.**

Nursing Action	Indicated	Contraindicated	Non-Essential
Contact the wound, ostomy, continence nurse (WOCN) about the surgery to determine ostomy placement.			
Include any family members or significant others in the teaching as the client requests.			
Reinforce teaching about the need to deep breathe and use the incentive spirometer every 1–2 hours.			
Remind the client that he will not be allowed to eat or drink anything until the ostomy begins to work.			
Reinforce teaching about the purpose of sequential compression/pneumatic devices after surgery.			

Thinking Exercise 6B-5

A 47-year-old female client had her first colonoscopy several weeks ago because she was at a high cancer risk due to ulcerative colitis for almost 11 years. She had a partial colectomy with an ascending colostomy this morning to remove colorectal cancer. What nursing actions are appropriate for the client's postoperative care at this time? **Select all that apply.**

_____ A. Help the client to get out of bed to a chair.

_____ B. Listen to abdominal bowel sounds every hour.

_____ C. Irrigate the colostomy using the prescribed solution.

_____ D. Teach the client how to change the ostomy pouch.

_____ E. Check the surgical dressing for bleeding or other drainage.

_____ F. Monitor the client's vital signs every 4 hours.

_____ G. Remind the client to use the incentive spirometer every 1 to 2 hours.

Thinking Exercise 6B-6

A 47-year-old female client has had ulcerative colitis for almost 11 years and was recently diagnosed with colorectal cancer. She had a partial colectomy with an ascending colostomy to remove the tumor and is visiting her surgeon for a 4-week follow-up visit. The nurse takes a brief client history and collects data for the surgeon before her examination. **For each client finding, use an X to indicate whether the client is progressing as expected or is <u>not</u> progressing as she should during her recovery.**

Client Data	Progressing	Not Progressing
Vital signs stable and without fever		
Is unable to do ostomy care including pouch changes		
Stoma is reddish without surrounding redness		
States she can never have sex with her husband again		
Ostomy draining mostly liquid stool		

Single-Episode Cases (6B-7 and 6B-8)

Thinking Exercise 6B-7

Pharmacology

A 52-year-old male client was started on sulfasalazine for an acute episode of ulcerative colitis. He tells the nurse that he is very embarrassed about "always having to get to the bathroom quickly," especially when he is in a business meeting. **Indicate which statements listed in the far-left column the nurse would include when reinforcing teaching about this medication. Note that not all health teaching statements will be used.**

Potential Health Teaching	Appropriate Health Teaching for the Sulfasalazine
"This drug is an antibiotic that is often given to clients who have an acute episode of inflammatory bowel disease."	
"You will need to take this drug for your entire life."	
"You shouldn't take this drug if you are allergic to sulfa or sulfa medications."	
"This drug should decrease your trips to the bathroom so you can feel a little more confident."	
"Be sure to drink lots of fluids to dilute your urine while on this drug."	

Thinking Exercise 6B-8

The nurse is caring for a 55-year-old female client who has had ulcerative colitis for over 15 years. For what medical complications does the nurse recognize that the client could be at risk? **Select all that apply.**

_____ A. Arthritis

_____ B. Anemia

_____ C. Hyperkalemia

_____ D. Hemorrhage

_____ E. Fistulas

_____ F. Fluid overload

_____ G. Polycythemia vera

Exemplar 6C. Urinary Incontinence (Medical-Surgical Nursing: Older Adult; Young Adult)

Unfolding Case (6C-1 Through 6C-6)

Thinking Exercise 6C-1

The nurse admits a 70-year-old obese female client who had a stroke a week ago to the rehabilitation unit in a skilled facility. The client has right-sided weakness and a history of diabetes mellitus, hypertension, and early dementia. She is able to communicate in short sentences but has trouble understanding what staff or family is saying. The transfer form states that the client needs help with all ADLs and she is incontinent of both bowel and bladder. The nurse contacts Rehabilitation Therapy for initial evaluation. **Highlight the client findings that are of immediate concern to the nurse at this time.**

Thinking Exercise 6C-2

The nurse admits a 70-year-old obese female client who had a stroke a week ago to the rehabilitation unit in a skilled facility. The client has right-sided weakness and a history of diabetes mellitus, hypertension, and early dementia. She is able to communicate in short sentences but has trouble understanding what staff or family is saying. The transfer form states that the client needs help with all ADLs and bed mobility skills. She is incontinent of both bowel and bladder. The nurse contacts Rehabilitation Therapy for initial evaluation. **Use an X to indicate for which potential complications the client is at risk while in the rehabilitation unit.**

Potential Complications	Risk to Client
Constipation	
Neurovascular compromise	
Pulmonary edema	
Skin breakdown	
Contractures	
Deep vein thrombosis	

Thinking Exercise 6C-3

The nurse admits a 70-year-old obese female client who had a stroke a week ago to the rehabilitation unit in a skilled facility. The client has right-sided weakness and a history of diabetes mellitus, hypertension, and early dementia. She is able to communicate in short sentences but has trouble understanding what staff or family is saying. The transfer form states that the client needs help with all ADLs and bed mobility skills. She is incontinent of both bowel and bladder. The nurse contacts Rehabilitation Therapy for initial evaluation. **Choose the *most likely* options for the information missing from the statements below by selecting from the lists of options provided.**

The nurse analyzes the assessment data and determines that the client ***most likely*** has _____1_____ or _____1_____ urinary incontinence, which are both common in clients who experience a stroke. Other risk factors that place the client at risk for urinary incontinence include _____2_____, _____2_____, and _____2_____.

Options for 1	Options for 2
Stress	Older age
Retentive	Impaired mobility
Urge	Malnutrition
Overflow	Diabetes mellitus
Functional	Hypertension

Thinking Exercise 6C-4

A 70-year-old obese female client who had a stroke was admitted to the rehabilitation unit in a skilled facility 2 weeks ago. The client has right-sided weakness and a history of diabetes mellitus, hypertension, and early dementia. She is able to communicate in short sentences but has trouble understanding what staff or family is saying. The physical therapist has begun to work with the client to learn to ambulate with a walker. The occupational therapist is working with her on ADL skills, including toileting because of her incontinence. The speech-language pathologist is helping the client improve her aphasia. **Place an X to show whether the nursing actions below are <u>Indicated</u> (appropriate or necessary), <u>Contraindicated</u> (could be harmful), or <u>Non-Essential</u> (makes no difference or is not necessary) to manage the client's urinary and bowel incontinence.**

Nursing Action	Indicated	Contraindicated	Non-Essential
Consult with the wound, ostomy, continence nurse (WOCN) to help plan the client's care.			
Place the client on a toileting schedule of every 1–2 hours while awake.			
Do not offer caffeinated beverages to the client.			
Teach the client how to do daily Kegel exercises.			
Administer oxybutynin to relax the bladder and prevent spasms.			
Insert an indwelling urinary catheter to prevent skin breakdown.			

Thinking Exercise 6C-5

A 70-year-old obese female client who had a stroke was admitted to the rehabilitation unit in a skilled facility 3 weeks ago. The client has right-sided weakness and a history of diabetes mellitus, hypertension, and early dementia. She is able to communicate in short sentences but has trouble understanding what staff or family is saying. The physical therapist has begun to work with the client to learn to ambulate with a walker. The occupational therapist is working with her on ADL skills, including toileting because of her incontinence. The client's bowel incontinence has improved, but she remains incontinent of urine. Today the assistive personnel (AP) reports that the client's buttocks and perineal area are very red and irritated. After assessment, the nurse determines that the client has skin excoriation and probable yeast infection. What nursing actions are ***most appropriate*** for the client at this time? **Select all that apply.**

______ A. Remind the AP to place a brief on the client while she is in bed.

______ B. Recommend the need for an antifungal topical drug.

______ C. Keep the client in bed until her skin heals from the excoriation.

______ D. Remind the AP to toilet the client every 1 to 2 hours while awake.

______ E. Tell the AP to restrict the client's fluids, especially after dinner.

______ F. Request an order for an indwelling urinary catheter.

______ G. Remind AP to toilet the client when she first awakens.

______ H. Remind AP to toilet the client immediately after each meal.

Thinking Exercise 6C-6

A 70-year-old obese female client who had a stroke was admitted to the rehabilitation unit in a skilled facility 6 weeks ago. The client has right-sided weakness and a history of diabetes mellitus, hypertension, and early dementia. She is able to communicate in short sentences but has trouble understanding what staff or family is saying. During her stay, the physical therapist worked with the client to learn to ambulate with a walker. The occupational therapist worked with her on ADL skills, including toileting because of her incontinence. The client is better able to communicate and will continue visits with the speech-language pathologist and physical therapist on an ambulatory basis after discharge to home with her daughter. The nurse collects data about the client's status to help with discharge planning. **For each assessment finding, use an X to indicate whether the intervention was Effective (helped to meet expected outcomes), Ineffective (did not help to meet expected outcomes), or Unrelated (not related to the expected outcomes).**

Assessment Finding	Effective	Ineffective	Unrelated
Has regular continent bowel movements every 1–2 days.			
Is beginning to communicate her need to go to the toilet.			
Walks independently with a roller walker and stand-by supervision.			
Performs most ADLs independently.			
Experienced a fall last night while in the bathroom.			
Has symptoms of seasonal allergies.			
Buttock and perineal skin intact and only slightly pink.			
Wears briefs during the day in case of incontinence episode.			

Single-Episode Cases (6C-7 and 6C-8)

Thinking Exercise 6C-7

Pharmacology

A 21-year-old male client experienced an acute spinal cord injury (SCI) resulting in quadriplegia. After surgical and medical stabilization, the client is admitted to the acute rehabilitation unit for intensive physical and occupational therapy. The nurse reviews the agency transfer information and notes that the client has a reflex (spastic) bladder and bowel with overflow incontinence. He has recently started bethanechol chloride to ensure bladder emptying. The client's mother states that the staff in the step-down unit taught them about the drug, but she is still unsure if he needs the drug because he does not like to take any medication. What health teaching will the nurse reinforce about bethanechol chloride? **Select all that apply.**

_____ A. "This drug helps to prevent bladder infection."

_____ B. "This drug is given at specific times so that the bladder can empty within about an hour."

_____ C. "This drug can cause side effects such as sweating and flushed skin."

_____ D. "Your son should not take this drug if he has asthma or heart disease."

_____ E. "This drug can cause excessive drowsiness and dizziness."

_____ F. "Let me know if your son has nausea or feels like his heart is racing."

_____ G. "We will be monitoring your son's urine for changes, such as cloudiness."

Thinking Exercise 6C-8

A 21-year-old male client experienced an acute spinal cord injury (SCI) resulting in quadriplegia. After surgical and medical stabilization, the client is admitted to the acute rehabilitation unit for intensive physical and occupational therapy. The nurse reviews the agency transfer information and notes that the client has a reflex (spastic) bladder and bowel with overflow incontinence. Which bowel training interventions will the nurse plan to manage the client's bowel elimination? **Select all that apply.**

_____ A. Schedule bowel emptying after a meal based on the client's usual bowel schedule.

_____ B. Administer regular oral laxatives and/or rectal suppository to help empty the bowel.

_____ C. Restrict the client's fluid intake to help prevent diarrhea.

_____ D. Encourage foods high in fiber to help prevent constipation.

_____ E. Manually remove the client's stool by disimpaction every evening before bedtime.

_____ F. Administer a mineral oil "cocktail" every morning after breakfast.

_____ G. Teach the client how to perform Kegel exercises several times a day.

Nutrition

7

Exemplar 7A. Cholecystitis/Cholecystectomy (Medical-Surgical Nursing: Young Adult; Middle-Age Adult)

Unfolding Case (7A-1 Through 7A-6)

Thinking Exercise 7A-1

A 30-year-old female client is brought to the local emergency department by her partner with report of intermittent nausea, vomiting, and diarrhea for the past 3 days; weakness; and abdominal pain that ranges from moderate to severe. Her partner states that the client has had these symptoms since they ate at a new Italian restaurant 3 nights ago. She also has been complaining to her partner about having achiness in many of her joints (arthralgias). The client's medical history includes Crohn's disease, psoriasis, and gastroesophageal reflux disease (GERD), for which she takes multiple medications. Her current vital signs include:

- Temperature = 100.4°F (38°C)
- Apical pulse = 94 beats/min
- Respirations = 22 breaths/min
- Blood pressure = 98/50 mm Hg

An abdominal ultrasound shows cholelithiasis and cholecystitis.

Highlight the client assessment findings that are of immediate concern to the nurse.

Thinking Exercise 7A-2

A 30-year-old female client is brought to the local emergency department by her partner with report of intermittent nausea, vomiting, and diarrhea for the past 3 days; weakness; and abdominal pain that ranges from moderate to severe. Her partner states that the client has had these symptoms since they ate at a new Italian restaurant 3 nights ago. She also has been complaining to her partner about having achiness in many of her joints (arthralgias). The client's medical history includes Crohn's disease and gastroesophageal reflux disease (GERD), for which she takes multiple medications. Her current vital signs include:

- Temperature = 100.4°F (38°C)
- Apical pulse = 94 beats/min
- Respirations = 22 breaths/min
- Blood pressure = 98/50 mm Hg

An abdominal ultrasound confirms cholelithiasis and cholecystitis.

Use an X to indicate which assessment findings are commonly associated with each client condition. Note that some assessment findings may be used for more than one client condition.

Assessment Finding	Cholelithiasis/Cholecystitis	Crohn's Disease	Dehydration
Nausea and vomiting			
Diarrhea			
Abdominal pain			
Weakness			
Arthralgias			
Tachycardia			
Fever			
Hypotension			

Thinking Exercise 7A-3

A 30-year-old female client is brought to the local emergency department by her partner with report of intermittent nausea, vomiting, and diarrhea for the past 3 days; weakness; arthralgias; and abdominal pain that ranges from moderate to severe. She currently has a low-grade fever, tachycardia, and hypotension. An abdominal ultrasound has confirmed cholelithiasis and cholecystitis. **Choose the *most likely* options for the information missing from the statements below by selecting from the lists of options provided.**

The nurse recognizes that the ***priority*** need for the client's care includes managing her ______1______, ______1______, and possible ______1______. Nursing care for the client would include administration of ______2______ and ______2______ medication.

Options for 1	Options for 2
Abdominal pain	An antibiotic
Dehydration	Oxygen therapy
Arthralgias	An anti-inflammatory
Diarrhea	An antiemetic
Electrolyte imbalance	An antihypertensive
Acid-base imbalance	An analgesic

Thinking Exercise 7A-4

A 30-year-old female client who had an abdominal ultrasound that confirmed cholelithiasis and cholecystitis last month had another episode of abdominal pain with severe nausea after eating a high-fat meal. She is referred to a general surgeon for consultation regarding the need for a laparoscopic cholecystectomy. The office nurse plans to reinforce preoperative teaching for the client. Which statements would the nurse include in the health teaching? **Select all that apply.**

_____ A. "You will have a few small abdominal incisions that will be covered with adhesive closure strips."

_____ B. "You will have a patient-controlled analgesia (PCA) pump to use after surgery to manage your pain."

_____ C. "You may have some nausea and possibly vomiting as a result of the anesthesia."

_____ D. "You'll need someone to drive you home on the day of surgery."

_____ E. "You'll need to avoid high-fat foods for a few weeks after surgery."

_____ F. "You'll need to make an appointment with the surgeon for a follow-up visit about 4 to 6 weeks after your surgery."

_____ G. "You'll need to avoid heavy lifting (over 10 lb [4.5 kg]) for 4 to 6 weeks after surgery."

_____ H. "You or your family will need to report any signs and symptoms of infection immediately to your surgeon."

Thinking Exercise 7A-5

A 30-year-old female client with cholelithiasis and cholecystitis had a laparoscopic cholecystectomy today and is transferred to the postanesthesia recovery unit. The nurse anticipates possible complications that may occur after surgery. **Indicate which nursing action listed in the far-left column is appropriate to help prevent, detect, or manage each potential postoperative complication. Note that not all nursing actions will be used.**

Nursing Action	Potential Postoperative Complication	Appropriate Nursing Action for Postoperative Complication
1 Teach the client to monitor for rigid boardlike abdomen.	Surgical wound infection	
2 Maintain bilateral sequential compression devices.	Nausea and vomiting	
3 Teach the client to observe for foul-smelling, purulent drainage.	Peritonitis	
4 Apply supplemental oxygen at 2 L/min.	Respiratory complications	
5 Administer an antiemetic medication.	Venous thromboembolism	
6 Teach the client to deep breathe and cough every 2 hours.		
7 Administer an analgesic medication.		

Thinking Exercise 7A-6

A 30-year-old female client with cholelithiasis and cholecystitis had a laparoscopic cholecystectomy 4 weeks ago. Today she visits the surgeon for a follow-up visit. The nurse performs a brief history and physical assessment prior to the surgeon's examination. **For each assessment finding, use an X to indicate whether the care for the client was <u>Effective</u> (helped to meet expected outcomes), <u>Ineffective</u> (did not help to meet expected outcomes), or <u>Unrelated</u> (not related to the expected outcomes).**

Assessment Finding	Effective	Ineffective	Unrelated
Abdominal incisions are closed and healed.			
No infection noted in abdominal incisions.			
States she has had several episodes of epigastric pain due to food intake.			
Breath sounds clear in all lung fields.			
Has had increasing problems with constipation since surgery.			
Bowel sounds present in all four quadrants.			
Has red rash on both arms.			
Has not had any signs or symptoms of deep venous thrombosis.			

Single-Episode Cases (7A-7 and 7A-8)

Thinking Exercise 7A-7

A 53-year-old female client had a traditional open exploratory laparotomy and cholecystectomy this morning. The client's history reveals that she had three previous abdominal operations during her lifetime: appendectomy, hysterectomy, and bowel resection. During her most recent operation, the surgeon removed multiple adhesions and explored her biliary ducts for stones or other obstruction. During postoperative client assessment, the nurse notes the presence of a T-tube connected to drainage, a Jackson-Pratt (J-P) drain, and a dry and intact bulky surgical dressing over the right epigastric area. The client has an IV of 5%D/RL infusion at 100 mL/hr and a nasogastric tube (NGT) connected to low continuous suction, which is draining yellowish-green liquid. **Choose the *most likely* options for the information missing from the statement below by selecting from the list of options provided.**

The nurse recognizes that the ***priority*** for the client's care is to implement actions that will help prevent postoperative ______________________ and ______________________.

Options
Incisional pain Respiratory complications Peritonitis Bowel obstruction Deep vein thrombosis GI bleeding

Thinking Exercise 7A-8

A 53-year-old female client had a traditional open exploratory laparotomy and cholecystectomy this morning. The client's history reveals that she had three previous abdominal operations during her lifetime: appendectomy, hysterectomy, and bowel resection. During her most recent operation, the surgeon removed multiple adhesions and explored her biliary ducts for stones or other obstruction. During postoperative client assessment, the nurse notes the presence of a T-tube connected to drainage, a Jackson-Pratt (J-P) drain, and a dry and intact bulky surgical dressing over the right epigastric area. The client has an IV of 5%D/RL infusion at 100 mL/hr and a nasogastric tube (NGT) connected to low continuous suction, which is draining yellowish-green liquid. The nurse is planning postoperative care. Which postoperative nursing actions would the nurse implement for the client? **Select all that apply.**

_____ A. Encourage oral fluids for the client to prevent dehydration.

_____ B. Observe the surgical dressing frequently for signs of bleeding or other drainage.

_____ C. Measure and document the amount and characteristics of J-P drainage every shift.

_____ D. Keep the T-tube bag below the level of the abdomen to promote gravity drainage.

_____ E. Encourage the client to use the incentive spirometer every 8 hours.

_____ F. Measure and document the amount and characteristics of NGT drainage every shift.

_____ G. Maintain sequential compression devices on both legs while in bed.

_____ H. Maintain the client in a flat supine position to help relieve pain.

_____ I. Teach the client how to perform leg and ankle exercises.

Exemplar 7B. Peptic Ulcer Disease (Medical-Surgical Nursing: Middle-Age Adult)

Unfolding Case (7B-1 Through 7B-6)

Thinking Exercise 7B-1

A 56-year-old male client visits the urgent care center for report of recent episodes of "stomach burning and pressure." He states that he had similar problems about 3 months ago, but antacids took care of it. However, for the past 2 weeks he has experienced intense upper abdominal pain and burning about 2 to 3 hours after most meals. He continues to take antacids but has noticed that eating more food also helps relieve the burning sensation. His medical history includes hypertension that is controlled with amlodipine, and multiple orthopedic injuries as a result of participation in high school and college athletics. For chronic pain that resulted from these injuries, the client alternates between taking acetaminophen and ibuprofen every day. **Highlight the client assessment findings that require follow-up by the nurse.**

Thinking Exercise 7B-2

A 56-year-old male client visits the urgent care center for report of recent episodes of "stomach burning and pressure." He states that he had similar problems about 3 months ago, but antacids took care of it. However, for the past 2 weeks he has experienced intense upper abdominal pain and burning about 2 to 3 hours after most meals. He continues to take antacids but has noticed that eating more food also helps relieve the burning sensation. His medical history includes hypertension that is controlled with amlodipine, and multiple orthopedic injuries as a result of participation in high school and college athletics. For chronic pain that resulted from these injuries, the client alternates between taking acetaminophen and ibuprofen. The urgent care provider prescribes omeprazole daily and famotidine as needed. The client is encouraged to see his primary health care provider for follow-up and possible diagnostic testing. **Choose the *most likely* options for the information missing from the statements below by selecting from the lists of options provided.**

The nurse recognizes that the client's signs and symptoms are associated with _____1_____. Common complications of this health problem include _____2_____, _____2_____, and _____2_____.

Options for 1	Options for 2
GI bleeding	Obstruction
Indigestion	Esophagitis
Peptic ulcer disease	Hemorrhage
Peritonitis	Gastroesophageal reflux disease
Cholecystitis	Perforation
Pancreatitis	Pancreatitis

Thinking Exercise 7B-3

A 56-year-old male client visits the urgent care center for report of recent episodes of "stomach burning and pressure." He states that he had similar problems about 3 months ago, but antacids took care of it. However, for the past 2 weeks he has experienced intense upper abdominal pain and burning about 2 to 3 hours after most meals. He continues to take antacids but has noticed that eating more food also helps relieve the burning sensation. His medical history includes hypertension that is controlled with amlodipine, and multiple orthopedic injuries as a result of participation in high school and college athletics. For chronic pain that resulted from these injuries, the client alternates between taking acetaminophen and ibuprofen. The urgent care provider prescribes omeprazole daily and famotidine as needed. The client is encouraged to see his primary health care provider for follow-up and possible diagnostic testing. Diagnostic testing for this client would ***most likely*** include which of the following tests? **Select all that apply.**

_____ A. Colonoscopy

_____ B. Esophagogastroduodenoscopy (EGD)

_____ C. *Helicobacter pylori (H. pylori)* testing

_____ D. Hematocrit

_____ E. Serum albumin

_____ F. Serum amylase and lipase

_____ G. International normalized ratio (INR)

_____ H. Chest x-ray

Thinking Exercise 7B-4

Pharmacology

A 56-year-old male client visited the urgent care center for report of recent episodes of "stomach burning and pressure." He stated that he had similar problems about 3 months ago, but antacids took care of it. However, for the previous 2 weeks he had experienced intense upper abdominal pain and burning about 2 to 3 hours after most meals. He continued to take antacids but noticed that eating more food also helped relieve the burning sensation. The urgent care provider prescribed omeprazole daily and famotidine as needed, and recommended follow-up with his primary care provider for diagnostic testing. After a diagnostic work-up, the client was diagnosed with a duodenal ulcer caused by *Helicobacter pylori* infection. The client's medications for this health problem include bismuth, omeprazole, and clarithromycin. **Use an X to show whether the health teaching listed below is <u>Indicated</u> (appropriate or necessary), <u>Contraindicated</u> (could be harmful), or <u>Non-Essential</u> (makes no difference or is not necessary) for the client's care at this time.**

Health Teaching	Indicated	Contraindicated	Non-Essential
"Take your medications exactly as directed by your primary health care provider."			
"You may have small amounts of alcohol, but avoid smoking and other tobacco products."			
"Be aware that bismuth may turn your stool darker."			
"Take omeprazole at dinner time with food."			
"Avoid drugs that can irritate your GI system, especially aspirin, ibuprofen, and other NSAIDs."			
"Avoid high-protein foods, which are difficult to digest."			

Thinking Exercise 7B-5

After a diagnostic work-up, a 56-year-old male client was diagnosed with a duodenal ulcer caused by *Helicobacter pylori* infection. After treatment with bismuth, omeprazole, and clarithromycin, he improved but continued to have upper abdominal burning pain at times. As a result, the client was scheduled to have an esophagogastroduodenoscopy (EGD). The nurse reinforces health teaching about the procedure. Which teaching will the nurse reinforce? **Select all that apply.**

_____ A. "This test will allow the doctor to see directly into your esophagus, stomach, and part of your small intestine (duodenum)."

_____ B. "You should have nothing by mouth for 6 to 8 hours before the procedure."

_____ C. "The procedure will be performed while you are under general anesthesia."

_____ D. "If you are allergic to shellfish such as clams, you cannot have this test."

_____ E. "Before the procedure, you'll need to remove any dentures or bridges."

_____ F. "After the procedure, you may experience belching or gas, which is expected."

_____ G. "After the procedure, you may have a sore throat, for which you can use warm gargles or ice."

_____ H. "After the procedure, you can have something to drink after your gag reflex returns."

Thinking Exercise 7B-6

After a diagnostic work-up, a 56-year-old male client was diagnosed with a duodenal ulcer caused by *Helicobacter pylori* infection. After treatment with bismuth, omeprazole, and clarithromycin, he improved but continued to have upper abdominal burning pain at times. The client had an esophagogastroduodenoscopy (EGD), which revealed two large duodenal ulcers. As a result, the client's drug regimen was changed. Today the client is visiting his primary health care provider for a 3-month follow-up. Before the client is examined by the provider, the nurse performs a brief assessment and documents the findings. **Highlight the client findings in the note below that demonstrates that the client is progressing well.**

Nurses' Notes

7/22/21 1400 Client states that he is feeling much better and has only occasional epigastric burning. Vital signs include: temperature = 98°F (36.7°C), pulse = 78 beats/min, respirations = 18 breaths/min, blood pressure = 158/88 mm Hg. Oxygen saturation = 97%. No adventitious breath sounds. Bowel sounds present in all 4 quadrants. States that the arthritis in his knees has recently worsened, but he has gained 14 lb (6.4 kg) in the past few months. ----------- *L.D. Santos, LPN*

Single-Episode Cases (7B-7 and 7B-8)

Thinking Exercise 7B-7

A 48-year-old female client is brought to the emergency department by her boyfriend because of two episodes of vomiting that contained blood. She has no history of GI health problems or other major health issues. Her boyfriend states that the client has a high-pressure job as a lawyer and has been trying to become a partner in the company. What collaborative interventions does the nurse anticipate to provide optimal care for the client at this time? **Select all that apply.**

_____ A. Inserting a nasogastric tube to connect to low continuous suction

_____ B. Ensuring that the client does not drink or eat anything

_____ C. Taking vital signs frequently to monitor for hypovolemic shock

_____ D. Drawing blood to assess complete blood cell count results

_____ E. Establishing two large-bore IV lines for fluids and possible blood transfusion

_____ F. Administering IV antibiotic therapy

_____ G. Placing the client in a semi-Fowler position of at least 30 degrees of elevation

Thinking Exercise 7B-8

A 59-year-old male client is admitted to the emergency department with report of acute abdominal pain, nausea, and vomiting. He has a history of peptic ulcer disease, for which he takes a proton pump inhibitor. The nurse documents the following client assessment data:

History and Physical	**Nurses' Notes**	Vital Signs	Laboratory Results

- Pain = 9/10
- Temperature = 101.4°F (38.6°C)
- Pulse = 102 beats/min
- Respirations = 28 breaths/min
- Blood pressure = 110/62 mm Hg
- Oxygen saturation = 95% (on room air [RA])
- Abdomen tender, particularly in the right and left upper quadrants

Highlight the client findings in the Nurses' Notes above that are of immediate concern to the nurse.

Mobility

8

Exemplar 8A. Sports Injury (Pediatric Nursing: School-Age Child)

Unfolding Case (8A-1 Through 8A-6)

Thinking Exercise 8A-1

An 11-year-old boy participating in soccer practice at school fell and twisted his right knee. The school health aide notified the child's mother, who took him to the pediatric urgent care center. The nurse at the center interviewed the mother and collected the initial data as documented below in the Nurses' Notes:

History and Physical	Nurses' Notes	Vital Signs	Laboratory Results

9/12/21 1630 Child fell during soccer practice and twisted his right knee. Right knee is swollen medially and painful when flexed. Abrasion present on lateral left leg. Both palms are reddened where he tried to balance himself during fall. Lower leg muscles of both legs unusually large. Mother states that his enlarged leg muscles are due to muscular dystrophy (MD), which was diagnosed last year. Additional medical history includes celiac disease, mild asthma, and several learning disabilities. In the 10th percentile for height and 15th percentile for weight. Vital signs: temperature, 98.4°F (36.9°C); heart rate, 92 beats/min; respirations, 22 breaths/min; blood pressure, 100/64 mm Hg. --*R.Garcia, LVN*

Place an X to indicate which client findings require immediate follow-up by the nurse at this time.

Client Finding	Requires Immediate Follow-Up
Abrasion on left leg	
Painful right knee	
Respirations = 22 breaths/min	
Swollen right knee	
History of muscular dystrophy (MD)	

Thinking Exercise 8A-2

An 11-year-old boy participating in soccer practice at school fell and twisted his right knee. The child's right knee is swollen medially and painful when flexed; an abrasion is present on the lateral left leg. His lower leg muscles of both legs are unusually large. The child's mother states that he was recently diagnosed with muscular dystrophy (MD). His medical history also includes celiac disease, mild asthma, and several learning disabilities. The child is in the 10th percentile for height and 15th percentile for weight. **Choose the *most likely* options for the information missing from the statements below by selecting from the list of options provided.**

The nurse recognizes that the child may have fallen due to ________________, which is common in children who have muscular dystrophy. His knee swelling and pain are probably the result of ______________________.

Options
Bone fracture
Muscle weakness
Knee arthritis
Muscle spasms
Ligament damage
Malnutrition

Thinking Exercise 8A-3

An 11-year-old boy participating in soccer practice at school fell and twisted his right knee. The child's right knee is swollen medially and painful when flexed; an abrasion is present on the lateral left leg. His lower leg muscles of both legs are unusually large. The child's mother states that he was recently diagnosed with muscular dystrophy (MD). His medical history also includes celiac disease, mild asthma, and several learning disabilities. The child is in the 10th percentile for height and 15th percentile for weight. What ***priority*** care will the child need to manage his sports injury **at this time**? **Select all that apply.**

_____ A. Apply a warm compress on the affected knee.

_____ B. Teach the child's mother the importance of keeping his right leg elevated.

_____ C. Apply an elastic wrap around the knee to reduce swelling.

_____ D. Administer an opioid, such as oxycodone, if needed for pain.

_____ E. Consult with the physical therapist to begin an exercise program.

_____ F. Remind the child to avoid weight bearing on the right leg.

_____ G. Assist the primary health care provider in applying a synthetic cast.

Thinking Exercise 8A-4

An 11-year-old boy participating in soccer practice at school fell and twisted his right knee 6 weeks ago. Although the swelling in his knee improved after conservative interventions, he continued to have pain and at times was unable to walk without a limp. As a result, the child had an arthroscopic procedure under general anesthesia to diagnose and repair any soft tissue damage. After the procedure, he was admitted to the same-day surgery recovery area. **Use an X to show whether the nursing actions listed below are Indicated (appropriate or necessary), Contraindicated (could be harmful), or Non-Essential (makes no difference or is not necessary) for the client's care at this time.**

Nursing Action	Indicated	Contraindicated	Non-Essential
Perform frequent neurovascular checks ("circ checks") of the client's right foot.			
Place the client in a high-Fowler bed position.			
Monitor the surgical dressing for drainage or blood.			
Take frequent vital signs until the client is fully awake.			
Determine the client's level of consciousness (LOC).			
Do not elevate the client's surgical leg to promote perfusion.			

Thinking Exercise 8A-5

Today an 11-year-old boy had an arthroscopic procedure to diagnose and repair ligament damage in his right knee following a sports injury 6 weeks ago. He is scheduled to be discharged with his mother to home later this afternoon. The nurse has been performing circulation checks ("circ checks") every 30 to 60 minutes, which have been normal. During a check at 1400, the nurse notes that the client's right pedal pulse is weaker than his left pulse for the first time since surgery. The child tearfully states that his knee is hurting "a lot more now" and his right foot "feels funny." **Choose the *most likely* options for the information missing from the statement below by selecting from the lists of options provided.**

The nurse's ***most appropriate*** action at this time is to ______1______ and continue monitoring the client's ______2______.

Options for 1	Options for 2
Loosen the surgical dressing	Level of consciousness
Distract the client with an iPad	Vital signs
Notify the registered nurse in charge	Surgical dressing
Elevate the client's surgical leg	Pain intensity level
Notify the orthopedic surgeon	Circulation status

Thinking Exercise 8A-6

An 11-year-old male had right knee ligament damage as a result of a fall during soccer practice 3 months ago. His medical history includes limb-girdle muscular dystrophy, mild asthma, celiac disease, and learning disabilities. Conservative interventions did not manage his injured knee pain, and he had arthroscopic surgery 4 weeks ago. Today his mother brought him to the surgeon for a follow-up visit. The nurse performs a brief history and physical assessment prior to the surgeon's examination. **For each client finding, use an X to indicate whether the care for the client was Effective (helped to meet expected outcomes), Ineffective (did not help to meet expected outcomes), or Unrelated (not related to the expected outcomes).**

Client Finding	Effective	Ineffective	Unrelated
Arthroscopic incisions are closed and healed			
No infection noted in arthroscopic incisions			
States he has been feeling more weak and tired when he plays sports			
Says that his right knee feels much better since his surgery			
Has increasing problems with constipation since surgery			
Mother says that she still notices a limp in his right leg at times			
States he has problems sleeping since he had his surgery			
Is getting better grades in school this term			

Single-Episode Cases (8A-7 and 8A-8)

Thinking Exercise 8A-7

An 8-year-old girl fell from a scooter onto an asphalt neighborhood road. When her grandfather went outside to check on her, he found her crying and holding her left ankle. When he helped her to a standing position, the child could not bear weight on it. On admission to the emergency department, the nurse notes that the child's left ankle is swollen and beginning to discolor. She is crying and says that it hurts when she tries to walk on it. She also states that her right wrist hurts. Both knees are scraped and bruised with dirt and pieces of stone in the wounds. **Highlight the client assessment findings that require follow-up by the nurse in coordination with the health care team.**

Thinking Exercise 8A-8

A 12-year-old male client had surgery this morning to repair severely torn ankle ligaments that resulted from playing football with friends. His right lower leg and foot are splinted and wrapped with a large compression bandage extending from the base of his toes to his knee. He will need to use crutches when he goes home to avoid weight bearing on his surgical foot. During his recovery from surgery while hospitalized, what nursing actions are **appropriate** for this client? **Select all that apply.**

_____ A. Teach the client how to use three-point crutch walking.

_____ B. Monitor the client's neurovascular status, including pedal pulse and sensation.

_____ C. Assess pain level and medicate with an analgesic as needed.

_____ D. Elevate the affected leg on one or two pillows.

_____ E. Administer subcutaneous heparin to prevent deep vein thrombosis.

_____ F. Ask his mother to stay in the waiting room while he is recovering from surgery.

_____ G. Keep the client NPO until he is fully awake and oriented.

Exemplar 8B. Fractured Arm/Cast Care (Pediatric Nursing: Preschool-Age Child)

Unfolding Case (8B-1 Through 8B-6)

Thinking Exercise 8B-1

A 4-year-old girl was riding her bicycle on the sidewalk in front of her house when she hit uneven concrete and lost her balance. Although she was wearing a helmet, elbow pads, and knee pads, she injured her left lower arm when she was projected over the bicycle handlebars. Her mother took her to the pediatric urgent care center for evaluation. On admission the nurse noted that the client had a large bruise and swelling on the radial side of her left lower arm. Her mother told the nurse that she does not want her daughter to have any "shots" because she does not believe in immunizations. **Highlight the client assessment findings that require follow-up by the nurse in coordination with the health care team.**

Thinking Exercise 8B-2

A 4-year-old girl was riding her bicycle on the sidewalk in front of her house when she hit uneven concrete and lost her balance. Although she was wearing a helmet, elbow pads, and knee pads, she injured her left lower arm when she was projected over the bicycle handlebars. Her mother took her to the pediatric urgent care center for evaluation. On admission the nurse noted that the client had a large bruise and swelling on the radial side of her left lower arm. Her mother told the nurse that she does not want her daughter to have any "shots" because she does not believe in immunizations. After x-ray confirmation of a displaced radial fracture, the primary health care provider informed the child's mother that a closed reduction and cast will be needed. **Choose the *most likely* options for the information missing from the statement below by selecting from the list of options provided.**

The nurse recognizes that the child will need a distraction during the treatment of her fracture, such as ______________________________, because this play activity is appropriate for her developmental age.

Options
Putting together a 500-piece puzzle
Playing a learning game on a personal electronic device
Using modeling clay to create animals
Making slime with her mother

Thinking Exercise 8B-3

A 4-year-old girl was riding her bicycle on the sidewalk in front of her house when she hit uneven concrete and lost her balance. Although she was wearing a helmet, elbow pads, and knee pads, she injured her left lower arm when she was projected over the bicycle handlebars. Her mother took her to the pediatric urgent care center for evaluation. On admission the nurse noted that the client had a large bruise and swelling on the radial side of her left lower arm. Her mother told the nurse that she does not want her daughter to have any "shots" because she does not believe in immunizations. After x-ray confirmation of a displaced radial fracture, the primary health care provider performed a closed reduction of her radius and applied a synthetic cast. **Choose the *most likely* options for the information missing from the statement below by selecting from the lists of options provided.**

The ***priority*** for nursing care of the child at this time is to provide ______1______ and manage the child's ______2______.

Options for 1	Options for 2
Frequent monitoring	Fracture
Emotional support	Anxiety
A trusting relationship	Pain
Discharge teaching	Apprehension

Thinking Exercise 8B-4

A 4-year-old girl was riding her bicycle on the sidewalk in front of her house when she hit uneven concrete and lost her balance. Although she was wearing a helmet, elbow pads, and knee pads, she injured her left lower arm when she was projected over the bicycle handlebars. Her mother told the nurse that she does not want her daughter to have any "shots" because she does not believe in immunizations. After x-ray confirmation of a displaced radial fracture, the primary health care provider performed a closed reduction of her radius and applied a synthetic cast. The nurse is reinforcing teaching with the child's mother prior to discharge from the emergency department. **Use an X to show whether each discharge teaching listed below is Indicated (appropriate or necessary), Contraindicated (could be harmful), or Non-Essential (makes no difference or is not necessary) for the client's care at home.**

Discharge Teaching	Indicated	Contraindicated	Non-Essential
"It's OK if your daughter's cast gets wet."			
"Remind your daughter to keep her arm down by her side most of the time."			
"To help with healing, offer your daughter foods high in protein."			
"Let your daughter play whenever she wants."			
"Check every day to determine if your daughter's cast is too tight or too loose."			
"Report changes in your daughter's left hand and fingers such as color changes, temperature changes, and increased pain."			
"I'd like to review why your daughter needs her preschool vaccines."			

Thinking Exercise 8B-5

A 4-year-old girl was riding her bicycle on the sidewalk in front of her house when she hit uneven concrete and lost her balance. Although she was wearing a helmet, elbow pads, and knee pads, she injured her left lower arm when she was projected over the bicycle handlebars and fractured her radius. The primary health care provider performed a closed reduction of her radius and applied a synthetic cast. Today the child is scheduled to have her cast removed after an x-ray confirmed bone healing. What actions will the nurse take in preparation for the cast removal? **Select all that apply.**

_____ A. Prepare the child for cast removal with the cast cutter to prevent anxiety.

_____ B. Administer an opioid to the child to prevent pain during the procedure.

_____ C. Tell the child's mother to expect that the child's skin will likely be very dry and flaky.

_____ D. Teach the child's mother to use mild soap and water on the affected arm.

_____ E. Remind the child's mother to use soothing lotion on the affected arm after cast removal.

_____ F. Encourage the child to return to her previous play activity, including riding her bicycle.

_____ G. Encourage the child to be independent in her daily activities.

Thinking Exercise 8B-6

A 4-year-old girl was riding her bicycle on the sidewalk in front of her house when she hit uneven concrete and lost her balance. Although she was wearing a helmet, elbow pads, and knee pads, she injured her left lower arm when she was projected over the bicycle handlebars. Her mother told the nurse that she does not want her daughter to have any "shots" because she does not believe in immunizations. After x-ray confirmation of a displaced radial fracture, the primary health care provider performed a closed reduction of her radius and applied a synthetic cast, which was removed 2 weeks later. Today the child is having her annual physical examination because she is turning 5 years of age next week. Before being examined by the provider, the nurse performs a brief assessment and documents the findings. **Use an X to indicate which client findings below demonstrate that the child is progressing well or is <u>not</u> progressing well with her arm injury and childhood development.**

Client Finding	Progressing Well	Not Progressing Well
Skin on both arms healthy, hydrated, and warm		
Lower left arm slightly smaller than lower right arm		
Has returned to riding her scooter and bicycle with training wheels		
Is very inquisitive and excited to start kindergarten next month		
Tells the nurse she looks forward to getting an allowance to help with daily chores		
Has gained 5 lb (2.3 kg) and 2 inches (5.1 cm) since her 4-year-old annual visit		
Has not received any recommended preschool immunizations		

Single-Episode Cases (8B-7 and 8B-8)

Thinking Exercise 8B-7

A 5-year-old boy was playing with friends on the playground when he fell off of the trampoline and landed on his right arm. His friend's mother called 911 because the child's right lower arm was misaligned and a bone end was jutting through the child's skin. His parents met him at the emergency department, where he had an x-ray to confirm a fractured radius and ulna. The child had surgery for fracture reduction and application of an external fixator. **Choose the *most likely* options for the information missing from the statement below by selecting from the list of options provided.**

The nurse recognizes that the client is at risk for several complications of his fracture or fracture management, especially ______________________ and ______________________.

Options
Osteoporosis
Compartment syndrome
Osteomyelitis
Bony malunion
Osteoarthritis

Thinking Exercise 8B-8

A 4-year-old girl was a rear seat passenger in her sister's car when she was in a motor vehicle accident. After examination by first responders, both sisters were taken to the emergency department for evaluation. The nurse prepares to assess the child, who is crying and asking for her mother. On examination, the nurse notes old bruising on her chest and an old scar on her right upper thigh. She also notes swelling of her right upper arm. X-ray results reveal three old rib fractures and a new right condylar fracture above the elbow. **Highlight the client assessment findings that are of immediate concern to the nurse.**

Metabolism

9

Exemplar 9A. Diabetes Mellitus (Medical-Surgical Nursing: Middle-Age Adult)

Unfolding Case (9A-1 Through 9A-6)

Thinking Exercise 9A-1

A 56-year-old female client is receiving skilled nursing care for neuropathic ulcers. The client has a history of diabetes mellitus type 2, for which she takes metformin, and hypertension, for which she takes atenolol and lisinopril. The client had several toes amputated over the past 2 years and was recently hospitalized for intravenous antibiotics because of a right lateral lower extremity ulcer. The nurse completes an initial shift assessment. **Highlight or place a check mark next to the client findings below that require immediate follow-up by the nurse.**

- Oriented × 3, follows all commands
- Reports blurry vision
- Lung fields clear throughout
- Bowel sounds present in all quadrants
- Reports nausea and abdominal discomfort
- Left large toe amputation
- Right lateral lower extremity ulcer with red edges and purulent exudate
- Reports not sleeping well the night before due to needing to urinate every 2 hours

Thinking Exercise 9A-2

A 56-year-old female client is receiving skilled nursing care for neuropathic ulcers. The client has a history of diabetes mellitus type 2, for which she takes metformin, and hypertension, for which she takes atenolol and lisinopril. The client had several toes amputated over the past 2 years and was recently hospitalized for intravenous antibiotics because of a right lateral lower extremity ulcer. After completing an assessment and documenting client findings, the nurse analyzes the client's clinical presentation, laboratory results, and intake and output records.

Physical Assessment	Laboratory Results
• Oriented × 3, follows all commands • Reports blurry vision • Lung fields clear throughout • Bowel sounds present in all quadrants • Reports nausea and abdominal discomfort • Left large toe amputation • Right lateral lower extremity ulcer with red edges and purulent exudate • Reports not sleeping well the night before due to needing to urinate every 2 hr	• Red blood cell (RBC) count = $4.9 \times 10^6/mm^3$ ($4.9 \times 10^{12}/L$ • White blood cell (WBC) count = $10{,}500/mm^3$ ($10.5 \times 10^9/L$) • Blood glucose = 380 mg/dL (20.9 mmol/L) • Serum sodium (Na^+) = 144 mEq/L (144 mmol/L) • Serum potassium (K^+) = 4.8 mEq/L (4.8 mmol/L) • Blood urea nitrogen (BUN) = 40 mg/dL (14.4 mmol/L) • Creatinine (Cr) = 0.9 mg/dL (79.4 mcmol/L)
Vital Signs	**Intake and Output**

• Temperature = 100.9°F (38.3°C)
• Heart rate (HR) = 105 beats/min
• Blood pressure (BP) = 136/40 mm Hg
• Respirations = 16 breaths/min
• Oxygen saturation = 96% (on room air [RA])
	• 12-hour urine output = 3500 mL
	• 12-hour fluid intake = 2200 mL
	• Meals eaten
	  • Breakfast = 100%
	  • Lunch = 150%—client asked for additional sandwich
	  • Dinner = 125%—client had additional protein shake

For each client finding below, determine if the finding is associated with hyperglycemia, dehydration, or infection. Some findings may be associated with more than one condition.

Client Finding	Hyperglycemia	Dehydration	Infection
Polyuria			
Nausea			
Tachycardia			
Nonhealing wound			
Polyphagia			

Thinking Exercise 9A-3

A 56-year-old female client is receiving skilled nursing care for neuropathic ulcers. The client has a history of diabetes mellitus type 2, for which she takes metformin, and hypertension, for which she takes atenolol and lisinopril. The client had several toes amputated over the past 2 years and was recently hospitalized for intravenous antibiotics because of a right lateral lower extremity ulcer. After analyzing the client's clinical assessment, laboratory results, and intake and output records, the nurse determines that client findings are consistent with several major health problems. **Use an X to identify the top two *priority* client health problems.**

Client Health Problems	Top Two Priority Client Health Problems
Fluid volume deficit related to hyperglycemia	
Lack of knowledge of dietary management for diabetes mellitus	
Ineffective therapeutic glucose management	
Impaired skin integrity related to neurologic and circulatory changes	
Infection related to nonintact skin secondary to diabetic ulcers	

Thinking Exercise 9A-4

A 56-year-old female client is receiving skilled nursing care for neuropathic ulcers. The client has a history of diabetes mellitus type 2, hypertension, amputation of several toes, and a recent hospitalization for intravenous antibiotics because of a right lateral lower extremity ulcer. After completing an assessment and documenting client findings, the nurse determined the client's priority health problems. **Complete the following sentences by choosing the *most likely* options for the missing information from the list of options provided.**

The desired outcomes for the client are that she will have ______________________ and ______________________. To meet these outcomes, the nurse collaborates with the health care team.

Options
Blood glucose maintained within 70 and 130 mg/dL (3.9 and 7.2 mmol/L)
Fasting blood glucose level of 100 to 125 mg/dL (5.6 to 6.9 mmol/L)
Pulse and blood pressure within usual limits
Oral mucosa that is pink and moist
Urine output at 30 mL/hr
Understanding of her treatment regimen

Thinking Exercise 9A-5

A 56-year-old female client is receiving skilled nursing care for neuropathic ulcers. The client has a history of diabetes mellitus type 2, hypertension, amputation of several toes, and a recent hospitalization for intravenous antibiotics because of a right lateral lower extremity ulcer. The client is prescribed:

- Continuous intravenous infusion of 0.9% normal saline at 150 mL/hr
- Regular subcutaneous insulin with a sliding scale dose to be administered with meals and prior to bed

This morning the client's finger stick blood glucose level was 266 mg/dL (14.8 mmol/L), and the nurse administered insulin at 0750 (7:50 a.m.) per the sliding scale below.

Finger Stick Blood Glucose (mg/dL)	Regular Subcutaneous Insulin (units)
<150	0
151–200	3
201–250	5
251–300	8
301–350	10
351–400	12
>400	15

Assistive personnel delivers the client's breakfast tray at 0840 (8:40 a.m.) and immediately requests the nurse to come to the client's bedside. Prior to implementing care, the nurse completes a focused assessment with the following results:

- Oriented × 2
- Pulls at sheets and attempts to climb out of bed
- Easily redirected and follows simple commands
- Skin is cool and clammy

Use an X to show whether the nursing actions below are Indicated (appropriate or necessary), Contraindicated (could be harmful), or Non-Essential (makes no difference or is not necessary) for the client's care at this time.

Nursing Action	Indicated	Contraindicated	Non-Essential
Obtain the client's current blood glucose level.			
Initiate oxygen therapy per nasal cannula.			
Administer subcutaneous insulin per the sliding scale.			
Help the client to drink 120 mL of fruit juice.			
Notify the primary health care provider.			
Administer 1 mg intramuscular glucagon.			
Reassess the glucose level 15 minutes after treatment is administered.			

Thinking Exercise 9A-6

A 56-year-old female client is preparing to be discharged after receiving skilled nursing care for neuropathic ulcers. The client has a history of diabetes mellitus type 2, hypertension, amputation of several toes, and a recent hospitalization for intravenous antibiotics because of a right lateral lower extremity ulcer. The nurse reinforces self-care management for diabetes mellitus including medications, diet, foot care, and exercise. Which client statements indicate that the client correctly **understood** the discharge teaching? **Select all that apply.**

_____ A. "I will hold my metformin dose if I choose to skip breakfast."

_____ B. "I will wash my feet, dry them thoroughly, and wear clean socks every day."

_____ C. "Eating foods high in protein, vitamins, and carbohydrates will help my ulcers heal."

_____ D. "It is okay for me to walk barefooted while inside my home."

_____ E. "I will make sure that I take my antidiabetic medications even when I am sick."

_____ F. "Aerobic exercise and resistance training may help lower my blood glucose levels."

_____ G. "My antidiabetic medications allow me to eat whatever I desire."

Single-Episode Cases (9A-7 and 9A-8)

Thinking Exercise 9A-7

A 49-year-old client arrives for a consultation appointment with a nephrologist. The client has a history of diabetes mellitus type 2, peripheral neuropathy, and hypertension. After obtaining initial vital signs, the nurse asks for a list of the client's current medications. The client provides a list but states that she doesn't know what they are for. **Indicate which medication action or indication listed in the far-left column is appropriate for each medication on the client's list. Note that not all actions or indications will be used.**

Medication Action or Indication	Client's Medication List	Appropriate Indication for Each Client Medication
1 Increases production of insulin from beta cells	Metformin 500 mg orally twice daily	
2 Stimulates insulin release, suppresses glucagon release, and reduces appetite	Exenatide 5 mcg subcutaneous injection twice daily before breakfast and dinner	
3 Improves neurologic conductivity in the eye	Gabapentin 300 mg orally every day before bed	
4 Increases glucose production by the liver	Glipizide 10 mg orally once daily with breakfast	
5 Relieves neuropathic pain	Lisinopril 10 mg orally once daily	
6 Promotes insulin secretion by the pancreas		
7 Decreases blood pressure and helps prevent kidney disease		
8 Decreases glucose production by the liver and increases tissue response to insulin		
9 Blocks beta-adrenergic receptors to decrease heart rate and blood pressure		

Thinking Exercise 9A-8

A 54-year-old male client who has a history of diabetes mellitus type 1, peripheral neuropathy, and retinopathy is transferred to a skilled nursing facility. On admission, the nurse implements a plan of care to prevent complications of diabetes mellitus and maintain client safety. Which nursing actions will the nurse include in this client's plan of care? **Select all that apply.**

_____ A. Coordinate meal-time insulin with food delivery.

_____ B. Ensure the path to the bathroom is well lit.

_____ C. Provide the client with a high-protein, high-fiber diet.

_____ D. Teach the client to recognize early signs of hypoglycemia.

_____ E. Assess the client's finger stick blood glucose level every 2 hours.

_____ F. Ensure the client wears properly fitting shoes when out of bed.

_____ G. Provide the client with a bedside commode.

_____ H. Schedule a sitter to be at the bedside during evening hours.

Exemplar 9B. Hypothyroidism (Medical-Surgical Nursing: Middle-Age Adult)

Unfolding Case (9B-1 Through 9B-6)

Thinking Exercise 9B-1

A 57-year-old female client was recently discharged home with home health services after a total left hip arthroplasty. The client's spouse lets a home health nurse into the residence for a follow-up visit. The nurse finds the client on the couch, next to a space heater and covered by multiple blankets. The client states, "I'm so cold. Can you get me more blankets?" The nurse obtains vital signs: temperature, 97.6°F (36.4°C); heart rate (HR), 58 beats/min; blood pressure (BP), 129/36 mm Hg; respirations, 14 breaths/min. Which focused questions will the nurse ask during the initial assessment? **Select all that apply.**

_____ A. "Do your children and grandchild visit you frequently?"

_____ B. "How has your energy level been?"

_____ C. "Have you experienced any changes in your muscles or joints?"

_____ D. "Do you feel warmer after taking a bath?"

_____ E. "Have you noticed any changes in your thinking processes?

_____ F. "Are you experiencing any shortness of breath?"

_____ G. "Have you been lying under those blankets all day?

_____ H. "Have you experienced any changes in your weight?"

Thinking Exercise 9B-2

A 57-year-old female client was recently discharged home with home health services after a total left hip arthroplasty. The client's spouse lets a home health nurse into the residence for a follow-up visit. The nurse finds the client on the couch, next to a space heater and covered by multiple blankets. The client states, "I'm so cold. Can you get me more blankets?" The nurse's initial assessment findings include:

- Vital signs: temperature, 97.6°F (36.4°C); heart rate (HR), 58 beats/min; blood pressure (BP), 129/36 mm Hg; respirations, 14 breaths/min
- Alert and oriented × 3
- Client reports feeling lethargic and more forgetful than normal
- Respirations equal and unlabored
- Lung fields clear throughout
- Client denies chest pain or shortness of breath, but states she has frequent headaches
- Skin cool and dry
- Bilateral hands and feet with nonpitting edema
- Client reports numbness and tingling in extremities as well as stiffness in joints
- Weight gain of 10 lb in past 6 months

For each client finding below, determine if the finding is associated with anemia, hypothyroidism, and/or heart failure. Note that some findings may be associated with more than one condition.

Client Finding	Anemia	Hypothyroidism	Heart Failure
Fatigue			
Generalized edema			
Frequent headaches			
Weight gain			
Numbness in extremities			

Thinking Exercise 9B-3

A 57-year-old female client was recently discharged home with home health services after a total left hip arthroplasty. The client's spouse lets a home health nurse into the residence for a follow-up visit. The nurse finds the client on the couch, next to a space heater and covered by multiple blankets. The client states, "I'm so cold. Can you get me more blankets?" The nurse completes an assessment and contacts the primary health care provider with recommendations for laboratory tests. Two days later, laboratory results are available:

Complete Blood Count	Thyroid Tests
• Red blood cells (RBCs) = 4.7 × 10^6/mm^3 (4.7 × 10^{12}/L) • White blood cells (WBCs) = 6500/mm^3 (6.5 × 10^9/L) • Hemoglobin = 10.1 g/L (101 g/mmol/L) • Hematocrit = 42% • Platelets = 250,000/mm^3 (250 × 10^9/L)	• Free thyroxine (T_4) = 0.6 ng/dL (7.8 pmol/L) • Thyroid-stimulating hormone (TSH) = 5.4 mIU/L • Brain natriuretic peptide (BNP) = 78 ng/L (78 mcg/L)

Complete the following sentences by choosing the *most likely* options for the missing information from the list of options provided.

The client is diagnosed with hypothyroidism. The top three ***priority*** problems for this client are activity intolerance related to _______________, weight gain related to _______________, and potential impaired skin integrity related to _______________ and _______________.

Options
Body image
Decreased metabolic rate
Decreased peristalsis
Dry skin
Fatigue
Decreased mobility
Weight loss

Thinking Exercise 9B-4

A 57-year-old female client was recently discharged home with home health services after a total left hip arthroplasty. During the client's first home health visit, the nurse's assessment and recommendations for diagnostic testing resulted in the client being diagnosed with hypothyroidism. Today the nurse consults with the interprofessional team in preparation for a follow-up visit with the client. **Use an X to show whether the nursing actions below are Indicated (appropriate or necessary), Contraindicated (could be harmful), or Non-Essential (makes no difference or is not necessary) for the client's plan of care.**

Nursing Action	Indicated	Contraindicated	Non-Essential
Teach the client about hormone replacement therapy.			
Encourage the client to integrate periods of rest during ADLs.			
Assist the client in bathing twice a day to decrease skin drying.			
Consult a registered dietitian nutritionist for diet and food option recommendations.			
Wear a cloth mask when outside the home to minimize risk of infection transmission.			

Thinking Exercise 9B-5

A 57-year-old female client was recently discharged home with home health services after a total left hip arthroplasty. During the client's first home health visit, the nurse's assessment and recommendations for diagnostic testing resulted in the client being diagnosed with hypothyroidism. The client has several questions during the nurse's second visit. **Indicate which nursing response listed in the far-left column is appropriate for the client's question. Note that not all actions will be used.**

Nurse's Responses	Client Questions	Appropriate Nurse's Response for Each Client Question
1 "Hypothyroidism can cause constipation. Increasing your fluid and fiber intake may minimize this issue."	"Will hormone replacement therapy help me lose weight?"	
2 "Hypothyroidism puts you at risk for a stroke. I will recommend that you have a brain scan."	Why did the registered dietarian nutritionist recommend a high-fiber diet with fresh fruits and raw vegetables?"	
3 "Thirty to 60 minutes before breakfast is the best time to take your medication."	"I feel like my brain isn't functioning correctly. Why am I having trouble thinking?"	
4 "Your weight should normalize when your hormone levels are corrected."	"What is the best time for me to take the prescribed levothyroxine dose?"	
5 "Mental slowness is a symptom of hypothyroidism and should improve with treatment."		
6 "You should take the dose at the same time each day and with food to decrease nausea."		
7 "Eating nutritional foods will help you lose weight."		

Thinking Exercise 9B-6

A 57-year-old female client was recently discharged home with home health services after a total left hip arthroplasty. During the client's first home health visit, the nurse's assessment and recommendations for diagnostic testing resulted in the client being diagnosed with hypothyroidism. The client was prescribed oral levothyroxine and provided with client education focused on the disease, potential complications, actions to minimize symptoms and reduce risks, and medication management. The home health nurse provides a follow-up visit 3 weeks later. **Highlight the client findings from the follow-up assessment (3 weeks later) below that indicate the client's condition has improved.**

Initial Assessment	Follow-up Assessment (3 Weeks Later)

• Vital signs:
  • Temperature = 97.6°F (36.4°C)
  • Heart rate (HR) = 58 beats/min
  • Blood pressure (BP) = 129/36 mm Hg
  • Respirations = 14 breaths/min
• Alert and oriented × 3
• Client reports feeling lethargic and being more forgetful than normal
• Respirations equal and unlabored
• Lung fields clear throughout
• Client denies chest pain or shortness of breath, but states she has frequent headaches
• Skin cool and dry
• Bilateral hands and feet with nonpitting edema
• Client reports numbness and tingling in extremities as well as stiffness in joints
• Weight gain of 10 lb in past 6 months
• Thyroid tests
  • Free thyroxine (T_4) = 0.6 ng/dL (7.8 pmol/L)
  • Thyroid-stimulating hormone (TSH) = 5.4 mIU/L
	• Vital signs:
	  • Temperature = 98.6°F (37°C)
	  • Heart rate (HR) = 66 beats/min
	  • Blood pressure (BP) = 124/32 mm Hg
	  • Respirations = 12 breaths/min
	• Alert and oriented × 3
	• Client reports feeling fatigue after completing ADLs
	• Respirations equal and unlabored
	• Lung fields clear throughout
	• Client denies pain or stiffness
	• Skin cool, dry, and without generalized edema
	• Client reports numbness and tingling in extremities
	• No change in weight in past 3 weeks
	• Thyroid tests
	  • Free T_4 = 0.8 ng/dL (10.4 pmol/L)
	  • TSH = 4.6 mIU/L

Single-Episode Case (9B-7)

Thinking Exercise 9B-7

A 55-year-old male client who resides in a long-term care facility has a history of hypothyroidism, heart failure, and early-onset Alzheimer disease. During shift change report, the nurse communicates that the client aspirated 6 days ago and was diagnosed with pneumonia. The nurse completes an initial assessment and identifies several complications of hypothyroidism. Which client findings will the nurse immediately report to the primary health care provider? **Select all that apply.**

_____ A. Cool, dry skin

_____ B. Last bowel movement 3 days ago

_____ C. Temperature = 95°F (35°C)

_____ D. Thin, coarse hair

_____ E. Respirations = 10 breaths/min

_____ F. Generalized edema on face, hands, and feet

_____ G. Stuporous

_____ H. Heart rate = 68 beats/min

10 Cellular Regulation: Breast Cancer *(Medical-Surgical Nursing: Middle-Age Adult)*

Unfolding Case (10-1 Through 10-6)

Thinking Exercise 10-1

A 48-year-old female client tells the nurse during her routine annual primary health care provider visit that she is concerned about her risk for breast cancer. Her mother and sister had the disease and were *BRCA2* positive. During the interview, the nurse notes that the client is not married and has never been pregnant. She states she is starting menopause and has frequent "hot flashes." The client reports that she consumes at least two or three glasses of wine every night to help her relax from her very stressful job as an accountant for a large company. Currently she lives alone but is within 25 miles of her parents' house. Both of her parents are living, but her father's health is declining owing to cardiovascular disease. What risk factors in this client's history does the nurse recognize are associated with breast cancer? **Select all that apply.**

_____ A. Alcohol consumption

_____ B. Stress

_____ C. Nulliparity (no pregnancies)

_____ D. Menopause

_____ E. Family history of breast cancer

_____ F. Female gender

_____ G. Father's health history

_____ H. Age

Thinking Exercise 10-2

A 48-year-old female client tells the nurse during her routine annual primary health care provider visit that she is concerned about her risk for breast cancer due to multiple factors, including a family history. Today an ultrasound and 3D mammography revealed a small lesion (0.9 cm) in her left breast. A needle biopsy confirmed early stage I breast cancer. **Choose the *most likely* options for the information missing from the statement below by selecting from the list of options provided.**

Based on the stage of the client's cancer, the nurse recognizes that she may select breast-conserving treatment, which includes ______________________________ and ______________________________.

Options
External beam radiation
Chemotherapy
Lithotripsy
Lumpectomy
Internal radiation
Breast reconstruction

Thinking Exercise 10-3

A 48-year-old female client at high risk for breast cancer had an ultrasound and 3D mammography that revealed a small lesion in her left breast. A needle biopsy confirmed early stage I breast cancer. **Choose the *most likely* options for the information missing from the statements below by selecting from the lists of options provided.**

The nurse recognizes that the ***priority*** for coordinated care of the client's cancer is to _______1_______. The nurse's role prior to the client's treatment would be to _______2_______.

Options for 1	Options for 2
Reduce pain and discomfort	Obtain informed consent for treatment
Minimize hospital stay	Discuss treatment options with the client
Prevent metastasis	Provide community resources
Provide emotional support	Consult with clergy or spiritual leader
Ensure that the client has health insurance	Reinforce client teaching

Thinking Exercise 10-4

A 48-year-old female client at high risk for breast cancer had an ultrasound and 3D mammography that revealed a small lesion in her left breast. A needle biopsy confirmed early stage I breast cancer. After an extensive discussion about treatment options with the primary health care provider, the client chose to have a lumpectomy to remove the lesion rather than have breast removal. She is now scheduled to have radiation therapy. **Indicate which client teaching listed in the far-left column is appropriate or <u>not</u> appropriate for the nurse to reinforce about radiation therapy.**

Client Teaching	Appropriate for Client	Not Appropriate for Client
1 "You will have an ink marking to outline the area that will be irradiated."		
2 "You will be hospitalized while receiving your radiation therapy."		
3 "You may wash the ink marking off of your skin once radiation therapy begins."		
4 "The irradiated skin will likely become irritated after about a week of radiation therapy."		
5 "Your radiation treatments may make you very tired."		
6 "Your family members will need to stay at least 6 feet from you on days when you have radiation."		

Thinking Exercise 10-5

Pharmacology

A 55-year-old female client was diagnosed 7 years ago (at the age of 48) with stage I breast cancer for which she had a left breast lumpectomy followed by external radiation therapy for 8 weeks. Today she had a breast ultrasound and 3D mammography that revealed a large tumor in her right breast. A biopsy confirmed stage III invasive breast cancer, for which she will receive doxorubicin, cyclophosphamide, and paclitaxel. Which nursing actions are appropriate for the client when she receives chemotherapy? **Select all that apply.**

_____ A. Monitor liver enzyme laboratory test values for increases.

_____ B. Teach the client to report jaundice and/or abdominal edema.

_____ C. Reassure the client that she will receive an antiemetic to decrease nausea and vomiting.

_____ D. Teach the client that she will likely experience alopecia.

_____ E. Teach the client to avoid crowds and people who have infections.

_____ F. Tell the client that she will need antibiotics while she is receiving chemotherapy.

_____ G. Remind the client that she will likely have fatigue for a few days after each drug treatment.

_____ H. Tell the client that these drugs will cure her breast cancer.

Thinking Exercise 10-6

A 55-year-old female client was diagnosed 7 years ago (at the age of 48) with stage I breast cancer. Recently, a breast ultrasound and 3D mammogram revealed a new, large tumor in her right breast. A biopsy confirmed stage III invasive breast cancer, for which she received doxorubicin, cyclophosphamide, and paclitaxel. Today she is visiting her oncologist for a follow-up visit after completing this chemotherapy. Before being examined by the provider, the nurse performs a brief assessment and documents the findings.

History and Physical	Nurses' Notes	Vital Signs	Laboratory Results

8/4/21 1015 Today the client states she is feeling much better; her last chemotherapy was completed 4 weeks ago. Vital signs: Temperature, 98°F (36.7°C); pulse, 76 beats/min and regular; respirations, 20 breaths/min; blood pressure, 118/74 mm Hg; oxygen saturation, 95%. Yesterday's lab work shows RBCs, WBCs, and platelets increased almost to normal ranges. Has lost 22 lb (10 kg) since beginning chemotherapy and still does not have a good appetite. States that her husband of 2 years has filed for divorce because he "can't handle her health issues." She is looking forward to having her follow-up testing to determine if her tumor has decreased in size. ----------------------------------P. Brown, LVN

Highlight the client findings in the Nurses' Notes that demonstrate that the client is progressing well.

Single-Episode Cases (10-7 and 10-8)

Thinking Exercise 10-7

A 46-year-old postmenopausal woman discovers a lump in her left breast. A breast biopsy reveals a large tumor that is classified as HER2 positive. As a result, the client chose to have a left radical mastectomy with breast reconstruction. She returns from the PACU with a Jackson-Pratt (J-P) drain and large intact surgical dressing. **Use an X to show whether the nursing actions below are Indicated (appropriate or necessary), Contraindicated (could be harmful), or Non-Essential (makes no difference or is not necessary) for the client's care at this time.**

Nursing Action	Indicated	Contraindicated	Non-Essential
Apply oxygen therapy at 2 L/min.			
Monitor the amount and color of the J-P drainage.			
Remind the staff to avoid taking blood pressures or drawing blood in the affected arm.			
Keep the client's head of the bed flat at all times.			
Elevate the affected arm on a pillow.			
Observe the surgical dressing for bleeding.			
Keep the client in bed for at least 48 hours.			
Begin to reinforce client teaching about how to perform postmastectomy exercises.			

Thinking Exercise 10-8

A 46-year-old postmenopausal female client who had a left mastectomy with breast reconstruction returns to the surgeon's office for a 6-week follow-up appointment. **For each assessment finding, use an X to indicate whether the treatment interventions were Effective (helped to meet expected outcomes), Ineffective (did not help to meet expected outcomes), or Unrelated (not related to the expected outcomes).**

Assessment Finding	Effective	Ineffective	Unrelated
Incisions show no sign of infection.			
Reports an inability to straighten her left elbow.			
Mastectomy and reconstruction incisions are healed without redness or drainage.			
Left arm is very swollen and much larger than the right arm.			
Reports frequent heart palpitations when she drinks caffeinated beverages.			

11 Infection

Exemplar 11A. Pneumonia (Medical-Surgical Nursing: Middle-Age Adult)

Unfolding Case (11A-1 Through 11A-6)

Thinking Exercise 11A-1

A 48-year-old female client visits the urgent care center with report of increasing shortness of breath. She tells the nurse that she has had a fever between 101° F (38.3° C) and 102°F (38.9°C), a moist cough, extreme fatigue, and generalized muscle aches for the last 5 days, which caused her to miss work at a local grocery store. Her boyfriend suggested that she go to urgent care because she was getting worse. What additional client assessment data are of **immediate concern** to the nurse? **Select all that apply.**

_____ A. Has premenstrual cramping that is worse this month

_____ B. Pulse rate = 94 beats/min

_____ C. Blood pressure (BP) = 92/48 mm Hg

_____ D. Expectorating thick mucus when coughing

_____ E. Reports lack of appetite

_____ F. Reports achiness in her chest when she coughs

_____ G. Oxygen saturation = 91% (on room air [RA])

_____ H. Respirations = 32 breaths/min

Thinking Exercise 11A-2

A 48-year-old female client visits the urgent care center with report of increasing shortness of breath. She tells the nurse that she has had a fever between 101° F (38.3°C) and 102°F (38.9°C), a moist cough, extreme fatigue, and generalized muscle aches for the last 5 days, which caused her to miss work at a local grocery store. Her current vital signs are: temperature, 102.8°F (39.3°C); pulse, 94 beats/min; respirations, 32 breaths/min; BP, 92/48 mm Hg; oxygen saturation, 91% (on RA). **Choose the *most likely* options for the information missing from the statements below by selecting from the lists of options provided.**

The nurse recognizes that the client's assessment findings suggest that the client *most likely* has ______1______. Based on her current vital signs, she also seems be ______2______.

Options for 1	Options for 2
Tuberculosis	Nauseated
Atelectasis	Dehydrated
Pneumonia	Hypertensive
Asthma	Bradycardic

Thinking Exercise 11A-3

A 48-year-old female client visits the urgent care center with report of increasing shortness of breath. She tells the nurse that she has had a fever between 101°F (38.3°C) and 102°F (38.9°C), a moist cough, extreme fatigue, and generalized muscle aches for the last 5 days, which caused her to miss work at a local grocery store. Her current vital signs are: temperature, 102.8°F (39.3°C); pulse, 94 beats/min; respirations, 32 breaths/min; BP, 92/48 mm Hg; oxygen saturation, 91% (on RA). After examination by the primary health care provider, the client was told that she needs to be admitted to the acute care hospital for management of her respiratory illness. **Choose the *most likely* options for the information missing from the statements below by selecting from the lists of options provided.**

The ***priority*** for the client's care in the hospital will be to treat her _____1_____ and increase her _____2_____. She will also require _____2_____ to manage _____1_____.

Options for 1	Options for 2
Tachycardia	Oxygenation
Infection	Blood pressure
Hypotension	IV fluids
Dehydration	Drug therapy
Tachypnea	Supplemental enteral nutrition

Thinking Exercise 11A-4

A 48-year-old female client was referred from the urgent care center for admission to the acute care hospital for treatment of her respiratory illness. Her most recent vital signs on hospital admission are: temperature, 103° F (39.4°C); pulse, 92 beats/min; respirations, 30 breaths/min; BP, 98/50 mm Hg; oxygen saturation, 90% (on RA). Based on the client findings, the nurse coordinates the client's care with the registered nurse and anticipates orders from the primary health care provider. **Use an X to show whether the primary health care provider's orders listed below are Indicated (appropriate or necessary), Contraindicated (could be harmful), or Non-Essential (makes no difference or is not necessary) for the client's care at this time.**

Primary Health Care Provider Order	Indicated	Contraindicated	Non-Essential
Obtain a sputum specimen for culture and sensitivity and chest x-ray stat.			
Start supplemental oxygen therapy via nasal cannula.			
Refer the client to physical therapy to help manage her fatigue.			
Provide access for IV fluid and antibiotic therapy.			
Place the client in a lateral position to prevent aspiration of secretions.			

Thinking Exercise 11A-5

A 48-year-old female client was referred from the urgent care center for admission to the acute care hospital for treatment of her respiratory illness. Her most recent vital signs on hospital admission at 2:00 p.m. (1400) are: temperature, 103°F (39.4°C); pulse, 92 beats/min; respirations, 30 breaths/min; BP, 98/50 mm Hg; oxygen saturation, 90% (on RA). Her chest x-ray and sputum analysis confirmed that the client has community-acquired streptococcal pneumonia, for which she is receiving her first dose of IV cefotaxime and 3 L/min of supplemental oxygen therapy via nasal cannula. At 7:30 p.m. (1930) the nurse notes that the client has rapid, more labored respirations with frequent coughing that is producing thick tenacious secretions. The client is alert and oriented, and able to speak between coughing episodes. She states that the last time she had this much coughing, the respiratory therapist (RT) gave her a nebulizer treatment, which "helped a lot." What nursing actions would the nurse implement at this time in coordination with the registered nurse (RN)? **Select all that apply.**

_____ A. Call the respiratory therapist to administer a nebulizer treatment.

_____ B. Contact the Rapid Response Team.

_____ C. Increase the supplemental oxygen flow.

_____ D. Administer the antitussive medication as prescribed PRN.

_____ E. Increase the rate of the client's IV fluids.

_____ F. Listen to the client's breath sounds to compare with previous findings.

_____ G. Ensure that the client is positioned in a high-Fowler position.

_____ H. Remind the client to drink additional fluids to thin secretions.

_____ I. Obtain the client's vital signs and note change from previous readings.

_____ J. Document the client findings and actions taken.

Thinking Exercise 11A-6

A 48-year-old female client was admitted to the acute care hospital for treatment of community-acquired streptococcal pneumonia 3 days ago. On admission she had a fever, productive cough, fatigue, and dyspnea. Today the nurse is preparing the client for discharge to home, where she will continue oral antibiotic therapy. **Highlight the client findings in the note below that demonstrate that the client is progressing well prior to hospital discharge.**

History and Physical	Nurses' Notes	Vital Signs	Laboratory Results

12/3/21 1015 Client states that she has only 2–3 coughing spells a day and has not coughed up any mucus since yesterday. VS: T = 99° F (37.2° C), P = 84, R = 22, B/P = 118/70, oxygen saturation = 95% (on room air). Continues to report extreme fatigue and anorexia. Understands that she needs to continue taking her antibiotic until the prescription is completed. Also able to demonstrate use of inhaler for home use to improve breathing. -- *S. Myers, LPN*

Single-Episode Cases (11A-7 and 11A-8)

Thinking Exercise 11A-7

A 55-year-old male client was admitted to the acute care hospital unit following a mild thrombotic stroke resulting in left-sided weakness and urinary incontinence. He was treated for atrial fibrillation with metoprolol and clopidogrel for several years. On assessment, the nurse finds the client has an IV for fluid replacement because he is currently NPO. The nurse is planning care for the client to prevent complications. **Place an X to show whether the nursing actions below are <u>Indicated</u> (appropriate or necessary), <u>Contraindicated</u> (could be harmful), or <u>Non-Essential</u> (makes no difference or is not necessary) for the client to prevent aspiration pneumonia.**

Nursing Action	Indicated	Contraindicated	Non-Essential
Remind assistive personnel to keep the client NPO.			
Maintain the client in a position with the head of the bed at 10 degrees or higher.			
Be sure that suction equipment is on hand and working.			
Consult with the speech-language pathologist (SLP) to perform a swallowing study.			
Mix liquid beverages with a thickening agent to prevent choking.			

Thinking Exercise 11A-8

A 36-year-old female client attended a birthday party with over 60 friends and family members a week ago. Today she visits the urgent care center with report of sudden onset shortness of breath, loss of taste and smell, anorexia, and a "runny" nose. The nurse interviews the client and collects the following data:

- No significant medical history
- Body mass index (BMI) = 28.6
- Temperature = 101.6°F (38.7°C)
- Pulse = 86 beats/min
- Respirations = 26 breaths/min
- Blood pressure = 122/78 mm Hg
- Oxygen saturation = 92% (on room air [RA])

Choose the *most likely* options for the information missing from the statements below by selecting from the lists of options provided.

The nurse suspects that the client ***most likely*** has _____1_____, which is a highly transmissible respiratory infection, and is at high risk for decreasing _____2_____. If the client is confirmed to have this health problem by means of a point-of-care test, she would probably be discharged or transferred to _____3_____.

Options for 1	Options for 2	Options for 3
Tuberculosis	Level of consciousness	Her home
Asthma	Appetite	The emergency department
COVID-19	Blood pressure	A rehabilitation setting
Influenza	Oxygenation	The intensive care unit

Exemplar 11B. Respiratory Syncytial Virus (Pediatric Nursing: Toddler)

Unfolding Case (11B-1 Through 11B-6)

Thinking Exercise 11B-1

A 16-month old female toddler is brought to the emergency department (ED) by her parents. Her mother tells the nurse that the toddler started having a "runny" nose and cough 2 days ago. This morning, she had a "little" fever, was very fussy, and seemed to have a couple of pauses in her breathing. Current vital signs include: axillary temperature, 100°F (37.8°C); apical pulse, 102 beats/min; respirations, 34 breaths/min; blood pressure, 76/50 mm Hg; oxygen saturation, 88%. The nurse auscultates occasional low-pitched wheezes in both lungs. The child is admitted to the acute care pediatric unit. **Highlight the client findings that are of immediate concern to the nurse.**

Thinking Exercise 11B-2

A 16-month old female toddler is brought to the ED by her parents. Her mother tells the nurse that the toddler started having a "runny" nose and cough 2 days ago. This morning, she had a "little" fever, was very fussy, and seemed to have a couple of pauses in her breathing. Current vital signs include: axillary temperature, 100°F (37.8°C); apical pulse, 102 beats/min; respirations, 34 breaths/min; blood pressure, 76/50 mm Hg; oxygen saturation, 88%. The nurse auscultates occasional low-pitched wheezes in both lungs. The child is evaluated for possible respiratory syncytial virus (RSV) bronchiolitis and/or bronchial asthma. **For each client assessment finding below, determine if the finding is associated with asthma, RSV bronchiolitis, or both of these respiratory diseases.**

Client Finding	Asthma	RSV
Low-grade fever		
Fussiness		
Low oxygen saturation		
Wheezing		
Cough		

Thinking Exercise 11B-3

A 16-month old female toddler is brought to the emergency department (ED) by her parents. Her mother tells the nurse that the toddler started having a "runny" nose and cough 2 days ago. This morning, she had a "little" fever, was very fussy, and seemed to have a couple of pauses in her breathing. Current vital signs include: axillary temperature, 100°F (37.8°C); apical pulse, 102 beats/min; respirations, 34 breaths/min; blood pressure, 76/50 mm Hg; oxygen saturation, 88%. The nurse auscultates occasional low-pitched wheezes in both lungs. The toddler was admitted to the acute care pediatric unit with respiratory syncytial virus (RSV) bronchiolitis and placed on supplemental high-humidity oxygen therapy via nasal cannula. What ***priority*** outcomes would guide the nurse in planning care? **Select all that apply.**

_____ A. Maintaining a patent airway

_____ B. Preventing infection transmission

_____ C. Maintaining hydration

_____ D. Managing pain

_____ E. Managing hypotension

_____ F. Managing fever

_____ G. Preventing respiratory failure

Thinking Exercise 11B-4

A 16-month old female toddler was admitted to the acute care pediatric unit with respiratory syncytial virus (RSV) bronchiolitis and placed on supplemental high-humidity oxygen therapy via nasal cannula. The nurse anticipates possible complications that may occur during the child's hospitalization, especially acute respiratory distress and dehydration. **For each nursing action below, use an X to**

indicate whether the action is *most appropriate* for preventing or detecting acute respiratory distress or dehydration.

Nursing Action	Acute Respiratory Distress	Dehydration
Weigh the child every day and report weight loss.		
Suction the child if thick secretions are present.		
Maintain the oxygen saturation at a minimum of 90% to 95%.		
Provide oral hydration fluids, such as Pedialyte.		
Report high-pitched wheezing to the registered nurse immediately.		
Document accurate intake and urinary output.		
Report tachypnea to the registered nurse immediately.		

Thinking Exercise 11B-5

A 16-month old female toddler was admitted to the acute care pediatric unit with respiratory syncytial virus (RSV) bronchiolitis and placed on supplemental high-humidity oxygen therapy via nasal cannula. The child's mother is concerned about transmission of RSV to other clients, visitors, and staff. Which interventions would the nurse implement to prevent RSV transmission? **Select all that apply.**

_____ A. Wash your hands frequently and thoroughly.

_____ B. Place the child on contact precautions.

_____ C. Wear a mask to help block droplets from sneezing and coughing.

_____ D. Administer antiviral medication as prescribed.

_____ E. Be aware that RSV is spread by the airborne route.

_____ F. Disinfect surfaces that have been contaminated by RSV secretions.

_____ G. Administer palivizumab to prevent transmission from the child to others.

Thinking Exercise 11B-6

A 16-month old female toddler was admitted to the acute care pediatric unit with respiratory syncytial virus (RSV) bronchiolitis and placed on supplemental high-humidity oxygen therapy via nasal cannula. As a result of the supportive care that the child received for almost a week, the primary health care provider determines that she can be discharged home. The nurse reinforces discharge teaching and documents the child's most recent assessment findings. **For each assessment finding, use an X to indicate whether the care for the child was Effective (helped to meet expected outcomes), Ineffective (did not help to meet expected outcomes), or Unrelated (not related to the expected outcomes).**

Assessment Finding	Effective	Ineffective	Unrelated
Has occasional low-pitched wheezing			
Temperature = 99°F (37.2°C)			
Oxygen saturation = 96% (on room air [RA])			
Respirations = 26 breaths/min			
Weight = 23 lb (10.4 kg)			
Urine output = 18 mL/hr			
Diarrheal stools due to teething			
No cough or rhinorrhea			

Single-Episode Case (11B-7)

Thinking Exercise 11B-7

The nurse interviews a grandmother who is the guardian of a 3-month-old male infant at the pediatric clinic. She brought her grandson in today for his monthly checkup and to inquire about whether he needs medication to help prevent respiratory syncytial virus (RSV) infection this winter. The baby was born prematurely and had the first stage of surgery for a congenital heart defect at 1 month of age. He will likely have additional operations in the future. The infant is currently being treated for gastroesophageal reflux disease (GERD) and has had a problem gaining weight because he "spits up" his formula a lot. **Choose the *most likely* options for the information missing from the statements below by selecting from the lists of options provided.**

The nurse recognizes that the infant is at high risk for RSV because he has _____1_____. The medication that is given to help prevent RSV in high-risk infants is a monoclonal antibody called _____2_____, which is typically given once a month from November through March.

Options for 1	Options for 2
Difficulty gaining weight	Ribavirin
A history of congenital heart defect	Remdesivir
GERD	Palivizumab
Been born prematurely	Methotrexate

Mood and Affect: Depression/Suicide Risk

(Mental Health Nursing: Older Adult)

12

Unfolding Case (12-1 Through 12-6)

Thinking Exercise 12-1

A 76-year-old female client who recently had a myocardial infarction is in a rehabilitation facility and refuses to attend physical therapy. The client states, "What's the point? I'll never be well enough to see my grandchildren." The nurse notes that the client's appetite has significantly declined over the past week, she has not had a visitor in several days, and she became agitated yesterday when asked to bathe. The nurse collects additional assessment data. **Highlight or place a check mark next to the client findings below that require follow-up by the nurse.**

- Oriented to person, place, and time
- Sitting in chair with slumped posture
- Avoids eye contact with nursing staff
- Reports feeling hopeless on most days over the past 3 weeks
- Heart rate (HR) = 72 beats/min
- Respirations = 14 breaths/min
- Lung fields clear throughout all lobes
- Moves all extremities with moderate strength
- Refuses to participate in ADLs or take meals in the dining hall
- Reports thinking about death frequently but denies thoughts of hurting herself

Thinking Exercise 12-2

A 76-year-old female client who recently had a myocardial infarction is in a rehabilitation facility and refuses to attend physical therapy. The client states, "What's the point? I'll never be well enough to see my grandchildren." The nurse notes that the client's appetite has significantly declined over the past week, she has not had a visitor in several days, and she became agitated yesterday when asked to bathe. Additional client findings include poor eye contact, slumped posture, insomnia, and impaired concentration. The client also refuses to participate in ADLs or have meals in the main dining room. She reports feelings of hopelessness on most days over the past 3 weeks, and verbalizes thinking about death frequently (but denies thoughts of hurting herself). The nurse analyzes client findings. **For each client finding below, determine if the finding is associated with anxiety, delirium, and/or depression. Note that some findings may be associated with more than one health problem.**

Client Finding	Anxiety	Delirium	Depression
Impaired cognition			
Reduced appetite			
Agitation			
Sleep disturbances			
Activity avoidance			

Thinking Exercise 12-3

A 76-year-old female client who recently had a myocardial infarction is in a rehabilitation facility and refuses to attend physical therapy. The client states, "What's the point? I'll never be well enough to see my grandchildren." The nurse notes that the client's appetite has significantly declined over the past week, she has not had a visitor in several days, and she became agitated yesterday when asked to bathe. Additional client findings include poor eye contact, slumped posture, insomnia, and impaired concentration. The client also refuses to participate in ADLs or have meals in the main dining room. She reports feelings of hopelessness on most days over the past 3 weeks and verbalizes thinking about death frequently (but denies thoughts of hurting herself). **Complete the following sentences by choosing the *most likely* option for the missing information from the lists of options provided.**

Based on the client's feelings of hopelessness for more than 2 weeks, as well as insomnia, poor concentration, and reduced appetite with weight loss, the nurse determines that the client is ***most likely*** experiencing __________1__________ . The nurse's ***priority*** is to closely monitor the client for __________2__________ to prevent client injury.

Options for 1	Options for 2
Mild depression	Hallucinations
Bipolar disorder	Social phobia
Major depressive disorder	Panic attack
Delirium	Suicidal thoughts
Major depressive episode	Somatic pain

Thinking Exercise 12-4

A 76-year-old female client who recently had a myocardial infarction is in a rehabilitation facility and refuses to attend physical therapy. The client states, "What's the point? I'll never be well enough to see my grandchildren." A thorough assessment determined feelings of hopelessness for more than 2 weeks as well as insomnia, poor concentration, and reduced appetite with weight loss. The client was diagnosed with major depressive episode and prescribed venlafaxine. The nurse collaborates with the health care team to develop a plan of care. **Use an X to show whether each nursing action below is Indicated (appropriate or necessary), Contraindicated (could be harmful), or Non-Essential (makes no difference or is not necessary) for the client's care at this time.**

Nursing Action	Indicated	Contraindicated	Non-Essential
Teach the client meditation and relaxation techniques.			
Encourage frequent oral care.			
Isolate the client from other rehabilitation clients.			
Remind the client that it may take several weeks for antidepressant drugs to begin working.			
Monitor the client for increasing blood pressure.			
Obtain consent for electroconvulsive therapy (ECT).			

Thinking Exercise 12-5

A 76-year-old female client in a rehabilitation facility was diagnosed with major depressive episode 3 days ago. The client was prescribed venlafaxine and encouraged to participate in group therapy. The client talks about dying and tells the nurse that she wants to end her own life. Which interventions will the nurse implement at this time to ensure client safety while she is experiencing suicidal thoughts? **Select all that apply.**

_____ A. Remove dangerous items from the client's room.

_____ B. Place the client in soft wrist restraints.

_____ C. Recommend increasing the client's antidepressant dosage.

_____ D. Implement a "no self-harm contract."

_____ E. Arrange for constant observation, with the client in full view at all times.

_____ F. Ask the client to describe her specific suicide plan.

_____ G. Demonstrate concern and advocate for the client.

_____ H. Allow the client to exercise in the courtyard alone.

Thinking Exercise 12-6

Four weeks ago, a 76-year-old female client in a rehabilitation facility was diagnosed with major depressive episode. The client was experiencing hopelessness, decreased appetite with weight loss, insomnia, social isolation, and impaired concentration. The client was treated with venlafaxine and group therapy. The nurse reassesses the client to evaluate if expected outcomes have been met. **For each client statement, use an X to indicate whether the client <u>is</u> progressing as expected or is <u>not</u> progressing as expected.**

Client Statements	Is Progressing	Is Not Progressing
"I am looking forward to seeing my grandchildren this afternoon."		
"Everything seems to run together in my mind. I don't know if it is day or night."		
"I need to take a nap after working so hard in physical therapy."		
"I feel comfortable sharing my hopes and fears in group therapy."		
"My clothes are not soiled. I can continue wearing them for several more days."		

Single-Episode Case (12-7)

Thinking Exercise 12-7

A home health nurse visits an 88-year-old male client who became widowed 6 months ago. The client lives alone and has chronic pain related to multiple health issues. A local charity provides meals three times each week, and a neighbor assists the client by picking up prescriptions and home supplies from the store a couple of times a month. The client appears disheveled, avoids eye contact with the nurse, and reports, "I should have died instead of my wife. She was always the strong one." Which questions will the nurse ask to evaluate the client's potential for suicide? **Select all that apply.**

_____ A. "Have you thought about harming or killing yourself?"

_____ B. "Do you prefer to have meals in your room instead of the dining hall?"

_____ C. "If you were to harm yourself, how would you do it?"

_____ D. "During the past month, have you often felt 'down,' depressed, or hopeless?"

_____ E. "Do you have access to the items you will need to carry out your suicide plan?"

_____ F. "What has kept you from harming yourself thus far?"

_____ G. "Do you think you can refrain from acting on your thoughts or impulses?"

_____ H. "How often do your children come to visit you?"

Stress and Coping 13

Exemplar 13A. Generalized Anxiety Disorder/Loss (Mental Health Nursing: Older Adult)

Unfolding Case (13A-1 Through 13A-6)

Thinking Exercise 13A-1

A home health nurse visits an 88-year-old male client who has a history of Alzheimer disease and chronic obstructive pulmonary disease (COPD). The client is alert, oriented to self only, and talkative, becoming short of breath frequently during the visit. Vital signs are: heart rate (HR), 65 beats/min; respirations, 16 breaths/min; blood pressure (BP), 136/48 mm Hg; oxygen saturation, 92% (on 4 L/min nasal cannula). The client has a large, barrel-shaped chest and a productive cough with thick, pale yellow sputum. The client's wife, who is 12 years younger and the primary caregiver for her spouse, is present for the visit. She fusses over the client by adjusting pillows behind his back and smoothing down the client's hair. She asks multiple questions about the client's medications, physical activity, and diet, but doesn't fully listen to the nurse's responses. She appears fidgety and responds, "Oh! I remember. Yes, I've got this." **Use an X to identify the three client findings from the list in the left column that require follow-up by the nurse.**

Client Finding	Client Finding That Requires Follow-up by the Nurse
Client's heart rate	
Shape and size of client's chest	
Spouse's behavior	
Client's sputum color and consistency	
Use of oxygen by the client	
Client's dyspnea	
Spouse's response to the nurse	
Client's orientation level	

Thinking Exercise 13A-2

A home health nurse visits an 88-year-old male client who has a history of Alzheimer disease and chronic obstructive pulmonary disease (COPD). The client is alert and talkative, becoming short of breath frequently during the visit. Vital signs are stable and the rest of the physical assessment is unremarkable. The client's wife, who is 12 years younger and the primary caregiver for her spouse, is present for the visit. She fusses over the client by adjusting pillows behind his back several times and smoothing down the client's hair. She asks multiple questions about the client's medications, physical activity, and diet, but doesn't fully listen to the nurse's responses. She appears fidgety and responds, "Oh! I remember. Yes, I've got this." **Complete the following sentences by choosing the *most likely* option for the missing information from the lists of options provided.**

To further analyze the situation, the nurse would ____1____ and ask the client's spouse to ____2____.

Options for 1	Options for 2
Ensure the client is safe	Call a friend to help care for her husband
Ask the client to take a deep breath	Repeat home health instructions
Establish rapport	Focus on her husband's health needs
Perform hand hygiene	Leave the examination area
Provide client privacy	Talk about her feelings

Thinking Exercise 13A-3

A home health nurse visits an 88-year-old male client who has a history of Alzheimer disease and chronic obstructive pulmonary disease (COPD). The client's wife, who is the client's primary caregiver, appears fidgety and frets about her husband's appearance. The nurse listens to the wife and learns that she is frequently anxious, has difficulty concentrating, and is unable to sleep through the night. She has church friends who visit weekly, but she has not attended services in several months because she feels unable to leave her husband alone for more than a short trip to the store. The wife begins to cry and states, "I've always been a worrier, but my husband was there to take care of things. Now I have to take care of everything. I don't trust anyone else to do it right." The nurse analyzes client findings to prioritize potential health problems for the client's wife. **Place an X to show whether the potential health problems below are Probable (most likely the explanation), Remote (unlikely, although possibly the explanation), or Improbable (not likely to be the explanation) based on the nurse's assessment findings.**

Potential Health Problems	Probable	Remote	Improbable
Ineffective coping			
Paranoia			
Anxiety disorder			
Social isolation			
Avoidant personality disorder			

Thinking Exercise 13A-4

A home health nurse visits an 88-year-old male client who has a history of Alzheimer disease and chronic obstructive pulmonary disease (COPD). The client's wife, who is the primary caregiver, appears fidgety and frets about her husband's appearance. The nurse listens to the spouse and learns that she is frequently anxious, has difficulty concentrating, and is unable to sleep through the night. She has church friends who visit weekly, but she has not attended services in several months because she feels unable to leave her husband alone for more than a short trip to the store. The wife begins to cry and states, "I've always been a worrier, but my husband was there to take care of me. Now I have to take care of everything. I don't trust anyone else to do it right." The nurse suspects that the wife has generalized anxiety disorder. **Complete the following sentences by choosing the *most likely* option for the missing information from the lists of options provided.**

Based on the nurse's suspected diagnosis, the nurse would plan interventions to meet desired client outcomes. The desired outcomes for older adults with anxiety disorders are to ________1________ and ________2________.

Options for 1	Options for 2
Identify effects of aging on stress and coping	Express feelings of spiritual comfort
Verbalize sources of conflicting values	Identify resources to reduce social isolation
Develop effective coping mechanisms	Experience fewer episodes of anxiety
Experience more social interactions	Verbalize grief and losses
Recognize emotional strengths and limitations	Maintain healthy emotional balance

Thinking Exercise 13A-5

A home health nurse visits an 88-year-old male client who has a history of Alzheimer disease and chronic obstructive pulmonary disease (COPD). The client's wife, who is the primary caregiver, appears fidgety and frets about her husband's appearance. The nurse listens to the spouse and learns that she is frequently anxious, has difficulty concentrating, and is unable to sleep through the night. She has church friends who visit weekly, but she has not attended services in several months because she feels unable to leave her husband alone for more than a short trip to the store. The wife begins to cry and states, "I've always been a worrier, but my husband was there to take care of things. Now I have to take care of everything. I don't trust anyone else to do it right." The nurse suspects that the wife has generalized anxiety disorder. Based on this health care problem, which interventions will the nurse include in this client's plan of care? **Select all that apply.**

_____ A. Eliminate the source of anxiety by institutionalizing the husband.

_____ B. Encourage participation in cognitive-behavioral therapy.

_____ C. Help the wife to recognize signs and symptoms of anxiety.

_____ D. Promote the use of defense mechanisms.

_____ E. Teach the wife relaxation techniques.

_____ F. Help the wife explore a variety of coping mechanisms.

_____ G. Recommend a prescription for benzodiazepine.

_____ H. Encourage the wife to verbalize thoughts and feelings.

Thinking Exercise 13A-6

A home health nurse follows up with an 88-year-old male client who has a history of Alzheimer disease. His wife is the primary caregiver and recently received a confirmed diagnosis of generalized anxiety disorder. The nurse reassesses the wife to evaluate whether expected outcomes were met. **For each statement by the client's wife, use an X to indicate whether the wife is progressing as expected or is <u>not</u> progressing as expected.**

Client Statement	Is Progressing	Is <u>Not</u> Progressing
"I pay a certified nursing assistant to care for my husband on Sunday mornings so that I can attend church."		
"I participate in group therapy with others who have spouses with Alzheimer disease."		
"I complete housework in the middle of the night when I cannot sleep."		
"I don't want to burden others, so I stopped allowing friends and family to visit."		
"I encourage my husband to do as much for himself as he can."		

Single-Episode Cases (13A-7 and 13A-8)

Thinking Exercise 13A-7

A 74-year-old female client was admitted to the telemetry unit 2 days ago for new-onset atrial fibrillation with a rapid ventricular response. The client, whose husband died 3 months ago, has been on bedrest owing to orthostatic hypotension and tachycardia. Although the client is oriented and can reposition herself independently, she is reluctant to participate in activities and appears detached from the current situation. Which statements by the client require follow-up by the nurse? **Select all that apply.**

_____ A. "I'm unable to brush my teeth. I simply don't have the energy."

_____ B. "I want these medications to start working so that I can get home to my cat."

_____ C. "I don't want any breakfast. Please don't allow any visitors today."

_____ D. "My husband is really smart with health issues. We should give him a call."

_____ E. "My heart broke when my husband died, but it will mend with time."

_____ F. "I'm a strong woman who will get through this difficult time."

_____ G. "I'm planning a trip to the beach with my friends this summer."

_____ H. "My children are right. I can't do anything right."

Thinking Exercise 13A-8

The nurse is caring for an 81-year-old male client who was recently admitted to a long-term care facility for more effective diabetic management and monitoring of complications. The client, who lived alone and drove himself to the Bingo Hall twice a week, is struggling with the new living arrangement. He feels a loss of control and has been acting inappropriately in front of the other residents. **Use an X to show whether each nursing action below is <u>Indicated</u> (appropriate or necessary), <u>Contraindicated</u> (could be harmful), or <u>Non-Essential</u> (makes no difference or is not necessary) for the client's care at this time.**

Nursing Actions	Indicated	Contraindicated	Non-Essential
Allow the client to make choices whenever possible.			
Ensure the same nurse is assigned to provide the client's bed bath each day.			
Explain the reasons when changes in the client's plan of care occur.			
Respect the client's right to refuse care and activities.			
Coordinate with the kitchen to provide the client's favorite foods.			

Exemplar 13B. Substance Use Disorder (Mental Health Nursing: Older Adult)

Unfolding Case (13B-1 Through 13B-6)

Thinking Exercise 13B-1

A nurse cares for a 70-year-old male client who is 26 hours after a transurethral resection of the prostate (TURP) procedure. The client has an indwelling urinary catheter with continuous bladder irrigation and IV morphine patient-controlled analgesia. While the nurse is assisting the client with hygiene activities prior to bed, the client states, "I usually have a glass of whiskey in the evening to help me sleep. I guess I'll take another shot of this pain pump to help me tonight." The nurse reviews the client's health history. **Highlight client data from the History and Physical below that require follow-up by the nurse.**

History and Physical | **Nurses' Notes** | **Vital Signs** | **Laboratory Results**

Health History

Benign prostatic hyperplasia

Hyperlipidemia

Osteoarthritis

Social History

Married with three adult children and several grandchildren

Retired primary school teacher

Denies alcohol use

Medications

Acetaminophen 650 mg orally every 12 hours

Atorvastatin 20 mg orally once daily

Tamsulosin 0.4 mg orally once daily

Thinking Exercise 13B-2

A nurse cares for a 70-year-old male client who is 26 hours after a transurethral resection of the prostate (TURP) procedure. The client has an indwelling urinary catheter with continuous bladder irrigation and IV morphine patient-controlled analgesia. While the nurse is assisting the client with hygiene activities prior to bed, the client states, "I usually have a glass of whiskey in the evening to help me sleep. I guess I'll take another shot of this pain pump to help me tonight." Which questions will the nurse ask to further assess the client's situation? **Select all that apply.**

_____ A. "When talking with others, do you ever underestimate how much you drink?"

_____ B. "Have you used prescription, over-the-counter, or recreational drugs to help you sleep?"

_____ C. "Does alcohol sometimes make it hard for you to remember parts of the day?"

_____ D. "Have you ever tried drinking warm milk as a substitute for your evening drink?"

_____ E. "Do you frequently have difficulty falling asleep or sleeping through the night?"

_____ F. "Have you ever increased your drinking after experiencing a loss in your life?"

_____ G. "Do you understand the purpose of the patient-controlled analgesia pump?"

_____ H. "Have you ever felt guilty about your drinking?"

Thinking Exercise 13B-3

A nurse cares for a 70-year-old male client who is 26 hours after a transurethral resection of the prostate (TURP) procedure. The client has an indwelling urinary catheter with continuous bladder irrigation and IV morphine patient-controlled analgesia. While the nurse is assisting the client with hygiene activities prior to bed, the client states, "I usually have a glass of whiskey in the evening to help me sleep. I guess I'll take another shot of this pain pump to help me tonight." The nurse further assesses the client and determines he frequently underestimates or denies drinking when speaking with others. He reports actually drinking three or four alcoholic beverages on each weekday and five or six alcoholic beverages on each weekend day. He also reports increasing his alcohol intake after the death of a friend and denies using any drugs to help him relax or sleep. **Complete the following sentence by choosing the *most likely* options for the missing information from the lists of options provided.**

The client's use of alcohol increases his risk for impaired ______1______ and ______1______, which may lead to ______2______ and ______2______.

Options for 1	Options for 2
Cardiac output	Dyspnea
Coordination	Falls
Hearing	Heart failure
Immunity	Medication misuse
Judgment	Pressure ulcers
Skin integrity	Social isolation

Thinking Exercise 13B-4

A nurse cares for a 70-year-old male client who is 26 hours after a transurethral resection of the prostate (TURP) procedure. The client has an indwelling urinary catheter with continuous bladder irrigation and IV morphine patient-controlled analgesia. The nurse's assessment indicates that he frequently underestimates or denies drinking when speaking with others. He reports actually drinking three or four alcoholic beverages on each weekday and five or six alcoholic beverages on each weekend day. He also reports increasing his alcohol intake after the death of a friend and denies using any drugs to help him relax or sleep. The client is diagnosed with alcohol use disorder and the nurse contributes to the plan of care. **Use an X to show whether each nursing action below is <u>Indicated</u> (appropriate or necessary), <u>Contraindicated</u> (could be harmful), or <u>Non-Essential</u> (makes no difference or is not necessary) for the client's care at this time.**

Nursing Action	Indicated	Contraindicated	Non-Essential
Withhold the client's dose of pain medication.			
Confront the client about his alcohol use and consequences.			
Encourage the client to agree to participate in a treatment program.			
Contact adult protective services to report elder abuse.			
Monitor the client for physiologic changes related to alcohol withdrawal.			

Thinking Exercise 13B-5

A nurse cares for a 70-year-old male client who had a transurethral resection of the prostate (TURP) procedure 3 days ago. The client's health history consists of benign prostatic hyperplasia, hyperlipidemia, and substance use disorder. The nurse's shift assessment identifies early signs of alcohol withdrawal including anxiety, bilateral lower extremity edema, and an increase in heart rate and blood pressure. Although the client is currently stable, the nurse recognizes that the client's condition may deteriorate quickly and therefore prepares to transfer care to the registered nurse. What essential information will the nurse include in a hand-off report to the registered nurse? **Select all that apply.**

_____ A. Family history of alcohol use disorders

_____ B. Current vital signs

_____ C. Last meal eaten

_____ D. Plans for inpatient rehabilitation

_____ E. As-needed medications administered

_____ F. Current mood and behavior

_____ G. Complete blood count (CBC) results

_____ H. Orientation assessment

Thinking Exercise 13B-6

A 70-year-old male client who had a transurethral resection of the prostate (TURP) procedure a week ago was treated for alcohol withdrawal syndrome. The client is stable and ready for discharge. A nurse evaluates the client after reinforcing discharge teaching and a referral to an outpatient treatment program. **For each client statement, use an X to indicate if the teaching was Effective (helped the client understand discharge teaching), Ineffective (did not help the client understand discharge teaching), or Unrelated (not related to discharge teaching).**

Client Statement	Effective	Ineffective	Unrelated
"I will be prescribed methadone to help me overcome my addiction."			
"It is my choice to participate in the alcohol treatment program."			
"Treatment may consist of individual, group, and family therapy."			
"I can't join Alcoholics Anonymous (AA) until after I complete the treatment program."			
"Eating a low-fat, high-protein diet will assist my recovery from alcoholism."			
"Decreasing my alcohol intake to only one glass a day is a positive step."			

Single-Episode Case (13B-7)

Thinking Exercise 13B-7

The nurse assesses a 67-year-old female client who has been receiving treatment for chronic pain over the past 5 years. The client, who is usually alert, oriented, and neatly dressed, appears disoriented and disheveled. The client's pupils are small and her vital signs are: heart rate (HR), 66 beats/min; respirations, 12 breaths/min; blood pressure (BP), 118/44 mm Hg; oxygen saturation, 93% (on room air [RA]). There are several expired bottles of pain pills scattered around the house and the nurse suspects the client has taken more than the prescribed dose. The nurse evaluates risk factors to more effectively assess the misuse of medication. Which client statements alert the nurse to risk factors associated with substance use disorder in older adults? **Select all that apply.**

_____ A. "My best friend died last week."

_____ B. "Last week I saw a news show about a new hip replacement technique."

_____ C. "The pain keeps getting worse. I can't stand it anymore."

_____ D. "I need to move because this big house is costing too much in upkeep."

_____ E. "I am so alone. All of my friends are gone and I am stuck here."

_____ F. "My ankles are more swollen than usual."

_____ G. "I would go back to drinking alcohol but I can't get anyone to buy it for me."

_____ H. "My sister asked me to knit her a blanket but I can't decide on a color."

Exemplar 13C. Elder Abuse/Neglect (Mental Health Nursing: Older Adult)

Unfolding Case (13C-1 Through 13C-6)

Thinking Exercise 13C-1

A 74-year-old male client who lives with his son is treated in the emergency department for an overdose of prescription medications. The client is stabilized and transferred to a medical-surgical unit for monitoring. While assisting in settling the client in his room, the nurse notes that the client is alert and oriented to self, positions himself in the bed, and denies any pain. Once he is settled, the nurse allows the client's son into the room and collects additional client data. **Highlight the client findings below that the nurse would report to the registered nurse.**

- Heart rate (HR) = 88 beats/min
- Blood pressure (BP) = 126/65 mm Hg
- Respirations (R) = 14 breaths/min
- Oxygen saturation = 94% (on room air [RA])
- Height = 5 feet 10 inches (1.8 m); weight = 122 lb (55.5 kg)
- Alert and oriented to self and place, confused to time and situation
- Follows simple commands
- Skin is warm and dry
- No skin tears, bruising, or wounds present
- Poor eye contact with son
- Avoids answering direct questions when son is in room

Thinking Exercise 13C-2

A 74-year-old male client who lives with his son is treated in the emergency department for an overdose of prescription medications. The client is stabilized and transferred to a medical-surgical unit for monitoring. While assisting in settling the client in a room, a nurse notes that the client is alert and oriented to self, positions himself in the bed, and denies any pain. Once he is settled, the nurse allows the client's son into the room and collects additional client data, including poor eye contact and evasiveness. The nurse also calculates that the client's body mass index (BMI) is lower than normal. The nurse reports client findings to the registered nurse, and a follow-up assessment is completed. Which statements by the client's son indicate risk factors for possible elder abuse and neglect by a family member? **Select all that apply.**

_____ A. "My father becomes agitated and confused at night when I need to sleep."

_____ B. "I work long hours and then come home to more work caring for my father."

_____ C. "He seems to enjoy a warm bath so I help him bathe in the evening hours."

_____ D. "I leave food out for him but it is always uneaten when I return home from work."

_____ E. "Locking him in his room is sometimes the only way I can keep him from hurting himself."

_____ F. "He listens to the radio and sometimes can recap stories from the shows."

_____ G. "I worry about him when I'm away, but I have no one to stay with him or check on him."

_____ H. "I love my father, but sometimes I get so frustrated with him."

Thinking Exercise 13C-3

A 74-year-old male client who lives with his son is treated in the emergency department for an overdose of prescription medications. The client is stabilized and transferred to a medical-surgical unit for monitoring. While assisting in settling the client in a room, a nurse notes that the client is alert and oriented to self, positions himself in the bed, and denies any pain. Once he is settled, the nurse allows the client's son into the room and collects additional client data, including poor eye contact and evasiveness. The nurse also calculates that the client's body mass index (BMI) is lower than normal. The nurse reports client findings to the registered nurse, and a follow-up assessment is completed. **Identify with an X the three *priority* health problems from the list on the left to be included in this client's plan of care.**

Potential Health Problems	Priority Health Problems
Decreased/impaired nutrition due to possible neglect	
Delayed growth due to inadequate caregiving	
Knowledge deficit about community support and resources for home care	
Poor self-esteem due to negative family interactions	
Acute pain due to physical injuries	

Thinking Exercise 13C-4

A 74-year-old male client who lives with his son is treated in the emergency department for an overdose of prescription medications. The client is stabilized and transferred to a medical-surgical unit for monitoring. While assisting in settling the client in a room, a nurse notes that the client is alert and oriented to self, positions himself in the bed, and denies any pain. Once settled, the nurse allows the client's son into the room and collects additional client data, including poor eye contact and evasiveness. The nurse also calculates that the client's body mass index (BMI) is lower than normal. The nurse contributes to the plan of care for the client. **Complete the following sentences by choosing the *most likely* option for the missing information from the list of options provided.**

The desired outcomes for this client are remaining free from injury, eating adequate nutrients to maintain health, feeling safe and secure at home, and practicing behaviors that promote self-confidence. Desired outcomes for the client's son are to ______________________________ and ______________________________.

Options
Demonstrate selection of appropriate foods and fluids Identify ways to compensate for personality deficits Perform the caregiver role with competence and confidence Use strategies and resources to promote stress reduction Verbalize understanding of prescribed medications

Thinking Exercise 13C-5

A 74-year-old male client who lives with his son is treated in the emergency department for an overdose of prescription medications. The client is stabilized and transferred to a medical-surgical unit for monitoring. While assisting in settling the client in a room, a nurse notes that the client is alert and oriented to self, positions himself in the bed, and denies any pain. Once settled, the nurse allows the client's son into the room and collects additional client data, including poor eye contact and evasiveness. The nurse also calculates that the client's body mass index (BMI) is lower than normal. Which actions will the nurse take to meet the desired outcomes for both the client and son? **Select all that apply.**

_____ A. Consult a registered dietitian nutritionist.

_____ B. Schedule for the client to be transferred to a long-term care facility.

_____ C. Teach the client's son healthy strategies to cope with caregiver stress.

_____ D. Consult a social worker to help identify community resources.

_____ E. Document all findings accurately and objectively.

_____ F. Encourage the client to not allow his son to visit during hospitalization.

_____ G. Provide privacy when addressing concerns with the client and the son.

_____ H. Confront the client's son with allegations of abuse.

Thinking Exercise 13C-6

A 74-year-old male client who lives with his son was treated in the emergency department for an overdose of prescription medications, stabilized, and transferred to a medical-surgical unit for monitoring 3 days ago. Interventions were implemented to address priority health problems. The health care team supports discharging the client back into the care of his son. After reviewing discharge instructions with the son, the nurse evaluates client outcomes. **For each client finding, use an X to indicate if interventions were Effective (helped to meet expectations), Ineffective (did not help to meet expected outcomes), or Unrelated (not related to the expected outcomes).**

Client Finding	Effective	Ineffective	Unrelated
Client eats 100% of meals and supplements.			
Client's son has joined a support group for caregivers of older adults.			
Client is oriented to person and place and follows basic commands.			
Client's son is afraid to use available respite care.			
Client states he is interested in going to the senior day care center.			

Single-Episode Case (13C-7)

Thinking Exercise 13C-7

The nurse cares for a 90-year-old male client who was admitted 3 days ago after a fall and has a history of dementia. After confirming discharge plans for the client, the wife stops the nurse in the hallway and states that she does not want her husband to come home because she is afraid of him. She explains that her husband is frequently confused and becomes agitated when she attempts to reorient him. She states, "My husband isn't the man I married. He's become very angry and says terrible things to me. He also hits and pushes me when I try to calm him down." **Use an X to show whether the nursing actions below are Indicated (appropriate or necessary), Contraindicated (could be harmful), or Non-Essential (makes no difference or is not necessary) for the client's care at this time.**

Nursing Action	Indicated	Contraindicated	Non-Essential
Ensure confidentiality when discussing concerns with the client and wife together.			
Consult the primary health care provider to evaluate the client's behavior and medication regimen.			
Assess the client's range of motion and strength to determine if he is physically capable of hitting his wife.			
Consult the case manager regarding alternatives for the client's discharge plan.			
Notify appropriate reporting agencies for suspected elder abuse.			

14 Reproduction

Exemplar 14A. Uterine Leiomyoma/Hysterectomy (Medical-Surgical Nursing: Middle-Age Adult)

Unfolding Case (14A-1 Through 14A-6)

Thinking Exercise 14A-1

A 48-year-old female client had a traditional open hysterectomy and a left salpingo-oophorectomy (LSO) this morning for multiple large uterine leiomyomas (fibroid tumors) and an enlarged left ovary. Her surgeon chose the traditional surgical approach rather than laparoscopy because the client is obese and has a history of hypertension and type 2 diabetes mellitus. On admission to the surgical unit from the postanesthesia care unit (PACU), the nurse reviews the PACU note and collects data as part of an initial admission assessment. **Use an X to indicate which client findings require immediate follow-up by the nurse.**

Client Finding in PACU	Client Finding on Surgical Unit	Client Finding Requiring Immediate Follow-up
Temperature = 99°F (37.2°C)	Temperature = 99°F (37.2°C)	
Apical pulse = 84 beats/min; strong and regular	Apical pulse = 100 beats/min; fairly strong and regular	
Respirations = 20 breaths/min	Respirations = 18 breaths/min	
Blood pressure = 122/78 mm Hg	Blood pressure = 102/54 mm Hg	
Oxygen saturation = 95% (on room air [RA])	Oxygen saturation = 95% (on room air [RA])	
Abdominal surgical dressing dry and intact	Abdominal surgical dressing dry and intact	
Mild abdominal distention	Moderate abdominal distention	
Bowel sounds absent × 4	Bowel sounds absent × 4	
Pain level = 7/10	Pain level = 9/10	
No nausea or vomiting	Reports feeling "a little nauseated"	
IV of D5/RL infusing at 80 mL/hr	IV of D5/RL infusing at 80 mL/hr	

Thinking Exercise 14A-2

A 48-year-old female client had a traditional open hysterectomy and a left salpingo-oophorectomy (LSO) this morning for multiple large uterine leiomyomas (fibroid tumors) and an enlarged left ovary. Her surgeon chose the traditional surgical approach rather than laparoscopy because the client is obese and has a history of hypertension and type 2 diabetes mellitus. On admission to the surgical unit from the postanesthesia care unit (PACU), the nurse reviews the PACU note and documents the following findings from the surgical unit assessment.

Client Finding in PACU	Client Finding on Surgical Unit Admission
Temperature = 99°F (37.2°C)	Temperature = 99°F (37.2°C)
Apical pulse = 84 beats/min; strong and regular	Apical pulse = 100 beats/min; weak and regular
Respirations = 20 breaths/min	Respirations = 18 breaths/min
Blood pressure = 122/78 mm Hg	Blood pressure = 102/54 mm Hg
Oxygen saturation = 95% (on room air [RA])	Oxygen saturation = 95% (on room air [RA])
Abdominal surgical dressing dry and intact	Abdominal surgical dressing dry and intact
Mild abdominal distention	Moderate abdominal distention
Bowel sounds absent × 4	Bowel sounds absent × 4
Abdominal pain level = 6/10 (patient-controlled analgesia [PCA] pump explained to client)	Abdominal pain level = 9/10
No nausea or vomiting	Reports feeling "a little nauseated"
IV of D5/RL infusing at 80 mL/hr	IV of D5/RL infusing at 80 mL/hr

Choose the *most likely* options for the information missing from the statements below by selecting from the lists of options provided.

When interpreting the admission assessment data, the nurse recognizes that the client is ***most likely*** experiencing ____1____ as evidenced by a(n) ____2____, ____2____, and ____2____.

Options for 1	Options for 2
Infection	Increased temperature
Paralytic ileus	Increased apical pulse
Internal bleeding	Increased abdominal pain level
Hypoxia	Decreased blood pressure
Cardiac dysrhythmias	Low oxygen saturation

Thinking Exercise 14A-3

A 48-year-old female client had a traditional open hysterectomy and a left salpingo-oophorectomy (LSO) this morning for multiple large uterine leiomyomas (fibroid tumors) and an enlarged left ovary. The client is obese and has a history of hypertension and type 2 diabetes mellitus. On admission to the surgical unit from the postanesthesia care unit (PACU), the nurse reviews the PACU note and documents the following findings from the surgical unit assessment.

Client Finding in PACU	Client Finding on Surgical Unit Admission
Temperature = 99°F (37.2°C)	Temperature = 99°F (37.2°C)
Apical pulse = 84 beats/min; strong and regular	Apical pulse = 100 beats/min; weak and regular
Respirations = 20 breaths/min	Respirations = 18 breaths/min
Blood pressure = 122/78 mm Hg	Blood pressure = 102/54 mm Hg
Oxygen saturation = 95% (on room air [RA])	Oxygen saturation = 95% (on room air [RA])

Continued

Client Finding in PACU	Client Finding on Surgical Unit Admission
Abdominal surgical dressing dry and intact	Abdominal surgical dressing dry and intact
Mild abdominal distention	Moderate abdominal distention
Bowel sounds absent × 4	Bowel sounds absent × 4
Abdominal pain level = 6/10 (patient-controlled analgesia [PCA] pump explained to client)	Abdominal pain level = 9/10
No nausea or vomiting	Reports feeling "a little nauseated"
IV of D5/RL infusing at 80 mL/hr	IV of D5/RL infusing at 80 mL/hr

Choose the *most likely* options for the information missing from the statement below by selecting from the list of options provided.

Based on the changes in the client's condition in the surgical unit, the nurse needs to plan care to meet the ***priority*** goals of preventing ______________________ and managing ______________________.

Options
Sepsis Bowel obstruction Hypovolemic shock Pain

Thinking Exercise 14A-4

A 48-year-old female client had a traditional open hysterectomy and a left salpingo-oophorectomy (LSO) this morning for multiple large uterine leiomyomas (fibroid tumors) and an enlarged left ovary. The client is obese and has a history of hypertension and type 2 diabetes mellitus. On admission to the surgical unit from the postanesthesia care unit (PACU), the nurse reviews the PACU note and documents the following findings from the surgical unit assessment.

Client Finding in PACU	Client Finding on Surgical Unit Admission
Temperature = 99°F (37.2°C)	Temperature = 99°F (37.2°C)
Apical pulse = 84 beats/min; strong and regular	Apical pulse = 100 beats/min; weak and regular
Respirations = 20 breaths/min	Respirations = 18 breaths/min
Blood pressure = 122/78 mm Hg	Blood pressure = 102/54 mm Hg
Oxygen saturation = 95% (on room air [RA])	Oxygen saturation = 95% (on room air [RA])
Abdominal surgical dressing dry and intact	Abdominal surgical dressing dry and intact
Mild abdominal distention	Moderate abdominal distention
Bowel sounds absent × 4	Bowel sounds absent × 4
Abdominal pain level = 6/10 (patient-controlled analgesia [PCA] pump explained to client)	Abdominal pain level = 9/10
No nausea or vomiting	Reports feeling "a little nauseated"
IV of D5/RL infusing at 80 mL/hr	IV of D5/RL infusing at 80 mL/hr

Diagnostic imaging tests confirmed a small clot in the client's abdominal cavity with no current active bleeding. Based on the changes in the client's condition, the nurse anticipates orders from the primary health care provider. **Use an X to show whether the potential orders listed below are Anticipated (appropriate or necessary), Contraindicated (could be harmful), or Non-Essential (makes no difference or is not necessary) for the client's care at this time.**

Potential Primary Health Care Provider Orders	Anticipated	Contraindicated	Non-Essential
Increase IV rate to 150 mL/hr.			
Obtain a complete blood count (CBC) and basic metabolic panel (BMP) stat.			
Monitor oral temperature every hour.			
Give regular insulin per sliding scale.			
Keep the client in a high-Fowler position.			
Maintain NPO status until further orders.			

Thinking Exercise 14A-5

A 48-year-old female client had a traditional open hysterectomy and a left salpingo-oophorectomy (LSO) 2 days ago for multiple large uterine leiomyomas (fibroid tumors) and an enlarged left ovary. The client is obese and has a history of hypertension and type 2 diabetes mellitus. Postoperatively the client was successfully treated for a small abdominal bleed. Since that time, she has been stable and is being prepared for discharge to home with her husband. The nurse reinforces health teaching prior to the client's discharge. Which health teaching will the nurse review with the client? **Select all that apply.**

_____ A. "Report any increased redness or drainage from your incision to your surgeon."

_____ B. "Contact your surgeon if you experience burning or frequency on urination."

_____ C. "Stay on bedrest for at least a week after you get home to prevent infection."

_____ D. "Avoid lifting anything more than 10 lb (4.5 kg) for the next 6 weeks."

_____ E. "Monitor your temperature and contact your surgeon if it goes above 100°F (37.8°C)."

_____ F. "When you shower, be sure to cover your incision and staples with plastic wrap."

_____ G. "If you experience any acute leg pain, swelling, or redness, contact your surgeon."

_____ H. "You will not have any more menstrual periods as a result of your surgery."

Thinking Exercise 14A-6

A 48-year-old female client had a traditional open hysterectomy and a left salpingo-oophorectomy (LSO) 4 weeks ago for multiple large uterine leiomyomas (fibroid tumors) and an enlarged left ovary. The client is obese and has a history of hypertension and type 2 diabetes mellitus. Today she is seeing her surgeon for a follow-up visit. The nurse collects and documents assessment data from the client prior to the surgeon's examination. **Highlight or place a check mark next to the assessment findings below that indicate that the client is progressing well.**

- Temperature = 98.8°F (37.1°C)
- Blood pressure = 166/94 mm Hg
- Oxygen saturation = 95%
- Incision clean, dry, and edges approximated
- Clear yellow urine
- Reports difficulty sleeping and excessive sweating at night
- No abdominal pain

Single-Episode Case (14A-7)

Thinking Exercise 14A-7

A 52-year-old female client had a laparoscopic total hysterectomy for menorrhagia due to fibroid tumors. After recovery in the postanesthesia care unit (PACU), the client is transferred to the short-stay surgical unit. The nurse reinforces postoperative health teaching for the client. Which statements by the nurse would be included in this client education? **Select all that apply.**

_____ A. "Be sure to use your incentive spirometer at least every 2 hours."

_____ B. "Exercise your legs and perform ankle pumps to help prevent leg clots."

_____ C. "You can't have anything to eat or drink for at least 8 hours."

_____ D. "Take deep breaths every hour to help expand your lungs."

_____ E. "Your abdomen will feel better if you stay in a sitting position in bed."

_____ F. "We will be helping you get out of bed to a chair soon."

_____ G. "You just have a couple of small adhesive bandages over your incisions."

_____ H. "You may have a scant amount of vaginal drainage for the next couple of days."

Exemplar 14B. Peripartum Care (Maternal-Newborn Nursing: Young Adult)

Unfolding Case (14B-1 Through 14B-6)

Thinking Exercise 14B-1

A 33-year-old woman suspects she is pregnant and visits her primary health care provider for confirmation. The office nurse takes the client's history and performs an initial assessment. The client tells the nurse that she has had nausea in the morning for several weeks, breast tenderness, amenorrhea, and abdominal enlargement. Earlier this week she took a home test, which indicated that she is pregnant. The nurse teaches the client about presumptive, probable, and positive signs of pregnancy. **Place an X next to each sign of pregnancy that would confirm positivity for pregnancy.**

Signs of Pregnancy	Positive Signs of Pregnancy
Morning nausea	
Audible fetal heartbeat	
Abdominal and breast striae	
Breast tenderness	
Amenorrhea	
Abdominal enlargement	
Ultrasound image of fetus	

Thinking Exercise 14B-2

A 33-year-old woman suspects she is pregnant and visits her primary health care provider for confirmation. The office nurse takes the client's history and performs an initial assessment. After verifying her pregnancy, the nurse collects additional data to determine her risk for common complications of pregnancy. **Complete the following sentences by choosing the *most likely* options for the missing information from the list of options provided.**

The nurse takes the client's blood pressure as a baseline because increased blood pressure during pregnancy may indicate ____________________________. The nurse also schedules the client for a glucose tolerance test because some pregnant women develop ____________________________ during pregnancy, which can lead to ____________________________ later in the woman's life.

Options
Preeclampsia/eclampsia
Diabetes mellitus type 1
Deep vein thrombosis
Diabetes mellitus type 2
Hyperemesis gravidarum
Gestational diabetes mellitus

Thinking Exercise 14B-3

A 33-year-old woman is admitted to the mother-baby suite in early labor at 40 weeks as a gravida 1, para 0. A check on labor progress reveals a 3-cm cervical dilation with 10% effacement. Her contractions are between 10 and 15 minutes apart and last for 20 to 45 seconds. The obstetrician prescribes external fetal monitoring to assess the fetal heart rate (FHR) during labor. Initially the FHR maintained a normal baseline and variability (with no late decelerations). However, an hour later the nurse notes that the client is beginning to have variable decelerations after her contractions causing a decrease in FHR. **Complete the following sentence by choosing the *most likely* options for the missing information from the lists of options provided.**

The nurse recognizes that the variable decelerations are ***most likely*** caused by _______1_______, and therefore the ***priority*** for client care is _______2_______.

Options for 1	Options for 2
Increasing contractions	Administering an analgesic
Umbilical cord compression	Continued fetal monitoring
Placental dysfunction	Repositioning to her left side
Position of the fetus	Administering supplemental oxygen

Thinking Exercise 14B-4

A 33-year-old woman is admitted to the mother-baby suite in early labor at 40 weeks as a gravida 1, para 0. The last three checks on labor progress have been the same, with a 4-cm cervical dilation and 15% effacement. Her contractions for the past 6 hours have been between 10 and 15 minutes apart and lasted for 30 to 50 seconds. External fetal monitoring is in place to assess the fetal heart rate (FHR) during labor. The nurse reports that the client is very tired and feeling frustrated that her labor is not progressing. After examination by the obstetrician and collaboration with the intrapartum team, the client is prepared to have an unplanned caesarean section. **Use an X to show whether the nursing actions listed below are Indicated (appropriate or necessary), Contraindicated (could be harmful), or Non-Essential (makes no difference or is not necessary) for the client's care at this time.**

Nursing Action	Indicated	Contraindicated	Non-Essential
Obtain blood for coagulation studies, complete blood count, and blood typing.			
Administer an enema.			
Ensure that informed consent is obtained.			
Shave the perineal area to remove excess hair.			
Insert an indwelling urinary catheter.			
Keep client NPO.			

Thinking Exercise 14B-5

A 33-year-old woman admitted to the mother-baby suite in early labor did not progress as usual. After almost 8 hours, the client had a 4-cm cervical dilation and 15% effacement. The client had an unplanned cesarean section with spinal anesthesia, and a healthy baby boy was successfully delivered. The nurse develops the client's postoperative plan of care. Which nursing actions will the nurse include for the client at this time? **Select all that apply.**

_____ A. Document the amount of urine output from the indwelling urinary catheter.

_____ B. Check the firmness, height, and position of the client's uterus frequently.

_____ C. Check lochia flow frequently for quantity, color, and presence of clots.

_____ D. Monitor the abdominal dressing for drainage and intactness.

_____ E. Monitor vital signs frequently.

_____ F. Assess the client's ability to move her legs and regain sensation.

_____ G. Remove the client's IV once she awakens.

_____ H. Administer prescribed analgesic medication for report of pain.

Thinking Exercise 14B-6

A 33-year-old woman had an unplanned cesarean section with spinal anesthesia, and a healthy baby boy was successfully delivered. Today she is visiting her obstetrician for a follow-up postpartum visit and to have her incisional staples removed. The nurse screens the client and collects assessment data before she is examined by her physician. **For each client finding, use an X to indicate whether the care for the client was Effective (helped to meet expected outcomes), Ineffective (did not help to meet expected outcomes), or Unrelated (not related to the expected outcomes).**

Nursing Action	Effective	Ineffective	Unrelated
Temperature = 98°F (36.7°C)			
Oxygen saturation = 97% (on room air [RA])			
Small incisional area in right lower abdominal quadrant reddened and oozing yellow drainage			
States that her seasonal allergies are especially annoying this year			
Has lost 22 lb since delivery			
States she feels tired most of the time because the baby is hungry every 2 hours			

Single Episode Cases (14B-7 and 14B-8)

Thinking Exercise 14B-7

A 31-year-old woman is 32 weeks pregnant (gravida 2, para 1) and tells the office nurse that she has been having "lots of little discomforts" as she has progressed during her pregnancy. The nurse provides health teaching about self-care interventions that the client can use. **Indicate which health teaching listed in the far-left column is appropriate for each of the client's discomforts of pregnancy. Note that not all health teaching statements will be used.**

Health Teaching Statement by Nurse	Client's Discomfort of Pregnancy	Health Teaching That Client Can Use to Manage Discomfort of Pregnancy
1 "Elevate your legs whenever you can."	Constipation	
2 "Avoid gas-forming and greasy foods."	Backache	
3 "Eat food high in fiber."	Ankle edema	
4 "Use good body mechanics."	Fatigue	
5 "Eat ginger several times a day."	Shortness of breath	
6 "Take naps during the day as needed."		
7 "Increase fluid intake to at least four glasses a day."		
8 "Sleep with several pillows at night."		

Thinking Exercise 14B-8

A 31-year-old woman is admitted to the maternity suite in early labor at 39 weeks as a gravida 2, para 1. The obstetrician prescribes external fetal monitoring to assess the fetal heart rate (FHR) during labor. The client becomes very anxious about having this device and asks why it is needed. The nurse provides health teaching to allay her anxiety. Which of the following statements about external fetal monitoring are correct and would be included by the nurse? **Select all that apply.**

_____ A. "The purpose of fetal monitoring is to continuously see the baby's heart rate during your labor."

_____ B. "The external device requires placement of two sensors on your abdomen—one over your fundus and one over the place where the fetal heart rate is the strongest."

_____ C. "I will be checking on the baby's heart rate every 10 minutes initially."

_____ D. "Your baby's heart rate is expected to change somewhat during contractions."

_____ E. "Continuously monitoring your baby's heart rate will let us know how much oxygen your baby is getting."

_____ F. "We will be recording the baby's heart rate on the monitor, which is referred to as tracings."

_____ G. "We will also be checking your vital signs during the stages of labor."

Exemplar 14C. Newborn Care (Maternal-Newborn Nursing: Newborn)

Unfolding Case (14C-1 Through 14C-6)

Thinking Exercise 14C-1

A 38-year-old woman had an unplanned cesarean section with spinal anesthesia, and a healthy baby girl weighing 8 lb 2 oz (3.7 kg) was successfully delivered. The nurse assesses the newborn using the Apgar scoring system. Which newborn findings would the nurse expect 1 minute after birth? **Select all that apply.**

_____ A. Heart rate = 124 beats/min

_____ B. Strong spontaneous cry

_____ C. Minimal flexion of extremities

_____ D. Prompt response to stimuli

_____ E. Body pink, extremities blue

_____ F. Flexed body posture

_____ G. Active spontaneous motion

Thinking Exercise 14C-2

A 38-year-old woman had an unplanned cesarean section with spinal anesthesia, and a healthy baby girl weighing 8 lb 2 oz (3.7 kg) was successfully delivered. The nurse assesses the newborn at intervals to determine Apgar score. At 5 minutes after birth, the nurse assesses the newborn to obtain the Apgar score. **For each client finding in the left column, provide the subscore in the right column. Add these subscores to obtain a total Apgar score at 5 minutes.**

Newborn Finding	Apgar Subscore
Heart rate = 98 beats/min	
Strong spontaneous cry	
Flexed body posture	
Prompt response to stimuli such as suction	
Body pink, extremities blue	
Total Apgar Score	

Thinking Exercise 14C-3

A 38-year-old woman had an unplanned cesarean section with spinal anesthesia, and a healthy baby girl weighing 8 lb 2 oz (3.7 kg) was successfully delivered. **Choose the *most likely* options for the information missing from the statement below by selecting from the lists of options provided.**

The nurse recognizes that the ***priority*** for the newborn is to support thermoregulation to prevent complications such as _____1_____ and _____1_____. To prevent becoming hypothermic, the newborn is kept _____2_____ until the newborn's temperature is stabilized.

Options for 1	Options for 2
Hypoglycemia	In a swaddling blanket
Tachycardia	In a receiving blanket
Hypotension	In a radiant warmer
Respiratory distress	In an incubator
Atrial fibrillation	Near the mother

Thinking Exercise 14C-4

A 38-year-old woman had an unplanned cesarean section with spinal anesthesia, and a healthy baby girl weighing 8 lb 2 oz (3.7 kg) was successfully delivered. The nurse obtains a newborn Apgar score of 10 at 15 minutes after birth and plans appropriate newborn care. **Use an X to show whether the nursing actions listed below are <u>Indicated</u> (appropriate or necessary), <u>Contraindicated</u> (could be harmful), or <u>Non-Essential</u> (makes no difference or is not necessary) for the client's care at this time.**

Nursing Action	Indicated	Contraindicated	Non-Essential
Provide the opportunity for the newborn to have skin-to-skin contact with the mother.			
Administer vitamin K to the newborn subcutaneously in the abdomen.			
Keep the umbilical cord moist and covered.			
Prepare the newborn for circumcision.			
Perform a heel stick on the newborn to test for phenylketonuria (PKU).			
Ensure that the mother's and newborn's identification bands match.			

Thinking Exercise 14C-5

A 38-year-old woman had an unplanned cesarean section with spinal anesthesia, and a healthy baby girl weighing 8 lb 2 oz (3.7 kg) was successfully delivered. The mother plans to breastfeed her baby but is afraid she may not be successful. The nurse reinforces health teaching provided by the lactation specialist to answer her questions. **Indicate which nursing response listed in the far-left column is appropriate for the client's question. Note that not all responses will be used.**

Nurse's Response	Client Question	Appropriate Nurse's Response for Each Client Question
1 "Breastfeeding is cheaper than buying milk formula."	"How often should I breastfeed the baby?"	
2 "Feed the baby on a 2- to 3- hour schedule."	"How do I make sure that the baby is latching onto my breast?"	
3 "Be sure that the baby's mouth covers the entire breast areola."	"How do I stop the baby from eating?"	
4 "Burp the baby halfway through the feeding."	"What is the main advantage of breastfeeding?"	
5 "Feed the baby when she cries."		
6 "Breastfeeding helps build a relationship with your baby and the milk is easily digested."		
7 "Put your finger in the corner of the baby's mouth."		

Thinking Exercise 14C-6

A 38-year-old woman had an unplanned cesarean section with spinal anesthesia, and a healthy baby girl weighing 8 lb 2 oz (3.7 kg) was successfully delivered. At the baby's 4-week checkup, the nurse collects assessment data. **For each newborn finding, use an X to indicate whether the client is progressing as expected or is not progressing as expected.**

Newborn Finding	Is Progressing	Is Not Progressing
Unable to hold head/chin up		
Grasp reflex is intact		
Focuses on surroundings		
Weight = 8 lb (3.6 kg)		
Holds hands closed most of the time		

Single-Episode Cases (14C-7 and 14C-8)

Thinking Exercise 14C-7

A 40-year-old woman had a healthy 9 lb (4.1 kg) baby boy by cesarean section this morning at 9 a.m. (0900). The lactation specialist met with the client to help her learn the best techniques for successful breastfeeding. In the evening, the client attempted to breastfeed but the baby was fussy and did not take much milk. The client requested that the baby be taken back to the nursery so she could rest through the night. The baby stayed with the client all day, during which she again struggled to breastfeed; the lactation specialist was off for the holiday weekend. As a result the baby cried most of the day. When the father came in for a visit, the client started to cry and said she was not a good mother because of problems feeding the baby. He called for the nurse to assess the situation. **Choose the *most likely* options for the information missing from the statement below by selecting from the lists of options provided.**

The nurse recognizes that the newborn ***most likely*** has ___________1___________ due to inadequate ___________2___________.

Options for 1	Options for 2
Constipation	Fluid intake
Dehydration	Bowel elimination
Infection	Fiber intake
Colic	Immune system

Thinking Exercise 14C-8

A 40-year-old woman had a healthy 9 lb (4.1 kg) baby boy by cesarean section this morning at 9 a.m. (0900). The lactation specialist met with the client to help her learn the best techniques for successful breastfeeding. In the evening, the client attempted to breastfeed but the baby was fussy and did not take much milk. The client requested that the baby be taken back to the nursery so she could rest through the night. The baby stayed with the client all day, during which she again struggled to breastfeed; the lactation specialist was off for the holiday weekend. As a result the baby cried most of the day. When the father came in for a visit, the client started to cry and said she was not a good mother because she had problems feeding the baby. He called for the nurse to assess the situation. What newborn assessment data would the nurse collect at this time? **Select all that apply.**

_____ A. Vital signs

_____ B. Weight

_____ C. Oxygen saturation

_____ D. Posterior fontanelle

_____ E. Number of diaper changes during day

_____ F. Mucous membranes

_____ G. Skin turgor

Clinical Judgment to Coordinate Care for Older Clients

PART 3

15 Perfusion

Exemplar 15A. Hypertension (Medical-Surgical Nursing: Older Adult)

Unfolding Case (15A-1 Through 15A-6)

Thinking Exercise 15A-1

A 69-year-old female client is participating in acute rehabilitation after a vehicular accident that resulted in a fractured arm, fractured clavicle, and several fractured ribs. The client has no recorded medical history. She claims to be healthy and only sees her primary health care provider every few years. Client findings from the nurse's shift assessment include:

- Alert and oriented
- Fidgety and restless
- Reports vision is "foggy around the edges"
- Heart rate (HR) = 88 beats/min
- Blood pressure (BP) = 164/88 mm Hg
- Respirations = 17 breaths/min
- Oxygen saturation = 94% (on room air [RA])
- Reports a headache at the back of her head, rated 6/10
- Respirations equal and unlabored
- Lung fields clear throughout
- Abdomen round and soft
- Bowel sounds present

Highlight the client findings that require follow-up by the nurse in collaboration with the health care team.

Thinking Exercise 15A-2

A 69-year-old female client is participating in acute rehabilitation after a vehicular accident that resulted in a fractured arm, fractured clavicle, and several fractured ribs. The client has no recorded medical history. She claims to be healthy and only sees her primary health care provider every few years. Client findings from the nurse's shift assessment include:

- Alert and oriented
- Fidgety and restless
- Reports vision is "foggy around the edges"
- Heart rate (HR) = 88 beats/min
- Blood pressure (BP) = 164/88 mm Hg
- Respirations = 17 breaths/min
- Oxygen saturation = 94% (on room air [RA])

- Reports a headache at the back of her head, rated 6/10 on a scale of 0 to 10
- Respirations equal and unlabored
- Lung fields clear throughout
- Abdomen round and soft
- Bowel sounds present

The nurse further assesses the client for risk factors of potential health issues associated with the client's findings. What additional information does the nurse need to analyze the client's findings? **Select all that apply.**

_____ A. Pupil size and reaction

_____ B. Smoking history

_____ C. Recent immunizations

_____ D. Peripheral pulses

_____ E. Facial symmetry

_____ F. Usual dietary intake

_____ G. History of migraines or headaches

_____ H. Usual sleep cycle

Thinking Exercise 15A-3

A 69-year-old female client is participating in acute rehabilitation after a vehicular accident that resulted in a fractured arm, fractured clavicle, and several fractured ribs. The client has no recorded medical history. She claims to be healthy and only sees her primary health care provider every few years. Client findings include signs of anxiety and visual changes but no neurologic deficits. The client reports an occipital headache, rated 6 on a scale of 0 to 10, and has a blood pressure (BP) of 154/88 mm Hg. The client shares that she works as a retail cashier and is the primary caregiver for her two school-age grandchildren. She says, "Life is busy and stressful. Fast food restaurants allow me to provide dinner each night." She usually sleeps only 4 to 5 hours a night, eats one meal a day, and drinks many caffeinated beverages to "keep going." The client also confesses to a 21 pack-year history of cigarette smoking but no health issues. **Complete the following sentences by choosing the *most likely* option for the missing information from the list of options provided.**

The client ***most likely*** has previously undiagnosed _____1_____. The nurse's ***priority*** is to implement a plan of care to prevent complications, including include heart failure, _____2_____, and _____2_____.

Options for 1	Options for 2
Anxiety disorder	Acute respiratory failure
Intracranial hemorrhage	Diabetes mellitus
Hypertension	Kidney disease
Migraines	Panic attack
Transient ischemic attack	Pneumonia
	Stroke
	Suicide

Thinking Exercise 15A-4

A 69-year-old female client is participating in acute rehabilitation after a vehicular accident that resulted in a fractured arm, fractured clavicle, and several fractured ribs. The client works as a retail cashier and is the primary caregiver for her two school-age grandchildren. She usually eats fast foods, sleeps only 4 to 5 hours a night, and drinks many caffeinated beverages to "keep going." The client's only health history is a 21–pack-year history of cigarette smoking. Current client findings include signs of anxiety and visual changes but no neurologic deficits. The client also reports an occipital headache, rated 6/10 on a scale of 0 to 10, and has a blood pressure (BP) of 164/88 mm Hg. The client is diagnosed with hypertension. The nurse collaborates with the health care team to revise the client's plan of care. **Use an X to show whether each nursing action below is <u>Indicated</u> (appropriate or necessary), <u>Contraindicated</u> (could be harmful), or <u>Non-Essential</u> (makes no difference or is not necessary) for the client's care at this time.**

Nursing Actions	Indicated	Contraindicated	Non-Essential
Consult a registered dietitian nutritionist to facilitate a low-fat and low-sodium diet.			
Provide client teaching focused on nutrition, exercise, and medication therapy.			
Monitor for therapeutic and side effects of antihypertensive medications.			
Collaborate with a physical therapist for passive range-of-motion activities when orthostatic hypotension occurs.			
Ensure that naloxone is on the unit in case of an overdose of antihypertensive medications.			

Thinking Exercise 15A-5

Pharmacology

A 69-year-old female client is participating in acute rehabilitation after a vehicular accident that resulted in a fractured arm, fractured clavicle, and several fractured ribs. The client works as a retail cashier and is the primary caregiver for her two school-age grandchildren. She usually eats fast food, sleeps only 4 to 5 hours a night, and drinks many caffeinated beverages to "keep going." The client's only health history is a 21–pack-year history of cigarette smoking. Current client findings include signs of anxiety and visual changes but no neurologic deficits. The client also reports an occipital headache, rated 6/10 on a scale of 0 to 10, and has a BP of 164/88 mm Hg. The client was diagnosed with hypertension, orders have been received, and the plan of care has been updated. Prior to administering the first dose of hydrochlorothiazide and amlodipine, the nurse obtains initial blood pressure (BP) and pulse rate. What additional nursing actions will the nurse implement related to the client's drug therapy? **Select all that apply.**

_____ A. Monitor the client's pulse and BP for tachycardia and hypotension.

_____ B. Ask the client to report side effects such as headache and dizziness.

_____ C. Monitor the client for upper and lower extremity edema.

_____ D. If ankle and foot edema occurs, remind the client to elevate her legs while sitting.

_____ E. Teach the client to expect increased voiding to rid the body of excessive fluid.

_____ F. Check for orthostatic BP changes, including standing, sitting, and lying BPs.

_____ G. Teach the client that she will need to increase her dietary intake of high-sodium foods.

_____ H. Monitor the client's intake and output while in the rehabilitation facility.

Thinking Exercise 15A-6

A 69-year-old female client is participating in acute rehabilitation after a vehicular accident that resulted in a broken arm, broken clavicle, and several broken ribs. The client works as a retail cashier and is the primary caregiver for her two school-age grandchildren. She usually eats fast food, sleeps only 4 to 5 hours a night, and drinks many caffeinated beverages to "keep going." The client's only health history is a 21 pack-year history of cigarette smoking. The client is diagnosed with hypertension. The nurse evaluates the client's understanding after reinforcing teaching related to the management of this chronic disorder. **For each client statement, use an X to indicate if the teaching was Effective (helped the client understand discharge teaching), Ineffective (did not help the client understand discharge teaching), or Unrelated (not related to the discharge teaching).**

Client Statement	Effective	Ineffective	Unrelated
"I will use the resources provided to begin a smoking cessation program."			
"Once my blood pressure is within normal limits, I can stop taking the medication."			
"I will add more fruits and vegetables to my diet and eat less fast food."			
"Spices, garlic, and onions can add flavor to my food without adding more sodium."			
"I will take my pulse for a full minute prior to taking my antihypertensive medications."			

Single-Episode Case (15A-7)

Thinking Exercise 15A-7

Pharmacology

An 82-year-old male client has a health history of hypertension and heart disease. The client manages his condition with diet, exercise, and several medications including atenolol, amlodipine, hydrochlorothiazide, and aspirin. A nurse evaluates the client's treatment plan for therapeutic and adverse effects. Which questions will the nurse ask related to drug therapy? **Select all that apply.**

_____ A. "Do you ever feel dizzy or lightheaded when rising from bed?"

_____ B. "Have you experienced any sexual dysfunction?"

_____ C. "Do you have any difficulty climbing the stairs in your home?"

_____ D. "Have you had any thoughts of hurting yourself?"

_____ E. "When is your next appointment with the ophthalmologist?"

_____ F. "What foods high in potassium do you eat on a daily basis?"

_____ G. "Have you experienced any palpitations or feelings that your heart is skipping?"

_____ H. "During the past month have you often felt down, depressed, or hopeless?"

Exemplar 15B. Stroke (Medical-Surgical Nursing: Older Adult)

Unfolding Case (15B-1 Through 15B-6)

Thinking Exercise 15B-1

A 77-year-old female client is recovering after an open reduction, internal fixation (ORIF) of the left hip 3 days ago. The client also has a history of type 2 diabetes mellitus and iron deficiency anemia. The client is retired and lives with her spouse of 52 years. At 7:30 a.m. (0730), the night nurse provides the hand-off report to the oncoming nurse at the bedside. The client participates in this report, denies pain, and shares that she is ready to move to a rehabilitation facility.

Thirty minutes later, the nurse returns to complete a shift assessment and notices the client is lethargic and oriented to self only. The client's speech is slurred, she is drooling from the left side of her mouth, and she has pale, cool skin. Vital signs are: heart rate (HR), 98 beats/min; blood pressure (BP), 160/92 mm Hg; respirations, 18 breaths/min; and oxygen saturation, 97% (on room air [RA]). **Identify the three most important client findings from the list below that require follow-up by the nurse.**

Client Finding	Priority Client Finding That Requires Follow-up by the Nurse
Level of consciousness	
Blood pressure	
Oxygenation status	
Pain	
Dysarthria	
Heart rate	

Thinking Exercise 15B-2

A 77-year-old female client is recovering after an open reduction, internal fixation (ORIF) of the left hip 3 days ago. The client also has a history of type 2 diabetes mellitus and iron deficiency anemia. The client is retired and lives with her spouse of 52 years. At 7:30 a.m. (0730), the night nurse provides the hand-off report to the oncoming nurse at the bedside. The client participates in this report, denies pain, and shares that she is ready to move to a rehabilitation facility.

Thirty minutes later, the nurse returns to complete a shift assessment and notices the client is lethargic and oriented to self only. The client's speech is slurred, she is drooling from the left side of her mouth, and she has pale, cool skin. Vital signs are: heart rate (HR), 98 beats/min; blood pressure (BP), 160/92 mm Hg; respirations, 18 breaths/min; and oxygen saturation, 97% (on room air [RA]). **For each client finding below, determine if the finding is associated with anemia, sepsis, hypoglycemia, and/or stroke. Each finding may be associated with more than one health problem.**

Client Finding	Anemia	Sepsis	Hypoglycemia	Stroke
Lethargy				
Slurred speech				
Confusion				
Pallor				

Thinking Exercise 15B-3

A 77-year-old female client is recovering after an open reduction, internal fixation (ORIF) of the left hip 3 days ago. The client also has a history of type 2 diabetes mellitus and iron deficiency anemia. At 7:30 a.m. (0730), the night nurse provides the hand-off report to the oncoming nurse at the bedside. The client participates in this report, denies pain, and shares that she is ready to move to a rehabilitation facility.

Thirty minutes later, the nurse returns to complete a shift assessment and notices the client is lethargic and oriented to self only. The client's speech is slurred, she is drooling from the left side of her mouth, and she has pale, cool skin. Vital signs are: heart rate (HR), 98 beats/min; blood pressure (BP), 160/92 mm Hg; respirations, 18 breaths/min; and oxygen saturation, 97% (on room air [RA]). The nurse completes a focused assessment to obtain additional information needed to prioritize the client's current condition. Additional client findings include:

- Temperature 98.8°F (37.1°C)
- Blurred vision
- Left-side hemiplegia
- Peripheral pulses: palpable 2+
- Denies chest pain and shortness of breath
- Difficulty clearing secretions
- Capillary blood glucose 188 mg/dL (10.4 mmol/L)
- Morning lab findings:

• Blood urea nitrogen (BUN) = 6.5 mg/dL (0.36 mmol/L) • Creatinine = 1.0 mg/dL (88 mmol/L) • Serum sodium = 142 mEq/L (142 mmol/L) • Hemoglobin A1c = 7.4%	• White blood cell (WBC) count = 8000/mm³ (8.0 × 10⁹/L) • Hemoglobin = 12 g/dL (7.4 mmol/L) • Hematocrit = 39% • Platelet count = 220,000/mm³ (220 × 10⁹/L)

Complete the following sentences by choosing the *most likely* option for the missing information from the list of options provided.

The client is ***most likely*** experiencing a _____1_____. The nurse must intervene immediately to prevent _____2_____.

Options for 1	Options for 2
Anemia	Aspiration pneumonia
Sepsis	Seizures
Hypoglycemia	Coma
Stroke	Respiratory failure
	Cold intolerance

Thinking Exercise 15B-4

A 77-year-old female client is recovering after an open reduction, internal fixation (ORIF) of the left hip 3 days ago. At 7:30 a.m. (0730), the night nurse provides the hand-off report to the oncoming nurse at the bedside. The client participates in this report, denies pain, and shares that she is ready to move to a rehabilitation facility.

Thirty minutes later, the nurse returns to complete a shift assessment and notices the client is lethargic and oriented to self only. The client's speech is slurred, she is drooling from the left side of her mouth, and she has pale, cool skin. The client is also experiencing left-side hemiplegia and blurred vision. The client's capillary blood glucose level is 188 mg/dL (10.4 mmol/L) and vital signs are: heart rate (HR), 98 beats/min; blood pressure (BP), 160/92 mm Hg; respirations, 18 breaths/min; and oxygen saturation, 97% (on room air [RA]).

The client is most likely experiencing a stroke. The nurse identifies potential complications during the acute phase of a stroke and interventions to prevent each complication. **Indicate which nursing or collaborative intervention listed in the far-left column is appropriate for each potential complication. Note that not all interventions will be used.**

Nursing Action	Potential Complication	Appropriate Nursing Action for Each Potential Complication
1 Explain what is happening, why interventions are implemented, and what can be expected.	Inability to communicate effectively	
2 Provide a notepad for the client to communicate in writing.	Anxiety due to loss of function or fear of disability	
3 Assess family strengths and resources.	Pulmonary infection due to impaired neuromuscular function and mobility	
4 Explore communication methods to determine what works best for the client.	Potential for falls related to hemiplegia	
5 Perform postural drainage and percussion therapy to mobilize bronchial secretions.		
6 Frequently remind the client to use the call light if the client needs to use the bathroom.		
7 Continuously monitor oxygen saturation levels and breath sounds; suction oral secretions as needed.		

Thinking Exercise 15B-5

A 77-year-old female client is recovering after an open reduction, internal fixation (ORIF) of the left hip 3 days ago. At 7:30 a.m. (0730), the night nurse provides the hand-off report to the oncoming nurse at the bedside. The client participates in this report, denies pain, and shares that she is ready to move to a rehabilitation facility.

Thirty minutes later, the nurse returns to complete a shift assessment and notices the client is lethargic and oriented to self only. The client's speech is slurred, she is drooling from the left side of her mouth, and she has pale, cool skin. The client is also experiencing left-side hemiplegia and blurred vision. The client's capillary blood glucose level is 188 mg/dL (10.4 mmol/L) and vital signs are: heart rate (HR), 98 beats/min; blood pressure (BP), 160/92 mm Hg; respirations, 18 breaths/min; and oxygen saturation, 97% on room air (RA). The client is most likely experiencing a stroke. Which actions will the nurse take? **Select all that apply.**

_____ A. Contact the Rapid Response or Stroke Team.

_____ B. Assist in completing the facility's approved stroke scale.

_____ C. Use a gait belt to ambulate the client to the bathroom.

_____ D. Contact the pharmacist to obtain an oral thrombolytic.

_____ E. Assess the client for allergies to contrast media.

_____ F. Report and document the time the symptoms began.

_____ G. Position to comfort with the head of bed flat.

_____ H. Assess the client for motor function and strength.

Thinking Exercise 15B-6

A 77-year-old female client had a stroke while recovering from an open reduction, internal fixation (ORIF) of the left hip. The client was treated medically and is ready to be discharged to an acute rehabilitation center. Prior to the transfer, the nurse reinforced teaching related to rehabilitation activities and the client's plan of care. **For each client statement, use an X to indicate if the teaching was Effective (helped the client understand discharge teaching), Ineffective (did not help the client understand discharge teaching), or Unrelated (not related to the discharge teaching).**

Client Statement	Effective	Ineffective	Unrelated
"Rehabilitation will teach me new ways to compensate for my loss of function."			
"I will remain in the rehabilitation center until I can complete ADLs independently."			
"I look forward to having a window in my room at the rehabilitation center."			
"The purpose of rehabilitation is for me to achieve the highest level of functioning possible with my deficits."			
"I am excited to learn how to use personal assistive devices to obtain more independence."			
"I will get to know several therapists who will take the place of a nurse during my rehabilitation."			

Single-Episode Cases (15B-7 Through 15B-8)

Thinking Exercise 15B-7

A 68-year-old client participates in acute rehabilitation after experiencing a stroke that resulted in expressive aphasia, dysphagia, and dyspraxia. The client has participated in rehabilitative therapies over the past 2 weeks. The nurse assesses the client to evaluate the client's progress toward meeting expected outcomes. **For each client finding, use an X to indicate whether the client is progressing as expected or is not progressing as expected.**

Client Finding	Is Progressing	Is Not Progressing
Uses picture boards to communicate effectively		
Experiences reflexive coughing during meals		
Voids 600 mL of dark amber urine in past 24 hours		
Requires verbal cues to initiate voluntary movements		
Reports feeling hopeful about recovery process		

Thinking Exercise 15B-8

A nurse prepares to discharge an 82-year-old male client who recently experienced a stroke with several right-sided deficits including impaired sensation, hemiplegia, and homonymous hemianopsia. The client participated in 3 weeks of acute rehabilitation and will be discharged to the care of his son. The son is married with three adult children and plans to arrange sleeping and living space for his father in one of his children's old bedrooms. Which statements will the nurse include in discharge teaching with the client and his son? **Select all that apply.**

_____ A. "You may need to remind your father to scan his affected visual field during activities."

_____ B. "Assistive devices for eating are only needed for clients who have dysphagia."

_____ C. "Help your father to assess his skin for redness, especially over bony prominences."

_____ D. "Do not apply a heating or cooling pad to the affected side of your body."

_____ E. "Adapting the home environment is not needed if you provide all of your father's care."

_____ F. "Position your father comfortably in bed if you will be gone for most of the day."

_____ G. "An indwelling urinary catheter may be used to protect his skin from breakdown."

_____ H. "I will provide resources for respite care so you are ready when relief is needed."

16 Mobility

Exemplar 16A. Parkinson Disease/Complications of Impaired Mobility (Medical-Surgical Nursing: Older Adult)

Unfolding Case (16A-1 Through 16A-6)

Thinking Exercise 16A-1

A 79-year-old male client with Parkinson disease (PD) is driven by his wife to the primary health care provider's office for his annual appointment. The nurse screens the client and collects client data prior to the provider's examination. **Highlight or place a check mark next to the client findings below that require follow-up by the nurse in collaboration with the health care team.**

- Lives at home with his wife, who cares for him
- Needs assistance with ADLs on days when his rigidity is worse
- Walks short distances in the house using a rollator walker
- Is alert and oriented × 2–3
- Wife states that he sometimes talks to himself and seems scared
- Has resting tremors in both arms and hands, but left hand is worse than the right (client is right-handed)
- Chokes at times when he eats
- Has fallen three times in the past week
- Has a stage 2 sacral pressure injury that is 2 cm × 1 cm without drainage
- Blood pressure (BP) (sitting) = 118/70 mm Hg; BP (standing) = 98/64 mm Hg
- Heart rate = 68 beats/min and regular
- Takes losartan for a 10-year history of hypertension
- Takes a carbidopa/levodopa combination for PD

Thinking Exercise 16A-2

A 79-year-old male client with Parkinson disease (PD) is driven by his wife to the primary health care provider's office for his annual appointment. The nurse screens the client and collects client data prior to the provider's examination. **For each client finding below, identify whether the finding is associated with Parkinson disease, orthostatic hypotension, or both health problems.**

Client Finding	Parkinson Disease	Orthostatic Hypotension
Needs assistance with ADLs on days when his rigidity is worse		
Has resting tremors in both arms and hands, but left hand is worse than the right (client is right-handed)		
Has fallen three times in the past week		
Chokes at times when he eats		
Blood pressure (BP) (sitting) = 118/70 mm Hg; BP (standing) = 98/64 mm Hg		
Wife states that he sometimes talks to himself and seems scared		

Thinking Exercise 16A-3

A 79-year-old male client with Parkinson disease (PD) is driven by his wife to the primary health care provider's office for his annual appointment. The nurse screens the client and collects client data prior to the provider's examination. Findings from the assessment include that the client has orthostatic hypotension, a pressure injury, muscle rigidity, and resting tremors. **Choose the *most likely* options for the information missing from the statement below by selecting from the list of options provided.**

Based on the client findings, the nurse recognizes that the ***priorities*** for the client's care at this time are ensuring _______________ and preventing additional ________________________.

Options
Nutrition and hydration Infection and sepsis Client safety Hallucinations and delusions Complications of impaired mobility

Thinking Exercise 16A-4

A 79-year-old male client with Parkinson disease (PD) is driven by his wife to the primary health care provider's office for a follow-up appointment. The nurse screens the client and collects client data prior to the provider's examination. Findings from the assessment include that the client has orthostatic hypotension, a pressure injury, muscle rigidity, and resting tremors. Based on these assessment findings and a physical examination, the primary health care provider adjusts the client's medications to help prevent orthostatic hypotension, which is likely contributing to his falls. **Use an X to show whether the nursing actions listed below are <u>Indicated</u> (appropriate or necessary), <u>Contraindicated</u> (could be harmful), or <u>Non-Essential</u> (makes no difference or is not necessary) for the client at this time.**

Nursing Action	Indicated	Contraindicated	Non-Essential
Refer the client to a registered dietitian nutritionist for food choices that are less likely to cause choking.			
Refer the wife to hospice care for the client.			
Remind the client and wife that he should get up slowly from the bed or chair.			
Suggest to the wife to keep a diary of the client's hallucinations or other mental and emotional changes.			
Teach the client how to care for the sacral pressure injury and report worsening or redness around the wound.			
Remind the wife to continue monitoring the client's blood pressure daily.			

Thinking Exercise 16A-5

A 79-year-old male client with Parkinson disease (PD) is driven by his wife to the primary health care provider's office for his annual appointment. The nurse screens the client and collects client data prior to the provider's examination. Findings from the assessment include that the client has orthostatic hypotension, a pressure injury, muscle rigidity, and resting tremors. Based on these assessment findings and a physical examination, the primary health care provider adjusts the client's medications to help prevent orthostatic hypotension, which is likely contributing to his falls. The nurse recognizes that the client is at risk for additional complications of impaired mobility and reinforces health teaching with the wife and client. Which health teaching would the nurse include? **Select all that apply.**

_____ A. "Remind the client to not rush when eating and to chew his food thoroughly."

_____ B. "Ensure that the client wears firm shoes to provide better support than soft slippers."

_____ C. "Perform active and active-assisted exercises as needed to maintain muscle tone and prevent contractures."

_____ D. "Remind the client to drink adequate fluids every day to prevent constipation and urinary tract infection."

_____ E. "Check that the client avoids too many high-fiber foods to prevent diverticular disease and diarrhea."

_____ F. "Ask the client to perform leg exercises such as marching in place and stretching before ambulating with his walker."

_____ G. "Be sure that the client takes a walk every day as tolerated to promote health and mobility."

Thinking Exercise 16A-6

A 79-year-old male client with Parkinson disease (PD) is driven by his wife to the primary health care provider's office for a 3-month follow-up appointment after his medication adjustment. The nurse screens the client and collects client data prior to the provider's examination. **For each client finding, use an X to indicate whether the client is progressing as expected or is <u>not</u> progressing as expected.**

Client Finding	Is Progressing	Is Not Progressing
Wife states that he has been choking less frequently in the past month on food or liquids.		
Blood pressure (BP) (sitting) = 130/76 mm Hg; BP (standing) = 124/72 mm Hg.		
Client walks every day inside and outside with his walker.		
Client has not fallen within the last 3 months.		
Client reports feeling sad and depressed most days.		
Stage 2 sacral pressure injury is smaller at 1.5 cm × 0.8 cm; no drainage or surrounding redness.		

Single-Episode Case (16A-7)

Thinking Exercise 16A-7

The nurse is caring for an 82-year-old female client recently admitted with moderate-stage Parkinson disease (PD) to a long-term care (LTC) facility. During the past 10 years while she lived at home with her daughter, the client becamc less independent in ADLs and recently fell several times. What client findings will the nurse expect when collecting admission assessment data? **Select all that apply.**

_____ A. Cogwheel rigidity

_____ B. Gait and balance disturbances

_____ C. Slurred speech

_____ D. Lack of facial expression

_____ E. Intentional hand tremors

_____ F. Tingling in lower extremities

_____ G. Visual disturbances

_____ H. Slowed movement

Exemplar 16B. Osteoarthritis/Total Knee Arthroplasty (Medical-Surgical Nursing: Older Adult)

Unfolding Case (16B-1 Through 16B-6)

Thinking Exercise 16B-1

The nurse is caring for a 66-year-old obese male client who worked on a farm for most of his life. Today he is being evaluated by his primary health care provider for increasing bilateral knee pain over the past year. The client's history includes hypertension, hyperlipidemia, and diabetes mellitus type 2, for which he takes a variety of medications, including amlodipine, lovastatin, and metformin. The nurse collects client data prior to the provider's examination. **Place an X next to each client finding in the left column that requires follow-up by the nurse in collaboration with the health care team.**

Client Finding	Client Finding That Requires Follow-up
Knee pain = 7/10 on a 0 to 10 pain rating scale	
Right knee reddened and swollen	
Height = 6 feet (1.8 m); weight = 265 lb (111.1 kg)	
Blood pressure = 154/90 mm Hg	
Blood glucose = 124 mg/dL (6.9 mmol/L)	
Right quadriceps have less tone than left quadriceps	

Thinking Exercise 16B-2

The nurse is caring for a 66-year-old obese male client who worked on a farm for most of his life. Today he is being evaluated by his primary health care provider for increasing bilateral knee pain over the past year; his current pain is described as a 7/10 on numeric intensity scale. His right knee is reddened and swollen, but he is independent in ADLs. The client's history includes hypertension, hyperlipidemia, and diabetes mellitus type 2, for which he takes a variety of medications, including amlodipine, lovastatin, and metformin. The nurse collects client data prior to the provider's examination. **Choose the *most likely* options for the information missing from the statement below by selecting from the lists of options provided.**

The nurse recognizes that the client's knee pain is ***most likely*** due to ______1______ as a result of ______2______, ______2______, and his ______2______.

Options for 1	Options for 2
Rheumatoid arthritis	Obesity
Psoriatic arthritis	Aging
Osteoarthritis	Hypertension
Gouty arthritis	Occupation
Rheumatism	Diabetes mellitus

Thinking Exercise 16B-3

The nurse is caring for a 66-year-old obese male client who worked on a farm for most of his life. Today he is being evaluated by his primary health care provider for increasing bilateral knee pain over the past year; his current pain is described as a 7/10 on numeric intensity scale. His right knee is reddened and swollen, but he is independent in ADLs. The client's history includes hypertension, hyperlipidemia, and diabetes mellitus type 2, for which he takes a variety of medications, including amlodipine, lovastatin, and metformin. **Choose the *most likely* options for the information missing from the statement below by selecting from the list of options provided.**

Based on an analysis of the client findings, the nurse recognizes that the ***priority*** health problems for the client at this time are ____________ and ____________.

Options
Inflammation
Acute pain
Neuropathic pain
Chronic pain
Joint deformity

Thinking Exercise 16B-4

The nurse is caring for a 66-year-old obese male client who worked on a farm for most of his life. Today he is being evaluated by his primary health care provider for increasing bilateral knee pain over the past year; his current pain is described as a 7/10 on numeric intensity scale. His right knee is reddened and swollen, but he is independent in ADLs. Based on client findings, the nurse reinforces health teaching about his disease process. **Use an X to show whether each health teaching below is <u>Indicated</u> (appropriate or necessary), <u>Contraindicated</u> (could be harmful), or <u>Non-Essential</u> (makes no difference or is not necessary) for the client at this time.**

Health Teaching	Indicated	Contraindicated	Non-Essential
"Use heat on both knees to help relieve pain and promote healing."			
"Use assistive-adaptive devices as needed (e.g., sock aids, shoehorns, dressing sticks, extenders)."			
"Seek out a weight reduction program to help reduce knee pain and promote general health."			
"Take acetaminophen when needed for pain."			
"Try to work on finding a new occupation that allows you to sit more."			
"Follow up with all physical therapy appointments as prescribed."			
"Wear good firm shoes to support your knees."			

Thinking Exercise 16B-5

The nurse is caring for a 67-year-old obese male client who worked on a farm for most of his life. He has been treated for knee pain for over a year using conservative measures, but his right knee has worsened. A recent right knee x-ray shows complete erosion of cartilage and bony spur formation. As a result, the client had a right total knee arthroplasty yesterday. The nurse is planning to reinforce health teaching for the client in preparation for discharge tomorrow. Which statements will the nurse include when reviewing postoperative teaching with the client? **Select all that apply.**

_____ A. "Ambulate several times every day using a walker."

_____ B. "Be sure to sleep with a pillow under your knees each night."

_____ C. "Do not put more weight on your affected leg than allowed and instructed."

_____ D. "Continue wearing your antiembolic stockings and taking your anticoagulant as prescribed at home."

_____ E. "Report any redness, swelling, and pain in either lower leg to your surgeon immediately."

_____ F. "Use a continuous passive motion machine every night while you are sleeping."

_____ G. "Inspect your surgical incision every day for increased redness, heat, or drainage; if any of these are present, call your surgeon immediately."

Thinking Exercise 16B-6

The nurse is caring for a 67-year-old obese male client who worked on a farm for most of his life. The client's history includes knee and hip osteoarthritis, hypertension, hyperlipidemia, and diabetes mellitus type 2. Six weeks ago he had a right total knee arthroplasty for severe chronic pain and is visiting his surgeon today for follow-up. The nurse collects client data prior to the surgeon's examination. **For each client finding, use an X to indicate whether the interventions were Effective (helped to meet expected outcomes), Ineffective (did not help to meet expected outcomes), or Unrelated (not related to the expected outcomes).**

Client Finding	Effective	Ineffective	Unrelated
Ambulates several times a day with a cane			
Incision healed without redness or drainage			
Right knee is slightly swollen and warm at times			
Reports new-onset toothache for the past few days			
Blood pressure = 126/80 mm Hg			
Reports no right knee pain but has "a little soreness"			

Single-Episode Cases (16B-7 and 16B-8)

Thinking Exercise 16B-7

A 73-year-old female client had a left total knee arthroplasty a month ago and is transitioning from ambulating with a walker to a cane. **Choose the *most likely* options for the information missing from the statements below by selecting from the lists of options provided.**

The nurse reinforces the teaching provided by the physical therapist about how to use a cane, including the need for the client to place the cane ________1________ when ambulating. To ensure proper cane height, the top of the cane should be at the level of the client's ________2________.

Options for 1	Options for 2
On either side	Antecubital space
On her left side	Greater trochanter
In front of her	Affected knee
On her right side	Fingertips

Thinking Exercise 16B-8

The nurse is interviewing and collecting assessment data on a 63-year-old female who visits the clinic because of painful joints that are beginning to interfere with her daily life. She states that she got arthritis from her mother and grandmother, and has always had "lousy" bones and joints. **Highlight the client findings in the Nurses' Notes below that require follow-up by the nurse.**

History and Physical	Nurses' Notes	Vital Signs	Laboratory Results

10/24/21 Reports severe intermittent pain in most of her hand joints, with right thumb base being the worst at 6/10 when picking up objects. Numerous enlarged bony nodules on most finger joints preventing the client from making a tight fist. Several finger nodules warm to touch. Chronic back pain (cervical and lumbosacral) for over 45 years with report of frequent crepitus when moving neck and shoulders. Minimal joint involvement in lower extremities, except for knees. Able to perform ADLs independently but beginning to have problems with opening containers, jars, and bottles. Job requires working long hours at a computer at home. Takes ibuprofen 800 mg orally every morning, which wears off by dinner time. States that if she takes too much of the drug, she gets nosebleeds. Is hoping to have other choices for decreasing pain and reducing deformity. -- R. J. Youseff, LPN

Exemplar 16C. Fractured Hip/Open Reduction, Internal Fixation (Medical-Surgical Nursing: Older Adult)

Unfolding Case (16C-1 Through 16C-6)

Thinking Exercise 16C-1

A 75-year-old female client residing in an assisted-living facility falls in her bathroom at 2:00 a.m. (0200) and yells for help. The assistive personnel finds the client wedged between the toilet and wall and calls the nurse, who assesses the client. **Highlight the client findings below that require immediate follow-up by the nurse.**

- Alert but unable to determine orientation due to severe pain
- Crying out and grabbing her right hip
- Right leg shorter than left and externally rotated
- Has history of severe osteoporosis for which she is prescribed risedronate
- Has been walking with a rollator walker or cane when ambulating before her fall
- Heart rate = 92 beats/min
- Respirations = 28 breaths/min
- Blood pressure = 162/90 mm Hg
- Oxygen saturation = 90% (on room air [RA])
- No other apparent injury noted

Thinking Exercise 16C-2

A 75-year-old female client residing in an assisted-living facility falls in her bathroom at 2:00 a.m. (0200) and yells for help. The assistive personnel finds the client wedged between the toilet and wall and calls the nurse, who assesses the client. The client is alert but the nurse is unable to determine her orientation because of severe pain. On inspection, the nurse notes that the client's right leg is shorter than the left leg and is externally rotated. The client has a long history of osteoporosis, and no other injury is apparent at this time. **Choose the *most likely* options for the information missing from the statements below by selecting from the lists of options provided.**

The nurse analyzes client findings and recognizes that the client ***most likely*** has a ________1________. This trauma can lead to complications including ________2________ and ________2________.

Options for 1	Options for 2
Dislocated hip	Infection
Dislocated knee	Bleeding
Fractured hip	Osteoarthritis
Fractured tibia	Pressure injury
Knee ligament injury	Neurovascular impairment

Thinking Exercise 16C-3

A 75-year-old female client residing in an assisted-living facility falls in her bathroom at 2:00 a.m. (0200) and is taken to the emergency department for evaluation and treatment. An examination and x-ray confirm an intertrochanteric fracture of the right hip. The nurse collaborates with the registered nurse to determine the client's priority for care. **Choose the *most likely* options for the information missing from the statement below by selecting from the list of options provided.**

In addition to monitoring for fracture complications, the ***priorities*** of care for the client are to manage ____________________ and assess for ______________________.

Options
Immobility
Infection
Pain
Delirium
Pressure injury

Thinking Exercise 16C-4

A 75-year-old female client residing in an assisted-living facility fell in her bathroom at 2:00 a.m. (0200) and was taken to the emergency department (ED) for evaluation and treatment. An examination and x-ray confirmed an intertrochanteric fracture of the right hip. The client's daughter joined her mother in the ED and discussed treatment options. The client had an emergent open reduction, internal fixation (ORIF) of the right hip that afternoon. After surgery, the nurse receives the report from the postanesthesia care unit (PACU) before transfer and develops an individualized postoperative plan of care in coordination with the registered nurse. **Indicate which nursing action listed in the far-left column is appropriate to help prevent, detect, or manage each potential postoperative complication. Note that not all nursing actions will be used.**

Nursing Action	Potential Postoperative Complication	Appropriate Nursing Action for Postoperative Complication
1 Turn the client and inspect skin every 1–2 hr.	Atelectasis	
2 Maintain bilateral sequential compression devices.	Nausea and vomiting	
3 Monitor the incision for redness and drainage.	Delirium	
4 Apply supplemental oxygen at 2 L/min.	Pressure injury	
5 Administer antiemetic medication.	Venous thromboembolism	
6 Teach the client to use incentive spirometry every 1–2 hr.		
7 Reorient the client frequently.		

Thinking Exercise 16C-5

A 75-year-old female client fell in an assisted-living facility and sustained a fractured right hip that was surgically repaired 2 days ago. The client is alert and oriented × 3, has stable vital signs, and has been out of bed several times today. She walked a few steps in her room with assistance of the physical therapist. The client's daughter tells the nurse that she wants to take her mother home instead of having her return to assisted living. Which health teaching will the nurse review with the daughter and client in preparation for discharge the next day? **Select all that apply.**

_____ A. "Be sure that you continue your anticoagulant until the follow-up surgeon visit."

_____ B. "Continue to wear compression stockings to help reduce the chance of a blood clot."

_____ C. "Contact the surgeon immediately if the incision becomes redder or begins to drain."

_____ D. "Do not bear weight on your affected surgical leg until the follow-up surgeon visit."

_____ E. "Sleep on your back or nonoperative hip, preferably with a pillow between your legs."

_____ F. "Avoid sitting or staying in one position too long to prevent pressure injury."

_____ G. "Ambulate with a cane when you return home to your daughter's house."

_____ H. "Allow your daughter to help you with ADLs until you get stronger."

Thinking Exercise 16C-6

A 75-year-old female client fell in an assisted-living facility and sustained a fractured right hip that was surgically repaired 5 weeks ago. She has been living with her daughter and receiving rehabilitation services at home. Today she has a follow-up appointment with her surgeon and sees the nurse prior to the surgical examination. **For each client finding, use an X to indicate whether the client is progressing as expected or is not progressing as expected.**

Client Finding	Is Progressing	Is Not Progressing
Temperature = 97.8°F (36.6°C)		
Surgical incision healed without redness or drainage		
Reports soreness in her incisional area but not severe pain		
Walks independently with a cane on her left side		
Performs ADLs without assistance		
Has no calf pain or redness		

Single-Episode Case (16C-7)

Thinking Exercise 16C-7

A 97-year-old male client was admitted to the hospital with a left femoral neck (hip) fracture and is placed temporarily in Buck's traction until a decision is made about his treatment plan. The client has a history of diabetes mellitus, stage 2 colorectal cancer, mild multi-infarct dementia, coronary artery disease, and chronic obstructive pulmonary disease (COPD). On assessment, the client is alert but oriented only to self. The nurse develops the client's plan of care in coordination with the registered nurse. What actions will the nurse include in his plan of care? **Select all that apply.**

_____ A. Check that the traction has at least 20 lb (9.1 kg) of weight to align the fracture.

_____ B. Maintain the client in a flat supine position at all times during his hospital stay.

_____ C. Ensure that a pressure-reducing surface is used for the client to prevent pressure injury.

_____ D. Keep all weights free hanging and not resting on the floor.

_____ E. Perform and document a neurovascular assessment of the lower extremities every 4 hours.

_____ F. Assess pin sites for redness, drainage, or odor that may indicate infection.

_____ G. Apply a restraint to the client to prevent him from getting out of bed because of delirium.

17 Sensory Perception: Cataracts
(Medical-Surgical Nursing: Older Adult)

Unfolding Case (17-1 Through 17-6)

Thinking Exercise 17-1

A 69-year-old female client was taken to the emergency department (ED) after a motor vehicle accident resulting from her going through a stop sign. After a thorough evaluation, the client was found to have no serious injuries but has multiple bruises on her chest and abdomen as a result of the car airbag. She states that she went through the stop sign because she has had some "problems" with one of her eyes. The nurse collects additional information from the client about her eye and vision concerns. **Place an X in the right column next to the client findings in the left column below that are of concern to the nurse and require follow-up.**

Client Finding	Client Finding That Requires Follow-up by the Nurse
History of diabetes mellitus type 2	
History of hypertension	
Was treated several years ago for depression after partner died	
Has worn glasses for almost 60 years	
Has new onset of decreased visual acuity	
Sees floaters and spots at times, especially in her left eye	
Sees better at night than during the day	

Thinking Exercise 17-2

A 69-year-old female client was taken to the emergency department (ED) after a motor vehicle accident. She states that she went through a stop sign because she has had some "problems" with visual acuity, including seeing floaters and spots, especially in her left eye. She says she seems to see better at night than during the day and has worn glasses for most of her life. **Choose the *most likely* options for the information missing from the statements below by selecting from the lists of options provided.**

The nurse recognizes that the client ***most likely*** has ________1________, a common problem of the eye associated with aging. The client needs to have a(n) ________2________ to accurately diagnose this problem.

Options for 1	Options for 2
Presbyopia	Physical examination
Glaucoma	Stronger eyeglasses
Cataracts	Corneal staining
Diabetic retinopathy	Eye examination
Macular degeneration	Lasik surgery

Thinking Exercise 17-3

A 69-year-old female client was taken to the emergency department (ED) after a motor vehicle accident. She states that she went through a stop sign because she has had some "problems" with visual acuity, including seeing floaters and spots, especially in her left eye. She says she seems to see better at night than during the day. The client has a history of diabetes mellitus type 2 and hypertension. **Choose the *most likely* options for the information missing from the statements below by selecting from the list of options provided.**

The ***priority*** for the client related to her visual changes is to ensure improvement in her ______________________________.

Options
Blood glucose control
Driving ability
Visual acuity
Blood pressure
Eyeglasses

Thinking Exercise 17-4

Pharmacology

A 69-year-old female client was driving and went through a stop sign because she has had some problems with visual acuity, including seeing floaters and spots, especially in her left eye. She says she seems to see better at night than during the day. The client visits her ophthalmologist, who diagnoses her with bilateral cataracts, the left eye being worse than the right eye. She is scheduled for cataract surgery next week. The nurse reinforces health teaching, including a review of multiple preoperative eyedrops that the client must instill as prescribed before surgery. Which health teaching about drug therapy is indicated for the client in preparation for cataract surgery? **Select all that apply.**

______ A. "You will have mydriatic eyedrops to put into your left eye to constrict your pupil."

______ B. "You will be using an antibacterial eyedrop to prevent infection after surgery."

______ C. "Make sure that all eyedrops are at room temperature when you use them."

______ D. "Instill all eyedrops into your lower eyelid by pulling down on it gently."

______ E. "You will likely have to use eyedrops that decrease inflammation from surgery."

______ F. "Look down toward the floor when you are instilling eyedrops."

______ G. "After you instill each eyedrop dose, close your eye gently and move it around."

______ H. "Wait at least 5 minutes between different types of eyedrops."

Thinking Exercise 17-5

A 69-year-old female client had a left cataract removal with insertion of an intraocular lens due to decreasing visual acuity, which had caused her to run a stop sign while driving. She has a history of diabetes mellitus type 2 and hypertension. What actions will the nurse include in this client's postoperative care? **Select all that apply.**

_____ A. Assess the client's pain level and offer a mild analgesic as needed.

_____ B. Teach the client to report severe intense eye pain to the surgeon immediately.

_____ C. Remind the client that she will need to instill several types of eyedrops after surgery.

_____ D. Teach the client the need to wear an eye patch over the affected eye as instructed.

_____ E. Reinforce the need to avoid rubbing the affected eye at any time.

_____ F. Follow the surgeon's instructions about any lifting restrictions.

_____ G. Remind the client to be sure to scan the immediate area by turning the head side to side.

_____ H. Remind the client to check her blood glucose after surgery.

Thinking Exercise 17-6

A 69-year-old female client had a left cataract removal with insertion of an intraocular lens 3 weeks ago because of decreasing visual acuity. She has a history of diabetes mellitus type 2 and hypertension. Today she has a follow-up appointment with her surgeon and sees the nurse prior to the surgical examination. **For each client finding, use an X to indicate whether the client is progressing as expected or is <u>not</u> progressing as expected.**

Client Finding	Is Progressing	Is Not Progressing
Temperature = 97.8°F (36.6°C)		
Blood pressure = 128/74 mm Hg		
No drainage from left eye		
Moderate redness in sclera		
Reports no severe eye pain		
Blood glucose = 195 mg/dL (10.8 mmol/L)		

Single-Episode Case (17-7)

Thinking Exercise 17-7

Pharmacology

A 75-year-old male client was recently diagnosed with glaucoma and early cataracts, which has not yet affected his vision. The ophthalmologist prescribed several types of eyedrops for him to use beginning immediately, with a follow-up visit in 6 months. The nurse teaches the client about the purpose of each drug. **Match the action of the ophthalmic drug in the left column with the drug name. Note that not all actions will be used.**

Drug Action	Drug Name	Appropriate Action for Each Prescribed Drug
1 Prevents eye infection	Latanoprost	
2 Constricts pupils of the eye	Timolol	
3 Increases ocular hypertension	Epinephrine	
4 Decreases aqueous humor formation		
5 Increases aqueous humor outflow		
6 Dilates pupils of the eye		

Infection: Pneumonia (Medical-Surgical Nursing: Older Adult) 18

Unfolding Case (18-1 Through 18-6)

Thinking Exercise 18-1

An 84-year-old male client lives in a long-term care facility for assistance managing health issues associated with chronic obstructive pulmonary disease (COPD) and history of lung cancer. The client is a widower and has an adult child who lives out of state. He has no history of dementia, performs ADLs with moderate assistance, and has a body mass index (BMI) of 19. He smokes cigarettes, uses a wheelchair to move around the facility, and refuses to participate in group activities because of chronic dyspnea. A nurse completes the client's daily assessment and notices that the client has new-onset confusion and stabbing pain in his right lateral chest. Additional client findings include:

- Vital signs: temperature, 102.1°F (38.9°C); heart rate (HR), 102 beats/min; blood pressure (BP), 128/63 mm Hg; respirations, 24 breaths/min; oxygen saturation, 86% (on 2 L/min oxygen via nasal cannula [NC])
- Barrel-shaped chest
- Productive cough with dark-red sputum
- Wheezes present on auscultation
- Reports shortness of breath
- Abdomen round, soft, nontender
- Moves all extremities
- Pulses palpable 2+
- Fingertips yellowed
- Shaking with chills

Identify with an X the most important client findings that require follow-up by the nurse.

Client Finding	Most Important Client Findings That Require Follow-up by the Nurse
Acute confusion	
Barrel-shaped chest	
Dark-red sputum	
Oxygen saturation = 86% (on 2 L/min oxygen via nasal cannula [NC])	
Yellowed fingertips	

Thinking Exercise 18-2

An 84-year-old male client lives in a long-term care facility for assistance managing health issues associated with chronic obstructive pulmonary disease (COPD) and a history of lung cancer. The client is a widower and has an adult child who lives out of state. He has no history of dementia, performs ADLs with moderate assistance, and has a body mass index (BMI) of 19. He smokes cigarettes, uses a wheelchair to move around the facility, and refuses to participate in group activities because of chronic dyspnea.

A nurse completes the client's daily assessment and notices that the client has new-onset confusion and stabbing pain in his right lateral chest. The client's vital signs are: temperature, 102.1°F (38.9°C); heart rate (HR), 102 beats/min; blood pressure (BP), 128/63 mm Hg; respirations, 24 breaths/min; oxygen saturation, 86% (on 2 L/min oxygen via nasal cannula [NC]). Additional client findings are visible shaking chills, dyspnea, and productive cough with dark-red sputum. **For each client finding below, determine if the finding is associated with chronic obstructive pulmonary disease (COPD), pneumonia, and/or lung cancer. Any client finding may be associated with more than one disease process.**

Client Finding	COPD	Pneumonia	Lung Cancer
Productive cough			
Dark-red sputum			
Dyspnea			
Wheezing			
Acute confusion			

Thinking Exercise 18-3

An 84-year-old male client lives in a long-term care facility for assistance managing health issues associated with chronic obstructive pulmonary disease (COPD) and history of lung cancer. He has no history of dementia, performs ADLs with moderate assistance, and has a body mass index (BMI) of 19. He smokes cigarettes, uses a wheelchair to move around the facility, and refuses to participate in group activities because of chronic dyspnea.

A nurse completes the client's daily assessment and notices that the client has new-onset confusion and stabbing pain in his right lateral chest. The client's vital signs are: temperature, 102.1°F (38.9°C); heart rate (HR), 102 beats/min; blood pressure (BP), 128/63 mm Hg; respirations, 24 breaths/min; oxygen saturation, 86% (on 2 L/min oxygen via nasal cannula [NC]). Additional client findings are visible shaking chills, dyspnea, and productive cough with dark-red sputum, possibly hemoptysis. **Complete the following sentences by choosing the *most likely* option for the missing information from the lists of options provided.**

The nurse determines that the client is ***most likely*** experiencing pneumonia as evidenced by his new-onset ____1____, ____1____, and ____1____. The nurse is most concerned with the client's ____2____ and ____2____ findings.

Options for 1	Options for 2
Confusion	Temperature
Dyspnea	Lung sounds
Fever	Orientation
Lateral chest pain	Oxygenation
Malnutrition	Pain
Productive cough	
Wheezing	

Thinking Exercise 18-4

An 84-year-old male client lives in a long-term care facility for assistance managing health issues associated with chronic obstructive pulmonary disease (COPD) and a history of lung cancer. The nurse completes the client's daily assessment and notices that the client has new-onset confusion and stabbing pain in his right lateral chest. The client's vital signs are: temperature, 102.1°F (38.9°C); heart rate (HR), 102 beats/min; blood pressure (BP), 128/63 mm Hg; respirations, 24 breaths/min; oxygen saturation, 86% (on 2 L/min oxygen via nasal cannula [NC]). Additional client findings are visible shaking chills, dyspnea, and hemoptysis. The client is diagnosed with pneumonia. The nurse prioritizes client problems and interventions to address each problem. **Indicate which nursing action listed in the far-left column is appropriate for each client problem. Note that all actions may not be used.**

Nursing Action	Client's Priority Problem	Appropriate Nursing Action for Each Priority Client Problem
1 Provide a high-calorie, low-protein diet to promote the immune system.	Inadequate oxygenation	
2 Assist the client in changing positions every 2 hours to help mobilize secretions.	Airway obstruction	
3 Place the client in a supine position to decrease pressure of abdominal organs on the diaphragm.	Inadequate nutrition	
4 Provide supplemental oxygen to keep saturation levels between 88% and 92%.		
5 Arrange for food options that are attractive and preferred by the client to enhance appetite.		

Thinking Exercise 18-5

An 84-year-old male client lives in a long-term care facility for assistance managing health issues associated with chronic obstructive pulmonary disease (COPD). The nurse completes the client's daily assessment and notices that the client has new-onset confusion and stabbing pain in his right lateral chest. The client's vital signs are: temperature, 102.1°F (38.9°C); heart rate (HR), 102 beats/min; blood pressure (BP), 128/63 mm Hg; respirations, 24 breaths/min; oxygen saturation, 86% (on 2 L/min oxygen via nasal cannula [NC]). Additional client findings are visible shaking chills, dyspnea, and hemoptysis. The client is diagnosed with pneumonia, and the nurse receives the following orders from the primary health care provider:

- Ciprofloxacin 400 mg IV every 12 hours
- Blood cultures × 2
- Supplemental oxygen to keep saturations at 88% to 92%
- Nutritional consultation
- Chest physiotherapy
- Sputum culture

Highlight the three orders above that the nurse would perform *first*.

Thinking Exercise 18-6

An 84-year-old male client lives in a long-term care facility for assistance managing health issues associated with chronic obstructive pulmonary disease (COPD) and undernutrition. The client was diagnosed with pneumonia based on new-onset confusion, visible shaking chills, dyspnea, stabbing right lateral chest pain, and hemoptysis. The client's vital signs were: temperature, 102.1°F (38.9°C); heart rate (HR), 102 beats/min; blood pressure (BP), 128/63 mm Hg; respirations, 24 breaths/min; oxygen saturation, 86% (on 2 L/min oxygen via nasal cannula [NC]).

Over the past 3 days, interventions were implemented including IV antibiotics, additional oxygen, and nutritional supplements. The nurse reassesses the client to evaluate if the client met expected outcomes. **For each client finding, indicate if the client's condition is progressing or is <u>not</u> progressing.**

Client Finding	Is Progressing	Is Not Progressing
Oxygen saturation = 93% (on 4 L/min via nasal cannula [NC])		
Drinks a protein shake between each meal		
Experiences dyspnea with activity and at rest		
Right pleural effusion present on chest x-ray		
Has dry, nonproductive cough		

Single-Episode Cases (18-7 and 18-8)

Thinking Exercise 18-7

A nurse cares for a 68-year-old female client who was cleaning her house gutters when she sustained a cervical spinal cord injury after falling. The client was stabilized and transferred to a long-term acute care facility 6 days ago with a tracheostomy with 40% supplemental oxygen and a gastrostomy tube for bolus feedings. Over the past 2 days, the client has tolerated a tracheostomy plug that allows the client to speak and eat a mechanical soft diet with thickened beverages. The nurse reviews the plan of care to decrease the client's risk potential for aspiration pneumonia. **Use an X to show whether each nursing action below is <u>Indicated</u> (appropriate or necessary), <u>Contraindicated</u> (could be harmful), or <u>Non-Essential</u> (makes no difference or is not necessary) for the client's care at this time.**

Nursing Action	Indicated	Contraindicated	Non-Essential
Ensure suction equipment is available at the bedside.			
Encourage the client to tilt her head back when swallowing.			
Keep the head of bed elevated during enteral feedings.			
Remove choking hazard foods such as hot dogs and grapes.			
Perform oral hygiene frequently.			

Thinking Exercise 18-8

A 72-year-old client was diagnosed 2 days ago with community-acquired pneumonia and prescribed azithromycin 250-mg tablet orally once a day. The nurse follows up with the client via a telehealth service. Which instructions will the nurse reinforce for this client who has pneumonia? **Select all that apply.**

_____ A. "Fatigue may persist for several weeks, so try to gradually increase your activity as you recover."

_____ B. "Take all of your antibiotics as prescribed. Do not stop when you begin to feel better."

_____ C. "You are very contagious, so do not leave your home and minimize visitors for the next 2 weeks."

_____ D. "Make sure to drink plenty of fluids. This will help to thin out your secretions so that you can cough them up."

_____ E. "Try to eat foods high in protein such as eggs, fish, lean meats, and nuts."

_____ F. "Stop immediately if your chest hurts when you attempt to cough up secretions."

_____ G. "Contact your primary health care provider about symptoms of nausea and vomiting while taking azithromycin."

_____ H. "Small frequent meals may be easier for you to eat because the act of eating can be very tiring."

19 Cognition

Exemplar 19A. Delirium (Mental Health Nursing: Older Adult)

Unfolding Case Study (19A-1 Through 19A-6)

Thinking Exercise 19A-1

A 77-year-old female client visits her primary health care provider with report of changes in urinary pattern and continence. Her medical history includes hypertension, gastroesophageal reflux disease (GERD), and osteoarthritis, all of which are being managed with drug therapy. The nurse collects data about the client prior to the provider's examination. **Highlight the client findings below that require follow-up by the nurse in collaboration with the provider.**

- Temperature = 97.8°F (36.5°C)
- Heart rate = 82 beats/min
- Blood pressure = 158/88 mm Hg
- Oxygen saturation = 95% (on room air [RA])
- Is alert and oriented × 3
- Is ADL independent and lives alone
- Has knee and hip pain most days from arthritis, which runs in her family
- States she has had a hard time recently controlling her bladder; feels like she has to void all the time
- Has nocturia 2 to 5 times every night, which makes her feel tired during the day
- Tries to drink plenty of water but is thinking she should restrict fluids to help with her bladder problem.

Thinking Exercise 19A-2

A 77-year-old female client visits her primary health care provider with report of changes in urinary pattern and continence. The client states she has had a hard time recently controlling her bladder and feels like she has to void all the time. She also has nocturia two to five times every night, which makes her feel tired during the day. The client's history includes hypertension, gastroesophageal reflux disease (GERD), and osteoarthritis, all of which are being managed with drug therapy. However, her blood pressure in the office was 158/88 mm Hg. As a result, the primary health care provider increased her amlodipine from 5 mg orally every day to 10 mg orally every day. The provider also prescribed oxybutynin chloride 5 mg orally twice a day for urge urinary incontinence.

During that same evening, the client experienced a fall at home and called her daughter, who brought her to the emergency department (ED). Her daughter tells the ED nurse that her mother seems very confused and keeps asking why there are bugs crawling on a vase in the living room. After an evaluation in the ED, the client was found to have no major injuries, but was admitted to the observational unit of the hospital. **Choose the *most likely* options for the information missing from the statement below by selecting from the lists of options provided.**

The nurse recognizes that the client is ***most likely*** experiencing ________1________ as a result of ______2______.

Option for 1	Option for 2
Delusions	Falling
Unsteadiness	Oxybutynin
Delirium	Amlodipine
Dizziness	Advanced age

Thinking Exercise 19A-3

A 77-year-old female client was admitted to the hospital for observation after experiencing a fall at home. Her daughter told the nurse that after the fall her mother was very confused and kept asking why there were bugs crawling on a vase in the living room. The client's drug regimen was recently changed because of hypertension (amlodipine increased from 5 mg to 10 mg daily). She was also prescribed to begin oxybutynin for urge urinary incontinence the day before hospital admission. The admitting nurse performs a focused assessment and notes the following:

- Temperature = 98°F (36.7°C)
- Heart rate = 72 beats/min
- Respirations = 20 breaths/min
- Blood pressure (BP) = 126/74 mm Hg
- Alert and oriented × 1 (person)
- Unable to follow conversation
- Bruising on left arm

The nurse is planning care for the client in coordination with the registered nurse. What ***priority*** problems would the nurse include in the plan of care? **Select all that apply.**

_____ A. Potential for falls

_____ B. Decreased visual acuity

_____ C. Hypertension

_____ D. Urinary incontinence

_____ E. Bowel incontinence

_____ F. ADL dependence

_____ G. Acute confusion

_____ H. Bradycardia

Thinking Exercise 19A-4

A 77-year-old female client was admitted to the hospital for observation after experiencing a fall at home. Her daughter told the nurse that after the fall her mother was very confused and kept asking why there were bugs crawling on a vase in the living room. The client's drug regimen was recently changed because of uncontrolled hypertension (amlodipine increased from 5 mg to 10 mg daily). She was also prescribed to begin oxybutynin for urge urinary incontinence the day before hospital admission. The admitting nurse performs a focused assessment and notes the following:

- Temperature = 98°F (36.7°C)
- Heart rate = 72 beats/min
- Respirations = 20 breaths/min
- Blood pressure (BP) = 126/74 mm Hg
- Alert and oriented × 1 (person)
- Unable to follow conversation
- Bruising on left arm

Use an X to show whether the nursing actions below are Indicated (appropriate or necessary), Contraindicated (could be harmful), or Non-Essential (makes no difference or is not necessary) for the client's care at this time.

Nursing Action	Indicated	Contraindicated	Non-Essential
Apply oxygen therapy at 2 L/min.			
Place a fall alarm on the client's mattress.			
Reorient the client frequently.			
Withhold oxybutynin until the client's delirium resolves.			
Apply a vest restraint to ensure that the client does not try to get out of bed.			
Remind assistive personnel to toilet the client every 2 hours.			

Thinking Exercise 19A-5

A 77-year-old female client was admitted to the hospital for observation after experiencing a fall at home. Her daughter told the nurse that after the fall her mother was very confused and kept asking why there were bugs crawling on a vase in the living room. The client's drug regimen was recently changed because of uncontrolled hypertension (amlodipine increased from 5 mg to 10 mg daily). She was also prescribed to begin oxybutynin for urge urinary incontinence the day before hospital admission. The primary health care provider wrote new orders as follows:

- Discontinue oxybutynin for urge incontinence
- Amlodipine 10 mg orally every morning
- Vital signs every 4 hours
- Continuous pulse oximetry
- Out of bed with assistance to bedside commode
- Toilet every 2 hours
- Diet as tolerated
- Continuous IV 5%D/0.45%NS at 80 mL/hr
- Fall precautions

The nurse plans to implement the above orders. **Place an X to indicate which three orders are the *highest priority* to implement first.**

Primary Health Care Provider's Orders	Orders That Are Priority for the Nurse to Implement First
Discontinue oxybutynin for urge incontinence	
Amlodipine 10 mg orally every morning	
Vital signs every 4 hours	
Continuous pulse oximetry	
Out of bed with assistance to bedside commode	
Toilet every 2 hours	
Diet as tolerated	
Continuous IV 5%D/0.45%NS at 80 mL/hr	
Fall precautions	

Thinking Exercise 19A-6

A 77-year-old female client was admitted to the hospital for observation after experiencing a fall at home. Her daughter told the nurse that after the fall her mother was very confused and kept asking why there were bugs crawling on a vase in the living room. The client's drug regimen was recently changed because of uncontrolled hypertension (amlodipine increased from 5 mg to 10 mg daily). She was also prescribed to begin oxybutynin for urge urinary incontinence before hospital admission, which caused delirium. She is scheduled for discharge home with her daughter, and the nurse documents the client's most recent assessment findings. **Use an X to indicate which client findings below demonstrate that the client is progressing or is not progressing.**

Client Finding	Is Progressing	Is Not Progressing
Has not experienced a fall while hospitalized		
Able to walk with minimal assistance		
Continues to have urge urinary incontinence		
Is alert and oriented × 2		
Has had no hallucinations while hospitalized		

Single-Episode Case (19A-7)

Thinking Exercise 19A-7

Pharmacology

A 84-year-old male client was admitted to the emergency department after a seizure at home. He is yelling, agitated, cursing loudly, and not oriented. The nurse takes a thorough history from the client's son, including a medication history. Which medications does the nurse recognize may be contributing to the client's delirium? **Select all that apply.**

_____ A. Antibiotics

_____ B. Benzodiazepines

_____ C. Diuretics

_____ D. Antidepressants

_____ E. Antihistamines

_____ F. Hypnotics

_____ G. Mydriatics

_____ H. Anticoagulants

Exemplar 19B. Alzheimer Disease (Mental Health Nursing: Older Adult)

Unfolding Case Study (19B-1 Through 19B-6)

Thinking Exercise 19B-1

A 72-year-old female client is admitted from her home to the memory care unit of a long-term care facility. The admitting nurse documents the following client findings. **Highlight the client findings that are of concern to the nurse.**

Health History	Nurses' Notes	Vital Signs	Laboratory Results

11-22-21 Client diagnosed with moderate-stage Alzheimer disease and depression. Alert and oriented × 1. Her partner states that she tends to wander often and tries to go outdoors. She sometimes takes an afternoon nap because she does not sleep well at night. Client has frequent anxiety, especially in unfamiliar places, and sometimes needs assistance with ADLs. Refuses to eat at times. She is able to ambulate without assistive device and recognizes her daughter and granddaughter. ---------------*M. A. Hollister, LVN*

Thinking Exercise 19B-2

A 72-year-old female client is admitted from her home to the memory care unit of a long-term care facility with a diagnosis of moderate-stage Alzheimer disease and depression. Her medical history includes an open reduction, internal fixation (ORIF) of her right ankle, hyperlipidemia, and atrial fibrillation. **Use an X to indicate which client findings are commonly associated with each client condition. Note that some findings may be used for more than one client condition.**

Client Finding	Alzheimer Disease	Depression
Partner states that she tends to wander often and tries to go outdoors.		
Sometimes takes an afternoon nap because she does not sleep well at night.		
Has frequent anxiety, especially in unfamiliar places.		
Sometimes needs assistance with ADLs.		
Refuses to eat at times.		

Thinking Exercise 19B-3

A 72-year-old female client is admitted from her home to the memory care unit of a long-term care facility with a diagnosis of moderate-stage Alzheimer disease and clinical depression. Her medical history includes an open reduction, internal fixation (ORIF) of her right ankle, hyperlipidemia, and atrial fibrillation. The admitting nurse documents the following client findings:

- Partner states that she tends to wander often and tries to go outdoors
- Sometimes takes an afternoon nap because she does not sleep well at night
- Has frequent anxiety, especially in unfamiliar places
- Sometimes needs assistance with ADLs
- Able to ambulate without assistive device
- Is able to recognize daughter and granddaughter
- Refuses to eat at times
- Alert and oriented × 1 (person only)

Choose the *most likely* options for the information missing from the statement below by selecting from the list of options provided.

The nurse identifies the ***priority*** needs of the client, which are to ____________________ and ____________________.

Options
Implement sleep hygiene Reorient the client to reality Maintain client safety Promote effective communication Ensure that basic needs are met

Thinking Exercise 19B-4

A 72-year-old female client is admitted from her home to the memory care unit of a long-term care facility with a diagnosis of moderate-stage Alzheimer disease (AD) and clinical depression. Her medical history includes an open reduction, internal fixation (ORIF) of her right ankle, hyperlipidemia, and atrial fibrillation. The admitting nurse documents the following client findings:

- Partner states that she tends to wander often and tries to go outdoors
- Sometimes takes an afternoon nap because she does not sleep well at night
- Has frequent anxiety, especially in unfamiliar places
- Sometimes needs assistance with ADLs
- Able to ambulate without assistive device
- Is able to recognize daughter and granddaughter
- Refuses to eat at times
- Alert and oriented $\times$ 1 (person only)

Indicate which nursing action listed in the far-left column is appropriate to help manage each client problem related to her dementia and depression. Note that not all nursing actions will be used.

Nursing Action	Client Health Problem	Nursing Action for Client Health Problem
1 Validate the client's statements rather than correcting them.	Potential for injury due to wandering	
2 Use an alarm device to notify staff when she tries to leave the unit.	Sleep disturbances	
3 Ask the client's partner what she likes to eat and drink.	Chronic confusion	
4 Assist the client with ADLs as needed.	Potential for inadequate nutrition	
5 Reorient the client to reality frequently.		
6 Keep the client active during the day, including walking.		

Thinking Exercise 19B-5

A 72-year-old female client was admitted from her home to the memory care unit of a long-term care facility a week ago with a diagnosis of moderate-stage Alzheimer disease and clinical depression. The client's partner states that she tends to wander often and tries to go outdoors, and that she does not sleep well at night. Today the client's partner visited and spent most of the day with her. The certified nursing assistant (CNA) told the nurse that the client cried for about 10 minutes after her partner left at 5:00 p.m. (1700). At 6:30 p.m. (1830), the CNA reported that the client was not in her room or in the unit. **Select the five actions that the nurse would take *at this time.***

_____ A. Search the entire memory unit again, including closets and other small areas.

_____ B. Report the incident to the local law enforcement agency.

_____ C. Report the incident to the charge nurse.

_____ D. Contact the other units in the long-term care facility and ask them to search for the client.

_____ E. Organize a search of the grounds of the long-term care facility.

_____ F. Check the alarm system to ensure that it is working properly.

_____ G. Ask visitors, staff, and other clients when they last saw or interacted with the client.

_____ H. Contact the responsible family member or guardian to inform them of the elopement.

_____ I. Complete a variance report regarding the elopement.

Thinking Exercise 19B-6

A 72-year-old female client was admitted from her home to the memory care unit of a long-term care facility a week ago with a diagnosis of moderate-stage Alzheimer disease (AD) and clinical depression. The client's partner states that she tends to wander often and tries to go outdoors and that she does not sleep well at night. Today the client's partner visited and spent most of the day with her. The certified nursing assistant (CNA) told the nurse that the client cried for about 10 minutes after her partner left at 5:00 p.m. (1700). At 6:30 p.m. (1830), the CNA reported that the client was not in her room or in the unit. After searching the unit and entire facility for over an hour, the staff found the client folding towels in the laundry room of the facility. The staff returned the client to the memory care unit so the nurse could assess her for injury. **Highlight the client findings in the Nurses' Notes below that indicate the client is safe and progressing.**

Nurses' Notes	**History and Physical**	**Vital Signs**	**Laboratory Results**

4/20/21 1930 CNA reported to nurse at 1830 that client was missing from her room and the unit. After searching the entire facility inside and outside, client was found folding towels in the laundry room while humming a song. Client stated that she felt very happy and wanted to do laundry. Alert and oriented × 2 (person and place). No apparent injuries. Incontinent of urine with perineal redness. Client had a shower and was assisted to prepare for bedtime. Barrier cream applied to perineum. ------------------------------ *S. M. Littleton, LVN*

Single-Episode Case (19B-7)

Thinking Exercise 19B-7

An 89-year-old male client has been a resident in a long-term care facility for over 7 years because of multiple medical problems, including late-stage Alzheimer disease. Recently the client has refused to eat when the staff tries to feed him. Even when he opens his mouth, he does not chew the food and it sits in his mouth. The client has lost 10 lb (22 kg) during the last month. **Select two actions that the nurse would take for the client's care *at this time.***

______ A. Refer the client to the speech-language pathologist for swallowing evaluation.

______ B. Consult with the registered dietitian nutritionist about changing his diet.

______ C. Obtain an order to have a gastrostomy tube for feeding inserted.

______ D. Check the client's advance directives to determine end-of-life care plan.

______ E. Obtain an order for an IV solution of 5%D/W via a peripheral catheter.

______ F. Obtain an order for total parenteral nutrition via a central line.

______ G. Discuss the client's situation with his family or guardian.

20 Elimination

Exemplar 20A. Chronic Kidney Disease (Medical-Surgical Nursing: Middle-Age Adult; Older Adult)

Unfolding Case (20A-1 Through 20A-6)

Thinking Exercise 20A-1

The nurse is assessing a 66-year-old male client who was brought to the urgent care clinic by his partner with new onset of symptoms including nausea, vomiting, and confusion. The nurse notes the following lab values and documents these assessment data. **Highlight the assessment findings below that are of immediate concern to the nurse.**

- History of diabetes mellitus type 2 and hypertension for over 20 years
- History of chronic kidney disease managed by diet and diuretic therapy for 6 years
- Reports feeling drowsy and disoriented
- Reports that urinary output greatly decreased over the past few days
- 3+ pitting edema in both ankles and feet
- Vital signs:
  - Temperature = 97.6°F (36.4°C)
  - Heart rate = 86 beats/min and regular
  - Respirations = 20 breaths/min
  - Blood pressure = 168/95 mm Hg
  - Oxygen saturation = 95% (on room air [RA])
- Lab test results:
  - Blood urea nitrogen (BUN) = 72 mg/dL (26.1 mmol/L)
  - Serum creatinine (Cr) = 7.8 mg/dL (689 mmol/L)
  - Potassium = 6.1 mEq/L (6.1 mmol/L)

Thinking Exercise 20A-2

The nurse is assessing a 66-year-old male client who was brought to the urgent care clinic by his partner with new onset of symptoms including nausea, vomiting, and confusion. The nurse notes the following lab values and documents these assessment data:

- History of diabetes mellitus type 2 and hypertension for over 20 years
- History of chronic kidney disease managed by diet and diuretic therapy for 6 years
- Reports feeling drowsy and disoriented
- Reports that urinary output greatly decreased over the past few days
- 3+ pitting edema in both ankles and feet
- Vital signs:
  - Temperature = 97.6°F (36.4°C)
  - Heart rate = 86 beats/min and regular
  - Respirations = 20 breaths/min
  - Blood pressure = 168/95 mm Hg
  - Oxygen saturation = 95% (on room air [RA])

- Lab test results:
  - Blood urea nitrogen (BUN) = 72 mg/dL (26.1 mmol/L)
  - Serum creatinine (Cr) = 7.8 mg/dL (689 mmol/L)
  - Potassium = 6.1 mEq/L (6.1 mmol/L)

Based on these client findings, select two potentially life-threatening complications that the nurse recognizes the client is most at risk for at this time.

_____ A. Heart failure

_____ B. Uremic frost

_____ C. Bone demineralization

_____ D. Hypothyroidism

_____ E. Cardiac dysrhythmias

_____ F. Asthma

_____ G. Stroke

Thinking Exercise 20A-3

The nurse is assessing a 66-year-old male client who was brought to the urgent care clinic by his partner with new onset of symptoms including nausea, vomiting, and confusion. The nurse notes the following lab values and documents these assessment data:

- History of diabetes mellitus type 2 and hypertension for over 20 years
- History of chronic kidney disease managed by diet and diuretic therapy for 6 years
- Reports feeling drowsy and disoriented
- Reports that urinary output greatly decreased over the past few days
- 3+ pitting edema in both ankles and feet
- Vital signs:
  - Temperature = 97.6°F (36.4°C)
  - Heart rate = 86 beats/min and regular
  - Respirations = 20 breaths/min
  - Blood pressure = 168/95 mm Hg
  - Oxygen saturation = 95% (on room air [RA])
- Lab test results:
  - Blood urea nitrogen (BUN) = 72 mg/dL (26.1 mmol/L)
  - Serum creatinine (Cr) = 7.8 mg/dL (689 mmol/L)
  - Potassium = 6.1 mEq/L (6.1 mmol/L)

Choose the *most likely* options for the information missing from the statement below by selecting from the lists of options provided.

The nurse recognizes that the ***priority*** needs for this client are to manage his _____1_____, which can lead to _____1_____, and _____2_____, which can lead to _____2_____.

Options for 1	Options for 2
Hypervolemia	Acute kidney injury
Oliguria	Dysrhythmias
Hyperkalemia	Shock
Tachycardia	Metabolic alkalosis
Azotemia	Stroke
Hypertension	Heart failure

Thinking Exercise 20A-4

The nurse is caring for a 66-year-old male client who was brought to the urgent care clinic by his partner with new onset of symptoms including nausea, vomiting, and confusion. He has a history of chronic kidney disease, which had been managed by diet and diuretic therapy. The client noticed that his urinary output greatly decreased over the previous few days. His blood pressure is elevated and he has 3+ pitting edema in both ankles and feet. The primary health care provider determines that the client needs emergent hemodialysis. **Use an X to show whether the nursing actions below are <u>Indicated</u> (appropriate or necessary), <u>Contraindicated</u> (could be harmful), or <u>Non-Essential</u> (makes no difference or is not necessary) for the client's care at this time.**

Nursing Action	Indicated	Contraindicated	Non-Essential
Apply oxygen therapy at 2 L/min.			
Prepare to assist with central line insertion.			
Explain the procedure to the client and his partner.			
Administer the prescribed opioid analgesic.			
Continue to assess vital signs frequently.			
Monitor the client's level of consciousness and orientation frequently.			

Thinking Exercise 20A-5

A 66-year-old male client has had chronic kidney disease (CKD) managed by diet and diuretic therapy for a number of years. As a result of his worsening CKD over the previous 2 weeks, the client received hemodialysis treatments before he began peritoneal dialysis (PD) at home. Today the nurse visits his home to observe the second PD treatment. Before the client begins the dialysate, the nurse notes slight redness and tan drainage around the abdominal catheter exit wound. During the inflow of the dialysate solution, the client reports unusual abdominal discomfort, which improved during dwell time. The nurse then observes the characteristics of the outflow (effluent) solution, which is cloudy with floating particles. What actions would the nurse take at this time? **Select all that apply.**

_____ A. Take the client's vital signs.

_____ B. Perform an abdominal assessment.

_____ C. Insert a urinary catheter.

_____ D. Remove the PD abdominal catheter.

_____ E. Take a culture of the PD catheter site drainage.

_____ F. Notify the client's primary health care provider.

_____ G. Call 911 immediately.

_____ H. Contact the home health nurse supervisor.

Thinking Exercise 20A-6

A 66-year-old male client has had chronic kidney disease (CKD) managed by diet and diuretic therapy for a number of years. As a result of his worsening CKD over the previous 2 weeks, the client received hemodialysis treatments before he began peritoneal dialysis (PD) at home. A home care nurse suspected that the client had peritonitis as a result of an infected PD catheter exit site infection, and the client was treated with IV fluid and antibiotic therapy. Today the client is returning to his primary health care provider for follow-up. The nurse assesses the client prior to examination by the provider. **Use an X to indicate which client findings below demonstrate that the client is progressing or is <u>not</u> progressing.**

Client Finding	Is Progressing	Is <u>Not</u> Progressing
Blood pressure = 128/80 mm Hg		
Alert and oriented		
3+ pitting edema of both ankles and feet		
Peritoneal dialysis catheter site clean and intact		
Serum creatinine = 1.8 mg/dL		

Single-Episode Cases (20A-7 and 20A-8)

Thinking Exercise 20A-7

The nurse is caring for a 75-year-old female client who was recently diagnosed with stage 4 (severe) chronic kidney disease (CKD). **Select four client findings that the nurse would expect.**

_____ A. Anemia

_____ B. Hypovolemia

_____ C. Hypocalcemia

_____ D. Hyperphosphatemia

_____ E. Metabolic acidosis

_____ F. Hypovolemia

_____ G. Infection

Thinking Exercise 20A-8

Pharmacology

The nurse is planning care for an 80-year-old male client with diabetes who has been diagnosed with chronic kidney disease (CKD), including managing common complications associated with the disease. **Indicate which nursing action listed in the far-left column is appropriate to help manage each client complication related to CKD. Note that not all nursing actions will be used.**

Nursing Action	CKD Complication	Nursing Action for Client Complication
1 Restrict fluids based on urinary output.	Hyperkalemia	
2 Administer an aluminum-based antacid.	Anemia	
3 Provide supplemental oxygen.	Hypervolemia	
4 Administer erythropoietin.	Hyperphosphatemia	
5 Infuse hypertonic glucose.		
6 Administer sodium polystyrene.		

Exemplar 20B. Intestinal Obstruction (Medical-Surgical Nursing: Older Adult)

Unfolding Case (20B-1 Through 20B-6)

Thinking Exercise 20B-1

The nurse is reviewing the assessment findings for a 73-year-old female client who has a possible intestinal obstruction.

Nurses' Notes | History and Physical | Imaging Test Reviews | Laboratory Results

10-4-21 Admitted from the local nursing home with severe abdominal pain and distention, vomiting, and obstipation. History of chronic obstructive pulmonary disease (COPD) and hypertension that has been well controlled. Current vital signs: temperature = 99°F (37.2°C); heart rate = 102 beats/min and regular; respirations = 26 breaths/min and slightly labored; blood pressure = 124/66 mm Hg; oxygen saturation = 92% (on room air [RA]). Bilateral fine crackles in lung bases. Bowel sounds absent in lower quadrants; hypoactive bowel sounds in upper quadrants.--*N. Brittingham, LPN*

Use an X to indicate which client findings listed in the left column would be of immediate concern to the nurse.

Client Finding	Client Finding of Immediate Concern to the Nurse
Severe abdominal pain and distention	
Vomiting	
Bilateral fine crackles in lung bases	
Decreased/absent bowel sounds	
Temperature = 99°F (37.2°C)	
Heart rate = 102 beats/min and regular	
Blood pressure = 124/66 mm Hg	

Thinking Exercise 20B-2

The nurse is analyzing the assessment findings for a 73-year-old female client who has a possible intestinal obstruction.

Nurses' Notes	History and Physical	Imaging Test Reviews	Laboratory Test Results

10-4-21 Admitted from the local nursing home with severe abdominal pain and distention, vomiting, and obstipation. History of chronic obstructive pulmonary disease (COPD) and hypertension that has been well controlled. Current vital signs: temperature = 99°F (37.2°C); heart rate = 102 beats/min and regular; respirations = 26 breaths/min and slightly labored; blood pressure = 124/66 mm Hg; oxygen saturation = 92% (on room air [RA]). Bilateral fine crackles in lung bases. Bowel sounds absent in lower quadrants; hypoactive bowel sounds in upper quadrants.--*N. Brittingham, LPN*

Use an X to indicate which client findings are commonly associated with each client condition. Note that some findings may be used for more than one client condition.

Client Finding	COPD	Intestinal Obstruction
Dyspnea		
Abdominal pain		
Bilateral fine crackles in lung bases		
Abdominal distention		
Below normal oxygen saturation		
Tachycardia		

Thinking Exercise 20B-3

As part of analyzing assessment findings for a 73-year-old female client who has a possible intestinal obstruction, the nurse prioritizes her current health needs.

Nurses' Notes	History and Physical	Imaging Test Reviews	Laboratory Test Results

10-4-21 Admitted from the local nursing home with severe abdominal pain and distention, vomiting, and obstipation. History of chronic obstructive pulmonary disease (COPD) and hypertension that has been well controlled. Current vital signs: temperature = 99°F (37.2°C); heart rate = 102 beats/min and regular; respirations = 26 breaths/min and slightly labored; blood pressure = 124/66 mm Hg; oxygen saturation = 92% (on room air [RA]). Bilateral fine crackles in lung bases. Bowel sounds absent in lower quadrants; hypoactive bowel sounds in upper quadrants.--*N. Brittingham, LPN*

Choose the *most likely* options for the information missing from the statement below by selecting from the lists of options provided.

The nurse recognizes that the client's ***priorities*** for care will be to prevent _____1_____ and monitor for potential _____2_____ that can result in peritonitis.

Options for 1	Options for 2
Diarrhea	Bowel impaction
Gastroenteritis	Volvulus
Shock	Intussusception
Fluid overload	Fistula
Colitis	Bowel perforation

Thinking Exercise 20B-4

The nurse is planning care for a 73-year-old female client who has an intestinal obstruction. She has severe abdominal pain and distention, vomiting, and obstipation. Her medical history includes chronic obstructive pulmonary disease (COPD) and hypertension. Her current vital signs are: temperature, 99°F (37.2°C); heart rate, 96 beats/min and regular; respirations, 28 breaths/min and slightly labored; blood pressure, 128/60 mm Hg; oxygen saturation, 90% (on room air [RA]). **Use an X to show whether the nursing actions below are Indicated (appropriate or necessary), Contraindicated (could be harmful), or Non-Essential (makes no difference or is not necessary) for the client's care at this time.**

Nursing Action	Indicated	Contraindicated	Non-Essential
Insert a nasogastric tube and connect to suction.			
Begin IV fluid administration.			
Obtain an electrocardiogram (ECG).			
Apply supplemental oxygen.			
Place the client in a flat supine position.			

Thinking Exercise 20B-5

The nurse is beginning to perform a shift assessment on a 73-year-old female client who has an intestinal obstruction. Yesterday she was admitted with severe abdominal pain and distention, vomiting, and obstipation. A nasogastric tube (NG) was inserted and connected to continuous low suction, an IV of normal saline was started, and oxygen at 2 L/min was administered via nasal cannula for her chronic obstructive pulmonary disease (COPD). This morning the nurse notes that the NG tube is clogged and there are no GI secretions in the drainage container. The nurse prepares to irrigate the NG tube to unclog it. Which nursing actions would the nurse include for this procedure? **Select all that apply.**

_____ A. Remove the nasal cannula and turn off the oxygen flow.

_____ B. Turn off the NG tube suction prior to the irrigation.

_____ C. Keep the client NPO at all times while the tube is in place.

_____ D. Check that the tube is secured with tape or special NG securement device.

_____ E. Instill 30 mL of normal saline in a large syringe into the NG tube.

_____ F. Reconnect the NG suction after instilling the normal saline.

_____ G. Place the client in a 30- to 60-degree sitting position.

Thinking Exercise 20B-6

A 73-year-old female client was treated for an intestinal obstruction in the local hospital 4 weeks ago. She has a history of chronic obstructive pulmonary disease (COPD) and hypertension. Today her primary health care provider visits her in the nursing home where she lives for follow-up. **Use an X to indicate which current client findings demonstrate that she is progressing or is not progressing.**

Client Finding	Is Progressing	Is Not Progressing
Abdomen soft, round, and nondistended		
No report of nausea or vomiting		
Respirations = 26 breaths/min and slightly labored		
Is alert and oriented × 3		
Heart rate = 88 beats/min		

Single-Episode Case (20B-7)

Thinking Exercise 20B-7

The nurse is planning care for an 81-year-old male client who yesterday had a colon resection for a tumor that was causing a partial intestinal obstruction. **Indicate the nursing action to take and parameter to monitor for each potential postoperative complication. Note that not all Actions and Parameters will be used.**

Action (A) to Take	A	Potential Condition	P	Parameter (P) to Monitor
A Encourage oral fluids as tolerated.		Deep vein thrombosis (DVT)		**1** Bowel sounds
B Keep the surgical dressing clean and dry.		Atelectasis		**2** Urinary output
C Maintain sequential compression stockings.		Wound infection		**3** Leg pain and swelling
D Perform active-assisted range-of-motion exercises.		Acute kidney injury (AKI)		**4** Blood pressure
E Introduce fluids to stimulate bowel function.		Paralytic ileus		**5** Breath sounds
F Apply supplemental oxygen.				**6** Abdominal incision
G Remind the client to use her incentive spirometer every 1–2 hours.				**7** Ability to perform ADLs

21 Metabolism

Exemplar 21A. Hypoglycemia (Medical-Surgical Nursing: Older Adult)

Unfolding Case (21A-1 Through 21A-6)

Thinking Exercise 21A-1

An 81-year-old female client was admitted 2 days ago with complications of a urinary tract infection. During the bedside shift report, the client is drowsy but participates by answering questions appropriately. The nurse's report includes the client's history of Addison disease, discontinuation of normal saline IV fluids this morning, and plans for the client's discharge with 14 more doses of trimethoprim/sulfamethoxazole. Forty-five minutes after the report, the nurse completes a shift change assessment and documents the following client findings. **Highlight the client findings below that require follow-up by the nurse.**

- Drowsy and confused to place and situation
- Reports blurry vision
- Respirations equal and unlabored
- Vital signs: heart rate = 88 beats/min; blood pressure = 98/44 mm Hg; respirations = 14 breaths/min; oxygen saturation = 96% (on room air [RA])
- Skin cool and diaphoretic
- Areas of skin hyperpigmentation present
- Reports join stiffness and pain rated 2/10

Thinking Exercise 21A-2

An 81-year-old female client was admitted 2 days ago with complications of a urinary tract infection. During the bedside shift report, the client is drowsy but participates by answering questions appropriately. The nurse's report includes the client's history of Addison disease, discontinuation of normal saline IV fluids this morning, and plans for the client's discharge with 14 more doses of trimethoprim/sulfamethoxazole. Forty-five minutes after the report, the nurse completes a shift change assessment. Abnormal client finding are mental confusion, blurred vision, and cool, diaphoretic skin. Vital signs are: heart rate, 88 beats/min; blood pressure, 98/44 mm Hg; respirations, 14 breaths/min; and oxygen saturation, 96% (on room air [RA]). **For each client assessment finding below, indicate if the finding is associated with infection, hypoglycemia, or stroke. Any finding may be associated with more than one disease process.**

Client Finding	Infection	Hypoglycemia	Stroke
Mental confusion			
Blurry vision			
Cool, diaphoretic skin			
Drowsiness			

Thinking Exercise 21A-3

An 81-year-old female client was admitted 2 days ago with complications of a urinary tract infection. During the bedside shift report the client is drowsy but participates by answering questions appropriately. The nurse's report includes the client's history of Addison disease, discontinuation of normal saline IV fluids this morning, and plans for the client's discharge with 14 more doses of trimethoprim/sulfamethoxazole. Forty-five minutes after the report, the nurse completes a shift change assessment. Abnormal client finding are mental confusion, blurred vision, and cool, diaphoretic skin. Vital signs are: heart rate, 88 beats/min; blood pressure, 98/44 mm Hg; respirations, 14 breaths/min; and oxygen saturation, 96% (on room air [RA]).

A capillary blood glucose test (finger stick blood glucose) reveals a blood glucose level of 56 mg/dL (3.108 mmol/L). The nurse assists the client in drinking a half-cup of fruit juice and reassesses the client 15 minutes later. Reassessed client findings are that she is alert and oriented, vision is clear, and skin is warm and dry. **Complete the following sentence by choosing the *most likely* options for the missing information from the lists of options provided.**

The client is ***most likely*** experiencing hypoglycemia not associated with diabetes mellitus. The ***priority*** for the nurse is to contact the primary health care provider and report the presence of ______1______, ______2______ when symptoms were present, and ______3______ of symptoms with the increase in blood glucose levels.

Options for 1	Options for 2	Options for 3
Addison disease	Blood pressure	Consistency
Family members	Blood glucose level	Deterioration
Hypoglycemia symptoms	Heart rate	Improvement
Urinary tract infection	Oxygen saturation	Inconsistency

Thinking Exercise 21A-4

An 81-year-old female client was admitted 2 days ago with complications of a urinary tract infection. During the bedside shift report the client is drowsy but participates by answering questions appropriately. The nurse's report includes the client's history of Addison disease, discontinuation of normal saline IV fluids this morning, and plans for the client's discharge with 14 more doses of trimethoprim/sulfamethoxazole. Forty-five minutes after the report, the nurse completes a shift change assessment. Abnormal client finding are mental confusion, blurred vision, and cool, diaphoretic skin. Vital signs are: heart rate, 88 beats/min; blood pressure, 98/44 mm Hg; respirations, 14 breaths/min; and oxygen saturation, 96% (on room air [RA]).

A capillary blood glucose test reveals a blood glucose level of 56 mg/dL (3.108 mmol/L). The nurse has the client drink a half-cup of fruit juice and reassesses the client 15 minutes later. The client is alert and oriented, vision is clear, and skin is warm and dry. After reporting results to the primary health care provider, the nurse prepares to implement care that prevents future hypoglycemia episodes and keeps the client safe if an episode occurs. **Use an X to show whether the nursing actions below are <u>Indicated</u> (appropriate or necessary), <u>Contraindicated</u> (could be harmful), or <u>Non-Essential</u> (makes no difference or is not necessary) for the client's care at this time.**

Nursing Action	Indicated	Contraindicated	Non-Essential
Administer 50 g of a carbohydrate.			
Consult a registered dietitian nutritionist.			
After administering a carbohydrate, recheck blood glucose in 15 minutes.			
Teach the client to check capillary blood glucose levels before each meal.			
Keep the client on bedrest until the episode resolves.			

Thinking Exercise 21A-5

An 81-year-old female client was admitted 2 days ago with complications of a urinary tract infection. The client has a history of Addison disease and was scheduled for discharge with 14 more doses of trimethoprim/sulfamethoxazole. The nurse recognized symptoms of hypoglycemia this morning, treated the client effectively, and received orders from the primary health care provider. Two hours later an assistive personnel (AP) finds the client unconscious and notifies the nurse. **Identify with an X the top three *priority* interventions that the nurse would implement at this time.**

Nursing Intervention	Top Three Priority Interventions
Help the client to drink a glass of milk and eat a sandwich.	
Draw blood to assess blood glucose and cortisol levels.	
Administer 50 mL of 50% glucose solution intravenously.	
Obtain capillary blood glucose level.	
Position the client in a side-lying position with the neck in a neutral position.	
Notify the primary health care provider.	

Thinking Exercise 21A-6

An 81-year-old female client was admitted 2 days ago with complications of a urinary tract infection. The client has a history of Addison disease and was scheduled for discharge with 14 more doses of trimethoprim/sulfamethoxazole. The nurse recognized symptoms of hypoglycemia this morning, treated the client effectively, and received orders from the primary health care provider. The client is at risk of future hypoglycemia episodes, and the nurse reinforces teaching to ensure client safety. Which client statements indicate correct understanding of teaching for nondiabetic hypoglycemia? **Select all that apply.**

_____ A. "Apples, spinach, and oat bran bread are complex carbohydrates."

_____ B. "I will carry hard candies in my purse in case my sugar drops while out of the house."

_____ C. "I will wear properly fitted shoes and inspect my feet daily."

_____ D. "Teaching my family signs of low blood sugar will help us identify them early."

_____ E. "My condition was caused by an allergy to trimethoprim/sulfamethoxazole."

_____ F. "I will meet with a physical therapist twice weekly to decrease my fall risk."

_____ G. "Drinking alcohol may increase my risk of hypoglycemia."

_____ H. "When my blood sugar levels begin to drop, I drink a glass of milk."

Single-Episode Case (21A-7)

Thinking Exercise 21A-7

A nurse assists with the care of a 72-year-old client who is receiving total parenteral nutrition (TPN) through a peripherally inserted central catheter (PICC). The nurse responds to the beeping IV pump and notices that the TPN bag is completely dry. Which actions will the nurse take? **Select all that apply.**

_____ A. Notify the registered nurse.

_____ B. Flush the PICC line with a heparin solution.

_____ C. Assess the client for signs of hypoglycemia.

_____ D. Contact the pharmacy for a new bag of TPN.

_____ E. Hang 0.9% normal saline solution.

_____ F. Obtain the client temperature.

_____ G. Check the client's blood glucose level.

_____ H. Administer a half-cup of orange juice.

Exemplar 21B. Cirrhosis (Medical-Surgical Nursing: Older Adult)

Unfolding Case (21B-1 Through 21B-6)

Thinking Exercise 21B-1

The daughter of a client who lives in an assisted living facility requests a nurse, stating, "My father is acting strange. He seems a bit confused." The nurse observes the client wandering around his living room without a shirt on. The client appears disoriented and agitated. He exhibits hand tremors and has a distended large abdomen with yellowish skin that is covered in spider angiomas. The nurse reviews the medical record. **Highlight information in the record that is relevant to the client's current assessment findings.**

Health History	**Nurses' Notes**	**Vital Signs**	**Laboratory Test Results**

Medical diagnoses

- Spinal disk herniation with diskectomy
- Osteoarthritis
- Hepatic cirrhosis

Social history

- Relationships—widowed, 1 adult child
- Work—retired military
- Alcohol use—prior use = 8–12 beers daily, quit 4 years ago
- Smoking—denies

Medications

- Lactulose 20 g orally three times a day
- Acetaminophen 500 mg orally twice a day
- Propranolol 40 mg orally daily

Thinking Exercise 21B-2

The daughter of a client who lives in an assisted living facility requests a nurse, stating, "My father is acting strange. He seems a bit confused." The nurse arrives and observes the client wandering around his living room without a shirt on. The client appears disoriented and agitated. He exhibits hand tremors and has a distended large abdomen with yellowish skin that is covered in spider angiomas. The client's medical record indicates that the client was previously diagnosed with hepatic cirrhosis secondary to alcohol use. He quit drinking 4 years ago. For which additional client findings will the nurse assess for to identify potential complications of cirrhosis? **Select all that apply.**

_____ A. Bradycardia

_____ B. Dizziness or light-headedness

_____ C. Black, tarry stools

_____ D. Hypertension

_____ E. Shortness of breath

_____ F. Oxygen saturation level <90%

_____ G. Increased weight

_____ H. Hemoptysis

Thinking Exercise 21B-3

The daughter of a client who lives in an assisted living facility requests a nurse, stating, "My father is acting strange. He seems a bit confused." The nurse arrives and observes the client wandering around his living room without a shirt on. The client appears disoriented and agitated. He exhibits hand tremors and has a distended large abdomen with yellowish skin that is covered in spider angiomas.

A focused assessment determines orientation to self only, symmetrical facial features, pupils equal and reactive to light, respirations unlabored, and lung fields clear throughout. The client's skin and sclera are jaundiced. Vital signs are: heart rate (HR), 115 beats/min; blood pressure (BP), 94/46 mm Hg; respirations, 18 breaths/min; oxygen saturation, 94% on room air [RA]; denies chest pain but reports light-headedness with position changes. Abdominal girth is 2 inches larger than the last measurement, and the client reports nocturnal dyspnea. The client's medical record indicates that the client was previously diagnosed with cirrhosis secondary to alcohol use. He quit drinking 4 years ago. **Complete the following sentences by choosing the *most likely* option for the missing information from the lists of options provided.**

The client is ***most likely*** experiencing complications of late-stage cirrhosis. The nurse is most concerned about the client's _______1_______ and the possibility of _______2_______.

Options for 1	Options for 2
Abdominal girth	Activity intolerance
Confusion	GI bleeding
Jaundice	Hepatic encephalopathy
Nocturnal dyspnea	Malnutrition
Vital signs	Respiratory failure

Thinking Exercise 21B-4

The daughter of a client who lives in an assisted living facility requests a nurse, stating, "My father is acting strange. He seems a bit confused." The nurse arrives and observes the client wandering around his living room without a shirt on. The client appears disoriented and agitated. He exhibits hand tremors and has a distended large abdomen with yellowish skin that is covered in spider angiomas.

A focused assessment determines orientation to self only, symmetrical facial features, pupils equal and reactive to light, respirations unlabored, and lung fields clear throughout. The client's skin and sclera are jaundiced. Vital signs are: heart rate (HR), 115 beats/min; blood pressure (BP), 94/46 mm Hg; respirations, 18 breaths/min; oxygen saturation, 94% on room air [RA]; denies chest pain but reports light-headedness with position changes. Abdominal girth is 2 inches larger than the last measurement, and the client reports nocturnal dyspnea. The client's medical record indicates that the client was previously diagnosed with cirrhosis secondary to alcohol use. He quit drinking 4 years ago. **Use an X to show whether each nursing action below is <u>Indicated</u> (appropriate or necessary), <u>Contraindicated</u> (could be harmful), or <u>Non-Essential</u> (makes no difference or is not necessary) for the client's care at this time.**

Nursing Action	Indicated	Contraindicated	Non-Essential
Administer the prescribed lactulose.			
Assist the client when ambulating to the bathroom.			
Provide the client with a meal high in calories, carbohydrates, and vitamins.			
Have the client lie in a supine position.			
Refer the client to Alcoholics Anonymous.			

Thinking Exercise 21B-5

Last evening a focused assessment of a client in an assisted living facility found that the client was oriented to self only and had symmetrical facial features, pupils were equal and reactive to light, respirations were unlabored, and lung fields were clear throughout. The client's skin and sclera were jaundiced. Vital signs were: heart rate (HR), 115 beats/min; blood pressure (BP), 94/46 mm Hg; respirations, 18 breaths/min; oxygen saturation, 94% on room air [RA]; denied chest pain but reported light-headedness with position changes. Abdominal girth was 2 inches larger than the previous measurement, and the client reported nocturnal dyspnea. The client's medical record indicated that the client had been previously diagnosed with cirrhosis secondary to alcohol use. He quit drinking 4 years ago.

This morning the client experiences an episode of syncope while on the toilet defecating a large amount of black tarry stool. After helping the client safely to a recliner, the nurse reassesses the client's vital signs: heart rate (HR), 122 beats/min; blood pressure (BP), 88/44 mm Hg; respirations, 23 breaths/min; oxygen saturation, 91% (on room air [RA]). The primary health care provider is notified, and transportation is arranged for the client to be admitted to the local hospital for possible GI bleeding. The client' daughter is concerned about her father's condition and has several questions. **Indicate which response by the nurse listed in the far-left column is appropriate for each question asked by the client's daughter. Note that all responses will not be used.**

Responses by the Nurse	Daughter's Questions	Appropriate Response by the Nurse for Each Question
1 "Liver disease can cause fluid to leak into the abdominal cavity, causing it to expand."	"What is causing my father to bleed?"	
2 "Bleeding episodes may be treated with a blood transfusion as well as medications to lower pressure in the liver and improve clotting."	"Why did he faint on the toilet?"	
3 "Alcoholic beverages are full of calories and sugar, which can lead to weight gain."	"Will he need blood transfusions?"	
4 "Poor nutrition leads to an ineffective clotting process called thrombocytopenia. This occurs in clients with cirrhosis and promotes GI bleeding."	"My father has always been skinny. Why has he gained so much weight in his belly?"	
5 "Blood transfusions may be needed if surgical interventions are not successful."		
6 "Syncope is a temporary loss of consciousness due to insufficient blood to the brain. The intestinal bleeding has caused a decrease in blood volume."		
7 "GI bleeding occurs when vessels in the esophagus, stomach, or intestines tear. Liver failure causes these vessels to bleed more easily."		

Thinking Exercise 21B-6

A client who lives in an assisted living facility was admitted to the hospital 5 days ago with GI bleeding secondary to esophageal varices. The client has a history of alcoholic cirrhosis, ascites, and hepatic encephalopathy. The client is ready for discharge, and his daughter is at the bedside to help transport him home. After reinforcing discharge instructions with the client and his daughter, the nurse evaluates their understanding. **For each statement by the client or his daughter, use an X to indicate if the teaching was Effective (helped the client understand discharge teaching), Ineffective (did not help the client understand discharge teaching), or Unrelated (not related to the discharge teaching).**

Statements by the Client or His Daughter	Effective	Ineffective	Unrelated
"We will consult the doctor before starting any herbal treatments."			
"I will eat a low-protein diet."			
"I will monitor my father for any signs of confusion or fatigue."			
"We will contact the community resources you provided."			
"I will sleep in my recliner because I'm most comfortable there."			

Single-Episode Case (21B-7)

Thinking Exercise 21B-7

A nurse cares for a 75-year-old client who has a history of choledocholithiasis and biliary obstruction. The client is diagnosed with biliary cirrhosis and is prescribed cholestyramine and furosemide to treat disease complications. Which actions will the nurse take to decrease the client's risk for further complications of cirrhosis and prescribed therapies? **Select all that apply.**

_____ A. Obtain daily weights.

_____ B. Monitor for heart palpitations.

_____ C. Strain all urine output.

_____ D. Request a nutritional consultation.

_____ E. Implement isolation precautions.

_____ F. Measure the abdominal girth daily.

_____ G. Monitor cholesterol levels.

_____ H. Apply a moisturizing lotion.

22 Coordinated Care
(Medical-Surgical Nursing: Older Adult)

Thinking Exercise 22-1

The nurse is planning assignments for residents in a long-term care (LTC) facility unit that has a census of 21 residents this morning. Nursing staff assigned to the unit include three assistive personnel (AP) who are all certified nursing assistants. One AP has been working on the unit for 4 years, but the other two AP have been working for less than 6 months. Each AP is assigned to care for seven residents. Which nursing activities or tasks would be appropriate for the nurse to assign to AP? **Select five activities or tasks that the nurse may assign to AP.**

_____ A. Maintaining accurate intake and output for a resident who has chronic kidney disease

_____ B. Feeding a resident with Parkinson disease who needs assistance with ADLs

_____ C. Providing an intermittent feeding to a resident through a gastrostomy tube

_____ D. Inserting a straight urinary catheterization for a resident who has a spinal cord tumor

_____ E. Taking vital signs for a resident who was admitted to the LTC unit this morning

_____ F. Performing passive range-of-motion exercises for a resident who is bedridden

_____ G. Providing oral suctioning of a resident with excessive oral secretions

_____ H. Applying a topical hydrocortisone cream for a resident who has a skin rash

Thinking Exercise 22-2

The nurse is reviewing the nurses' notes for a 77-year-old male client with a left cerebral stroke recently admitted to the rehabilitation unit.

Nurses' Notes	History and Physical	Imaging Test Reviews	Laboratory Test Results

11-6-21 1045 77-year-old male admitted with left cerebral stroke from Community Hospital this morning. Has right-sided weakness with arm worse than leg. Not able to grasp with right hand; family states he is right-handed. Unable to communicate his needs and cannot answer questions appropriately. Transfer form states that he has some difficulty swallowing and requires soft foods. Unable to perform ADLs at this time. -- *S. A. Thomas, LPN*

Based on the client's assessment findings in the Nurses' Notes, the nurse recognizes that the client will need referrals to members of the interdisciplinary team. To which health care team members will the nurse refer this client to meet his rehabilitation goals at this time? **Select all that apply.**

_____ A. Social worker

_____ B. Case manager

_____ C. Physical therapist

_____ D. Speech-language therapist

_____ E. Clergy

_____ F. Occupational therapist

_____ G. Orthotist

_____ H. Registered dietitian nutritionist

Thinking Exercise 22-3

The nurse is caring for a 70-year-old male client who is scheduled to have a below-the-knee amputation tomorrow morning. He has had diabetes type 2, peripheral vascular disease, peripheral neuropathy, and early stage chronic kidney disease. When the nurse interviews the client to determine if he is prepared for his elective surgery, he states that he is not sure about where his leg will be amputated and what kind of anesthesia he is going to have. **Choose the *most likely* options for the information missing from the statements below by selecting from the lists of options provided.**

As a result of the nurse's conversation with the client, the nurse recognizes that the ______1______ was/were not adequate. Therefore the nurse contacts the ______2______ to ensure that the client understands the surgical procedure prior to having his amputation.

Options for 1	Options for 2
Preoperative preparation	Nurse manager
Physician's orders	Social worker
Informed consent	Anesthesiologist
Preoperative checklist	Surgeon

Thinking Exercise 22-4

The oncoming day nurse receives the report from the night shift nurse in the long-term care facility. The night nurse includes information about these five residents who need follow-up on the day shift:

- **Resident 1:** An 88-year-old woman with Parkinson disease who fell last night in her room while walking to the bathroom with her walker; no apparent injury and vital signs stable
- **Resident 2:** An 81-year-old man who has had several embolic strokes; was admitted yesterday for rehabilitative therapies
- **Resident 3:** A 69-year-old woman who has moderate-stage Alzheimer disease; found wandering outside last evening; no apparent injury
- **Resident 4:** A 90-year-old woman with diabetes who has a new stage 2 sacral pressure injury and refuses to eat; history of depression
- **Resident 5:** A 70-year-old woman with a history of hypertension who was seen last evening in the emergency department for a transient ischemic attack (TIA); returned to the unit with no current neurologic symptoms

Choose the *most likely* options for the information missing from the statement below by selecting from the list of options provided.

The day nurse organizes and prioritizes care by planning to assess ______________ and ______________ ***first*** to ensure safety.

Options
Resident 1 Resident 2 Resident 3 Resident 4 Resident 5

Thinking Exercise 22-5

The oncoming day nurse receives the report from the night shift nurse in the long-term care facility. The night nurse includes information about these five residents who need follow-up on the day shift:

- **Resident 1:** An 88-year-old woman with Parkinson disease who fell last night in her room while walking to the bathroom with her walker; no apparent injury and vital signs stable
- **Resident 2:** An 81-year-old man who has had several embolic strokes; was admitted yesterday for rehabilitative therapies
- **Resident 3:** A 69-year-old woman who has moderate-stage Alzheimer disease; found wandering outside last evening; no apparent injury
- **Resident 4:** A 90-year-old woman with diabetes who has a new stage 2 sacral pressure injury and refuses to eat; history of depression
- **Resident 5:** A 70-year-old woman with a history of hypertension who was seen last evening in the emergency department for a transient ischemic attack (TIA); returned to the unit with no current neurologic symptoms

Indicate which nursing action listed in the far-left column is appropriate for each assigned resident's care at this time. Note that not all actions will be used.

Nursing Action	Resident	Appropriate Nursing Action for Resident
1 Perform a finger stick blood glucose (FSBG).	Resident 1	
2 Determine the client's mental status and compare with baseline.	Resident 2	
3 Assess the client's level of consciousness for change from baseline.	Resident 3	
4 Perform a skin assessment for integrity.	Resident 4	
5 Monitor the client's blood pressure every 4 hours today.	Resident 5	
6 Confirm that the client will begin physical and occupational therapy today.		
7 Perform a neurologic assessment for new symptoms.		

Thinking Exercise 22-6

A 72-year-old female client who had a total hip arthroplasty is scheduled to be discharged tomorrow from the acute care hospital to a rehabilitation unit. The nurse assists with discharge planning and client transfer. Indicate which client discharge activities are **appropriate** and which ones are **not appropriate** for the nurse to perform from the list provided below.

Potential Client Discharge Activity	Appropriate for the Nurse to Perform	Not Appropriate for the Nurse to Perform
Assist in completing the agency transfer form.		
Reinforce discharge health teaching.		
Obtain informed consent.		
Perform medication reconciliation.		
Check on client transportation to the rehabilitation facility.		
Notify the client's family or designee about the planned transfer.		

Thinking Exercise 22-7

A 78-year-old female client is admitted to the community hospital with probable lower GI bleeding from diverticulitis. The primary health care provider orders a transfusion of packed red blood cells, which the RN hung 30 minutes ago at 10 a.m. (1000). The RN asks the LPN to take vital signs frequently per agency protocol and monitor the client for any significant changes in her condition. When assessing the client at 11:30 a.m. (1130), the LPN notes a change in respiratory rate from 20 to 28 breaths/min, and her apical pulse rate has increased to 100 beats/min. Her other vital signs remain unchanged. The client states that she feels like she "can't get enough air" and her breathing is labored. What ***priority*** actions will the LPN implement at this time? **Select all that apply.**

_____ A. Position the client into a flat supine position.

_____ B. Prepare to administer oxygen via nasal cannula.

_____ C. Document the client's assessment findings.

_____ D. Report the client's findings to the RN immediately.

_____ E. Stop the blood transfusion immediately.

_____ F. Contact the respiratory therapist to provide a breathing treatment.

_____ G. Contact the laboratory to draw blood for hemoglobin and hematocrit.

Thinking Exercise 22-8

The nurse is in charge today for a 48-bed long-term care unit and reviews the nursing staff assigned to the unit:

- An LPN who graduated 3 months ago and has worked on the unit for a month as a medication nurse
- Six certified nursing assistants (CNAs); four CNAs are experienced, one CNA was hired yesterday, and one CNA has worked on the unit for less than a month

The nurse also reviews the 24-hour report and notes that two admissions are scheduled for today from the local hospital. One admission has been a resident for several years, but the other resident is new to the facility. Three of the current residents on the unit have gastrostomy tubes, one resident is on long-term oxygen for chronic obstructive pulmonary disease (COPD), and one resident has an old tracheostomy that needs occasional suctioning. As a result of this review, the nurse assigns care to the nursing staff. Which nursing care activities would the charge nurse ***most likely*** assign to the new LPN graduate today? **Select all that apply.**

_____ A. Administering medications for all residents on the unit

_____ B. Helping to supervise resident care provided by the CNA staff

_____ C. Helping with resident showers

_____ D. Performing head-to-toe assessments for some of the residents

_____ E. Admitting the two new residents

_____ F. Monitoring the gastrostomy continuous tube feedings

_____ G. Suctioning the resident's tracheostomy as needed

_____ H. Maintaining oxygen therapy for the resident who has COPD

Pharmacology (Medical-Surgical Nursing: Older Adult)

23

Thinking Exercise 23-1

The nurse reviews the postoperative medications ordered for a 75-year-old female client admitted to the orthopedic unit from the postanesthesia care unit (PACU) with an open reduction, internal fixation (ORIF) of the right ankle.

Current Medications	**History and Physical**	**Imaging Test Reviews**	**Laboratory Test Results**

Amlodipine 10 mg orally once daily

Simvastatin 20 mg orally once daily

Losartan 50 mg orally once daily

Alendronate 35 mg orally once weekly (Monday)

Lorazepam 1 mg orally twice daily

Hydrocodone/acetaminophen (5/25) 2 tablets every 4 hours as needed for postoperative pain

Zolpidem 5 mg orally at bedtime daily

The nurse documents the client's vital signs on admission to the orthopedic unit as follows:

- Temperature = 98°F (36.7°C)
- Heart rate = 64 beats/min
- Respirations = 16 breaths/min
- Blood pressure = 98/52 mm Hg
- Oxygen saturation = 95% (on room air [RA])

Which of the client's medications would the nurse hold at this time based on the client's current vital signs? **Select two medications that the nurse would hold.**

_____ A. Amlodipine

_____ B. Simvastatin

_____ C. Losartan

_____ D. Alendronate

_____ E. Lorazepam

_____ F. Hydrocodone/acetaminophen (5/25)

_____ G. Zolpidem

Thinking Exercise 23-2

An 83-year-old female client is discharged to home after a 5-day hospital stay for atrial fibrillation and unstable angina. The home care nurse reviews her postdischarge medications, which include:

- Nitroglycerin 0.4 mg sublingually as needed × 3
- Clopidogrel 75 mg orally once daily
- Levothyroxine 150 mcg orally before breakfast
- Venlafaxine ER 75 mg orally once daily
- Hydrochlorothiazide (HCTZ) 12.5 mg once daily

Choose the *most likely* options for the information missing from the statement below by selecting from the list of options provided.

The nurse recognizes ***priority*** health teaching needs, including reinforcing the need for the client to have laboratory testing to monitor ____________________ levels due to being on levothyroxine and ____________________ levels due to being on HCTZ.

Options
Hematocrit
Electrolyte
Platelets
Prothrombin
Thyroid-stimulating hormone
Troponin

Thinking Exercise 23-3

A 78-year-old female client with a history of gastroesophageal reflux disease (GERD) and penicillin allergy is diagnosed with *Helicobacter pylori* infection. Her primary health care provider prescribes clarithromycin-based triple therapy for 14 days. Her new drugs include:

- Clarithromycin 500 mg orally twice daily
- Metronidazole 500 mg orally twice daily
- Pantoprazole 40 mg orally once daily

What health teaching will the nurse reinforce for the client related to her drug therapy? **Select all that apply.**

_____ A. "Take all of the drugs that are prescribed for the full 14 days."

_____ B. "Report new-onset prolonged diarrhea to your primary health care provider."

_____ C. "Report any feeling of fluttering or palpitations while on these drugs."

_____ D. "Take all of these drugs on an empty stomach before breakfast."

_____ E. "Be sure to get a bone scan before and after the drug therapy."

_____ F. "Have the magnesium level in your blood checked before and after taking these drugs."

_____ G. "Be aware that pantoprazole may make you more likely to develop pneumonia."

_____ H. "Avoid alcohol while you are taking these drugs to prevent interaction."

Thinking Exercise 23-4

A 65-year-old female client was diagnosed with probable rheumatoid arthritis. After a thorough evaluation by the primary health care provider, the client was placed on hydroxychloroquine 200 mg orally once a day, methotrexate (MTX) 10 mg orally once a week, and folic acid 400 mcg orally once a day. Which health teaching related to the drug therapy will the nurse reinforce for the client at this time? **Select all that apply.**

_____ A. "Take your new medications with food or milk."

_____ B. "Be sure to avoid large crowds in public places."

_____ C. "Be sure to have frequent eye examinations to detect any changes."

_____ D. "Avoid children and adults who have infections."

_____ E. "Follow up with all lab testing to detect any changes from baseline."

_____ F. "Take MTX the same day each week to ensure the needed serum drug level."

_____ G. "Expect to see improvement from these drugs in 3 to 6 weeks."

_____ H. "When you begin feeling better, you can discontinue the medications."

Thinking Exercise 23-5

The nurse is caring for a 78-year-old female client who resides in an assisted-living facility. Five days ago the client reported having a productive cough and "night sweats." She also experienced weakness and chest discomfort. Diagnostic testing confirmed bacterial pneumonia for which she was prescribed the following medications:

- Azithromycin 500 mg orally once daily on day 1, then 250 mg orally once daily on days 2 to 5
- Guaifenesin 200 mg orally every 4 hours
- Acetaminophen 650 mg orally every 6 hours PRN for chest discomfort or temperature higher than 100.4°F (38°C)

Today the nurse is collecting client data to evaluate how well she recovered from pneumonia. **For each client finding, use an X to indicate if the interventions were Effective (helped to meet expected outcomes), Ineffective (did not help to meet expected outcomes), or Unrelated (not related to the expected outcomes).**

Client Finding	Effective	Ineffective	Unrelated
States she is feeling stronger today			
Temperature = 97.2°F (36.2°C)			
States that she has no more "night sweats"			
Has a productive cough			
Reports frequent indigestion after meals			
Reports having no chest discomfort			

Thinking Exercise 23-6

An 80-year-old male client returned from the acute care hospital to the long-term care setting after having a bowel resection for colorectal cancer. His antidiabetic medications were changed postoperatively owing to poor glucose control. The new orders for insulin include:

- NPH insulin 22 units subcutaneously before breakfast every day
- NPH insulin 8 units subcutaneously at bedtime every day
- Point-of-care blood sugars (finger stick blood glucose [FSBG]) 4 times a day before meals and at bedtime
- Regular insulin (aspart) per sliding scale based on FSBG before meals and at bedtime:

<70 mg/dL	Follow agency HYPOglycemia guidelines
70–139 mg/dL	0 units
140–180 mg/dL	2 units
181–240 mg/dL	3 units
241–300 mg/dL	4 units
301–350 mg/dL	6 units
351– 400 mg/dL	8 units
More than 400 mg/dL	10 units and notify primary health care provider

The client's FSBG this morning before breakfast is 198 mg/dL. **Choose the *most likely* options for the information missing from the statements below by selecting from the lists of options provided.**

Based on the client's morning FSBG value, the nurse would give _____1_____ units of NPH insulin and _____1_____ units of regular insulin at 7:30 a.m. (0730). Because of the peak action of NPH insulin, the nurse would monitor the client for hypoglycemia beginning at _____2_____.

Options for 1	Options for 2
3	10:00 a.m. (1000)
6	11:30 a.m. (1130)
8	12:30 p.m. (1230)
10	2:00 p.m. (1400)
22	3:30 p.m. (1530)

Thinking Exercise 23-7

An 82-year-old male client residing in a long-term care facility has a history of Parkinson disease and heart disease. He also has a long history of low back pain, for which he has had four back operations. The nurse reviews the client's medication list. **Match each of the client's drugs (Column A) with its correct drug class (Column C) from the choices provided in Column B.**

A. Client's Drugs	B. Drug Class	C. Correct Drug for Drug Class
1 Fluoxetine	Antiepileptic drug	
2 Gabapentin	Cardiac glycoside	
3 Baclofen	Dopaminergic drug	
4 Digoxin	Nonsteroidal anti-inflammatory drug	
5 Carbidopa/levodopa	Antispasmodic drug	
6 Celecoxib	Antidepressant drug	

Answer Key

CHAPTER 3 Perfusion

Answers With Rationales for Thinking Exercises

Exemplar 3A. Bradycardia/Pacemaker (Medical-Surgical Nursing: Older Adult)

Thinking Exercise 3A-1

Answers

History and Physical	**Nurses' Notes**	**Vital Signs**	**Laboratory Results**

82-year-old female residing in an independent living senior center

Heart rate (HR), 55 beats/min

Medications:

- Acetaminophen 650 mg orally every 4–6 hours PRN
- Aspirin (ASA) 325 mg orally daily
- Atenolol 50 mg orally daily
- Calcium carbonate 1000 mg chewable tabs every 4–6 hours PRN
- Clopidogrel 75 mg orally daily
- Nifedipine ER 30 mg orally daily

Recent physical assessment (2 weeks ago):

- Alert and oriented × 3
- Lung fields clear throughout
- Denies chest pain or shortness of breath
- Bowel sounds present × 4
- Reports constipation, encouraged to drink more fluids
- Denies incontinence or difficulty voiding
- Right forearm skin tear, 2 mm × 4 mm, scant serous drainage

Rationales

The client's heart rate is 55 beats/min. Her heart rate is less than 60 beats/min, indicating bradycardia. Some of the client's current medications can cause bradycardia and are therefore relevant to the client's condition. Atenolol belongs to a class of drugs known as beta-adrenergic blockers and works on the heart and blood vessels to lower the heart rate, lower the blood pressure, and decrease the work of the heart. Nifedipine belongs to a class of drugs known as calcium channel blockers and lowers the blood pressure by relaxing blood vessels so that the heart does not have to pump as hard. Both medications can cause bradycardia. Acetaminophen, aspirin, and calcium carbonate tabs have no impact on the client's heart rate or current condition. The client lost consciousness while on the toilet. The client's report of constipation as well as her age are relevant. Individuals who are constipated may strain to defecate, causing an increase in intra-abdominal pressure called vasovagal reflex or the Valsalva maneuver. Bradycardia and hypotension occur as a result of the vasovagal reflex and result in light-headedness, nausea, sweating, and syncope (fainting). The vasovagal reflex is especially problematic in older adults, who frequently have impaired circulation. The client's living situation and skin tears are not relevant to the client's bradycardia and episode of syncope. The client's other assessment findings are all normal.

CJ Cognitive Skill

Recognize Cues

Reference

Linton & Matteson, 2020, pp. 200, 683

Thinking Exercise 3A-2

Answers

B, D, E, F

Rationales

The nurse would ask questions related to the client's medications and symptoms prior to the episode of syncope. Assessing the client for symptoms of light-headedness or dizziness when going from a lying or sitting position to a standing position will determine if the client is at risk for orthostatic hypotension (Choice B). This condition is a common side effect of the antihypertensive medications the client is taking and increases the client's risk for syncope. Identifying the client's heart rate prior to taking medications would provide a baseline rate for the nurse to compare with the client's current heart rate (Choice D). Straining to defecate and symptoms of nausea or sweating will provide the nurse with client findings that support a vasovagal reflex as a potential cause of the syncope episode (Choices E and F). The other questions do not provide the nurse with information to determine the significance of the client's health history.

CJ Cognitive Skill

Analyze Cues

Reference

Linton & Matteson, 2020, pp. 200, 683, 688

Thinking Exercise 3A-3

Answers

This client is ***most likely*** experiencing <u>bradycardia</u>, which refers to a heart rate slower than 60 beats/min. The ***most likely*** explanation for this client's slow heart rate is <u>antihypertensive drugs</u>. If the heart rate is too slow, the brain and other organs may not get enough oxygen, causing symptoms of dizziness and fainting. Additional symptoms may include <u>fatigue</u>, <u>chest pain</u>, and <u>confusion</u>.

Rationales

The normal heart rate for an adult is 60 to 100 beats/min. Bradycardia refers to a slow heart rate that is less than 60 beats/min; tachycardia refers to a fast heart rate that is greater than 100 beats/min. Bradycardia symptoms are confusion, fatigue, dizziness, syncope, and chest pain. Heart rates vary and are influenced by several factors including age, body build and size, blood pressure, drugs, emotions, blood loss, exercise, body temperature, and pain. The client presents with several factors related to bradycardia: age (82 years old) and drugs (atenolol and nifedipine). Because bradycardia is an acute symptomatic change, the most likely explanation for the slow heart rate is the prescribed drug therapy.

CJ Cognitive Skill

Prioritize Hypotheses

Reference

Williams, 2018, pp. 358–360

Thinking Exercise 3A-4

Answers

Nursing Action	Indicated	Contraindicated
Administer oxygen via nasal cannula.		X
Teach the client to rise slowly from lying or sitting positions.	X	
Hold the client's atenolol dose.		X
Encourage the client to exercise daily.	X	
Assess orthostatic vital signs.	X	
Administer a laxative each morning.		X

Rationales

The client's episode of syncope is most likely related to a vasovagal reflex secondary to constipation and the client's antihypertensive medications. Assessing orthostatic vital signs and teaching the client to rise slowly from lying and sitting positions are indicated to evaluate and manage side effects of antihypertensive medications. Management of constipation will minimize future vasovagal episodes. Interventions for constipation include eating high-fiber foods, drinking more fluids, and exercising daily. Laxatives can be used safely for occasional constipation but should not be administered daily as they can interfere with normal elimination. Beta-blocking drugs (atenolol) should not be held or stopped abruptly. The client's oxygen saturation is 96% on room air (RA). Although it would likely not cause the client any harm, there is no indication that supplemental oxygen via nasal cannula is needed.

CJ Cognitive Skill

Generate Solutions

Reference

Linton & Matteson, 2020, pp. 688, 748–749

Thinking Exercise 3A-5

Answers

B, C, E, G, H

Rationales

The hand-off report focuses on changes in the client's status, actions taken, and treatments or tests scheduled. The client is experiencing a third-degree heart block. The registered nurse's initial responsibility is to determine if the client is tolerating this cardiac rhythm (asymptomatic) or not tolerating the rhythm (symptomatic). Reporting heart rate, blood pressure, respiratory rate, and oxygen saturation with the percentage of any supplemental oxygen being provided will assist the registered nurse in evaluating the client's current status (Choice C). The client's current level of consciousness and orientation status are also important client findings related to cardiac output and perfusion (Choice E). The registered nurse also needs to know what interventions have been implemented because of the client's change in status. Any PRN medications that were administered would be reported (Choice B). Atropine may be administered for third-degree heart block, especially if a client is symptomatic. A temporary pacemaker (transcutaneous, epicardial, or transvenous) may also be used while awaiting the insertion of a permanent pacemaker. If a temporary pacemaker is in use, the nurse would report the pacer settings to the registered nurse (Choice H). Although scheduled medications are not usually reported during nursing care hand-offs, the client may be scheduled for an invasive pacemaker procedure. The nurse's decision to call attention to the client's clopidogrel and heparin doses allows the registered nurse to more effectively evaluate the client's risk (Choice G). Activity level, immunizations, and family history do not provide any immediate and essential information for the registered nurse.

CJ Cognitive Skill

Take Action

Reference

Linton & Matteson, 2020, pp. 609–614, 628–632

Thinking Exercise 3A-6

Answers

Client Finding	Is Progressing	Is Not Progressing
An ECG tracing presents pacemaker spikes.	X	
The client reports dyspnea and chest pain during physical therapy.		X
A medical identification card describing the pacemaker is in the client's wallet.	X	
The client reports light-headedness when rising from a chair.		X
Heart rate is 72 beats/min during occupational therapy.	X	
The client takes her pulse rate for a full minute each morning.	X	

Rationales

An ECG is used to monitor the proper pacemaker functioning. A pacemaker "spike" on the ECG tracing demonstrates the impulse generated by the pacemaker. Although the nurse is not expected to evaluate the pacemaker's settings, identifying spikes on the ECG strip is an indication that the pacemaker is functioning. The client's heart rate should be at the set pacemaker rate or higher than the set pacemaker rate. A heart rate below the pacemaker's set rate would indicate that the pacemaker is not functioning properly. Clients with permanent pacemakers are taught how to count the pulse for 1 full minute and keep a record to share with the primary health care provider. They are also instructed to carry an identification card describing the type of pacemaker implanted. The client's ability to take his pulse and the identification card in his wallet are both positive findings. Dyspnea, light-headedness, and chest pain are symptoms of decreased cardiac output. These symptoms indicate the client is not progressing, and they should be communicated to the primary health care provider.

CJ Cognitive Skill

Evaluate Outcomes

Reference

Linton & Matteson, 2020, pp. 631–632

Thinking Exercise 3A-7

Answers

A, B, C

Rationales

The client is experiencing orthostatic or postural hypotension—a sudden drop in systolic blood pressure when going from a lying or sitting position to a standing position. The client reports light-headedness when standing because the body is not compensating for the change in position, resulting in an inadequate amount of oxygenated blood being supplied to the brain. The nurse would position the client back in the chair or bed and stay with the client until the light-headedness subsides (Choice A). The client would be expected to get out of bed for meals, for hygiene activities, and to use the bathroom. Therefore the client should be reminded to call for assistance (Choice B), and a bedpan would not be used. Clients with orthostatic vital signs, especially older adults, are often dehydrated. The nurse would assess for other symptoms of dehydration before recommending the administration of additional fluids because of the client's history of cardiac disease (Choice C). There is no indication that the client needs a permanent pacemaker or that the client has a urinary tract infection. Orthostatic hypotension is a common side effect of beta blockers; the client is not having adverse or toxic effects from the digoxin dose.

CJ Cognitive Skill

Take Action

Reference

Linton & Matteson, 2020, pp. 532–533, 688

Exemplar 3B. Heart Failure (Medical-Surgical Nursing: Older Adult)

Thinking Exercise 3B-1

Answers

- Oriented to person, place, and time
- Irregular heart rhythm
- Dyspnea when resting
- Auscultated crackles in basal lung fields
- Hemoglobin = 15 g/dL (150 g/L)
- Hematocrit = 50%
- Prothrombin time = 18 seconds
- International normalized ratio (INR) = 2.5

Rationales

The client has a history of heart failure and is experiencing symptoms associated with left-sided heart failure. Clients with heart failure frequently experience dyspnea and may sometimes experience chest pain with activity and exertion. Both shortness of breath and chest pain should resolve with rest. Experiencing dyspnea or angina while at rest is a sign of worsening heart failure. Auscultated crackles in basal lung fields is a sign that fluid has leaked from pulmonary capillaries into the interstitial space and alveoli, causing beginning pulmonary edema. If untreated, the client's exchange of oxygen and carbon dioxide will be further impaired and the body will be unable to supply oxygenated blood to vital organs. The nurse would follow up on these client findings. The client's irregular heart rate is expected for a diagnosis of atrial fibrillation. The client's laboratory results demonstrate therapeutic values for warfarin and no signs of bleeding. Laboratory results should be monitored on a regular schedule. There is no need for the nurse to follow up on these results at this time.

CJ Cognitive Skill

Recognize Cues

Reference

Linton & Matteson, 2020, pp. 646–648

Thinking Exercise 3B-2

Answers

Client Finding	Heart Failure	Atrial Fibrillation	Hyperlipidemia
Ejection fraction <45%	X	X	
Dyspnea	X	X	
Palpitations		X	
Activity intolerance	X	X	
Low-density lipoprotein = 160 mg/dL (4.14 mmol/L)			X

Rationales

Atrial fibrillation is an irregular cardiac rhythm that results in the "quivering" of the heart muscle. Manifestations of atrial fibrillation are palpitations, angina, and decreased cardiac output. Heart failure (the inability of the heart to meet the metabolic needs of the body) also causes decreased cardiac output (the amount of blood ejected from the heart each minute). Ejection fraction (EF) is a measurement of how much blood the left ventricle pumps out with each contraction. The normal EF is 55% to 70%. The EF would be lower than normal for both heart failure and atrial fibrillation. When the cardiac output and the EF are low, blood not being pumped out of the heart backs up into the pulmonary vasculature, causing dyspnea. Activity intolerance is also associated with heart failure and atrial fibrillation due to impaired tissue perfusion and oxygenation. Lipid panels to evaluate hyperlipidemia include cholesterol, triglycerides, and lipoproteins (high-density lipoproteins and low-density lipoproteins). Depending on the laboratory range for normal low-density lipoprotein (LDL) levels, her LDLs should be less than 130 mg/dL (3.36 mmol/L). An LDL level of 160 mg/dL (4.14 mmol/L) is considered hyperlipidemia.

CJ Cognitive Skill

Analyze Cues

Reference

Linton & Matteson, 2020, pp. 612, 619–620, 646–649

Thinking Exercise 3B-3

Answers

The client is ***most likely*** experiencing <u>left ventricular dysfunction</u>. Based on the client findings, he has hypoxemia, activity intolerance, and fluid overload. These symptoms are complications of <u>pulmonary congestion</u> and decreased <u>cardiac output</u>.

Rationales

The most likely explanation for the client's symptoms is left ventricular dysfunction or left-sided heart failure. The client has a history of atrial fibrillation and hyperlipidemia, which are risk factors for heart failure. The client is also experiencing hypoxemia, activity intolerance, and fluid overload, all complications associated with heart failure. Hypoxemia is a complication of pulmonary congestion and decreased cardiac output. Activity intolerance is a result of neuromuscular fatigue due to impaired tissue perfusion and oxygenation. Fluid overload occurs when the kidneys' compensation mechanism retains too much fluid for the already damaged heart.

CJ Cognitive Skill

Prioritize Hypotheses

Reference

Linton & Matteson, 2020, pp. 646–651

Thinking Exercise 3B-4

Answers

Expected Outcome	Client Problem	Appropriate Outcome for Each Client Problem
1 The client performs ADLs without fatigue.	Hypoxemia	**3** Respiratory rate and oxygen saturation are within normal limits.
2 Intake and output are equal, and no peripheral edema is present.	Activity intolerance	**1** Performs ADLs without fatigue.
3 Respiratory rate and oxygen saturation are within normal limits.	Increased fluid volume	**2** Intake and output are equal, and no peripheral edema is present.
4 The client denies dizziness, chest pain, and dyspnea.		
5 The client participates in physical therapy three times daily.		

Rationales

Hypoxemia is a complication of inadequate oxygen diffusion secondary to pulmonary congestion and impaired cardiac output related to ventricular dysfunction. A respiratory rate and oxygen saturation within normal limits would demonstrate that the client is receiving adequate oxygen (Outcome 3). Activity intolerance is a result of fatigue, a common manifestation of heart failure. The desired outcome is for the client to perform ADLs without fatigue, dyspnea, and chest pain (Outcome 1). Fluid retention occurs as the kidneys attempt to compensate for decreased cardiac output and becomes a fluid volume complication as the workload of the heart increases. The increased fluid volume increases pulmonary and central venous pressures, resulting in pulmonary congestion, peripheral edema, and abdominal engorgement. The desired outcome is an equal intake and output fluid balance and no peripheral edema (Outcome 2).

CJ Cognitive Skill

Generate Solutions

Reference

Linton & Matteson, 2020, pp. 646–651

Thinking Exercise 3B-5

Answers

A, B, E, F, G

Rationales

The client is experiencing hypoxemia; therefore the nurse would administer supplemental oxygen to increase the amount of oxygenated blood available to organs throughout the body. Oxygen should be administered via mask if tolerated and as needed to keep oxygen saturation levels greater than 90% or other goal specified by the primary health care provider (Choice A). The nurse would schedule frequent rest periods and pace activities to help the client conserve energy (Choice B). Anxiety commonly occurs in clients experiencing shortness of breath secondary to heart failure. Acknowledging the client's anxiety and explaining nursing actions in a calm manner may reduce the client's anxiety (Choice E). Nausea, anorexia, and visual disturbances are signs of digoxin toxicity and would be reported to the primary care provider (Choice F). Changes in weight over a short period of time indicate changes in the body's fluid volume. Obtaining and monitoring daily weights would assist the nurse in identifying early signs of fluid overload (Choice G). The client is not experiencing an infectious disease and does not need to be placed in an isolation room. Repositioning the client every 2 hours while in bed prevents skin breakdown but does not address the client's oxygen needs nor the client's fatigue with ADLs. In addition, there is no indication that he cannot turn and reposition himself.

CJ Cognitive Skill

Take Action

Reference

Linton & Matteson, 2020, pp. 646–651

Thinking Exercise 3B-6

Answers

Client Finding	Effective	Ineffective	Unrelated
Chooses low-sodium food options for each meal	X		
Denies dyspnea or chest pain when ambulating with physical therapy	X		
Had a bowel movement this morning			X
Gained 3 lb (1.4 kg) of weight since yesterday		X	
Respirations =15 breaths/min; oxygen saturation = 95% (on room air [RA])	X		

Rationales

Decreasing salt intake would reduce fluid retention by the kidneys; therefore clients with heart failure are taught to avoid salty foods and table salt and how to read food labels for sodium content. That the client is choosing low-sodium food options indicates that he understood nutritional teaching related to heart failure. Ambulating without experiencing dyspnea or chest pain indicates that the client is tolerating ADLs and that interventions were effective. The client's respiratory rate and oxygen saturation are also within normal limits, which is a desired outcome for heart failure interventions. One kilogram of weight is equal to almost 1 liter of fluid. This significant increase in fluid retention in 24 hours is a sign of recurrent heart failure and indicates interventions were not effective. The client's bowel patterns are unrelated to complications of heart failure.

CJ Cognitive Skill

Evaluate Outcomes

Reference

Linton & Matteson, 2020, pp. 646–651

Thinking Exercise 3B-7

Answers

Health Teaching	Prescribed Medications	Appropriate Teaching for Each Prescribed Medication
1 "Eat foods high in potassium including bananas and orange juice."	Captopril	**4** "Contact your primary health care provider if you experience a dry cough or dizziness."
2 "Perform good oral hygiene to prevent dry mouth."	Digoxin	**3** "Take your radial pulse for 1 minute at the same time each day."
3 "Take your radial pulse for 1 minute at the same time each day."	Furosemide	**1** "Eat foods high in potassium including bananas and orange juice."
4 "Contact your primary health care provider if you experience a dry cough or dizziness."	Atenolol	**6** "Do not abruptly discontinue this medication."
5 "Keep the drug in a dark container to avoid air and light exposure."		
6 "Do not abruptly discontinue this medication."		

Rationales

Captopril, an angiotensin-converting enzyme (ACE) inhibitor, reduces aldosterone secretion and prevents the formation of angiotensin II. This decreases fluid volume by preventing the kidneys from retaining fluid. A dry cough is the most common side effect, but the nurse would also want to educate the client to rise slowly and report dizziness associated with hypotension and dehydration (Teaching 4). Digoxin belongs to a class of drugs known as cardiac glycosides and is used to increase cardiac output in clients who have heart failure and atrial fibrillation. Digoxin lowers the heart rate; therefore the nurse would assess the client's apical heart rate for 1 minute prior to administering the medication and reinforce teaching for the client to take his radial pulse rate for 1 minute each day (Teaching 3). Furosemide is a loop diuretic that promotes the excretion of fluid volume by blocking the absorption of salt in the kidneys. As fluids are excreted, potassium is also excreted. Therefore the client would be encouraged to eat foods high in potassium (Teaching 1). Atenolol belongs to a class of drugs known as beta blockers, and works on the heart and blood vessels to lower the heart rate, lower the blood pressure, and decrease the work of the heart. Beta-adrenergic blockers should not be stopped abruptly because that may cause a rebound hypertension effect (Teaching 6). Clients taking $alpha_2$ antagonist drugs should be encouraged to perform good oral hygiene. Clients taking nitroglycerin tablets would be taught to keep the drug in a dark container to avoid air and light exposure.

CJ Cognitive Skill

Take Action

Reference

Linton & Matteson, 2020, pp. 620–627, 683–684

Thinking Exercise 3B-8

Answers

Medication	Dose, Frequency, Route	Drug Class	Indication
Aspirin	325 mg once a day orally	Salicylate	**Decreases platelet aggregation**
Atorvastatin	20 mg once a day orally	HMg-CoA reductase inhibitor	**Decreases cholesterol**
Digoxin	0.125 mg once a day orally	**Cardiac glycoside**	Increases myocardial contractile force and cardiac output
Warfarin	2.5 mg once a day orally	**Anticoagulant**	Reduces risk of embolic stroke

Rationales

Aspirin has many properties, but the most common use is to reduce the ability of platelets to aggregate, or stick together. This assists in the prevention of a thrombus or blood clot. Atorvastatin belongs to a class of drugs known as lipid-lowering drugs. This medication, also known as a "statin," reduces cholesterol and treats hyperlipidemia by decreasing the synthesis of LDL and increasing its excretion. Digoxin belongs to a class of drugs known as cardiac glycosides and is used to increase cardiac output in clients who have heart failure and atrial fibrillation. Digoxin has a positive inotropic effect—it causes an increase in the strength or force of myocardial contractions. Warfarin is an anticoagulant agent and interferes with blood clotting. The medication is prescribed to prevent blood clots associated with several disorders. In this client it is used to prevent clots in the left ventricle due to pooling or stasis blood secondary to atrial fibrillation that could cause an embolic stroke.

CJ Cognitive Skill

Analyze Cues

Reference

Linton & Matteson, 2020, pp. 620–629

Thinking Exercise 3B-9

Answers

A, B, D, F

Rationales

Decreasing salt intake will reduce fluid retention by the kidneys. Clients with heart failure are taught to avoid salty foods and table salt and how to read food labels for sodium content (Choice A). Changes in weight over a short period of time indicate changes in the body's fluid volume. Clients who have heart failure are taught to weigh themselves every day to monitor for fluid changes, especially fluid retention (Choice B). Clients are taught to contact the primary health care provider immediately if they experience a rapid weight gain of 3 pounds in 1 week or 1 to 2 pounds in 1 day, as this is a sign of recurrent heart failure (Choice D). Clients with heart failure frequently experience dyspnea and may sometimes experience chest pain with activity and exertion. Both shortness of breath and chest pain should resolve with rest. Experiencing dyspnea or angina while at rest is a sign of heart failure exacerbation. The client must be taught to contact the primary health care provider if this occurs (Choice F). Although the client may experience shortness of breath with activity, the client is encouraged to maintain independence with ADLs. The client's wife should not perform all activities for her husband. Clients prescribed beta blockers including metoprolol are taught to monitor vital signs before and sometimes after administration of the medication. Clients who stop taking a beta blocker abruptly are at risk for rebound hypertension and tachycardia. Therefore clients are taught to continue taking the medication as ordered and contact the primary health care provider when vital signs are abnormal or the client feels dizzy, light-headed, or confused. Clients are not encouraged to drink alcohol, and there is no research that indicates red wine will prevent further cardiac issues.

CJ Cognitive Skill

Evaluate Outcomes

Reference

Linton & Matteson, 2020, pp. 646–651

CHAPTER 4 **Clotting: Deep Vein Thrombosis** *(Medical-Surgical Nursing: Middle-Age Adult)*

Answers With Rationales for Thinking Exercises

Thinking Exercise 4-1

Answers

A and D

Rationales

The nurse would follow up with the client's report of pain (Choice A). Although the client indicates that the pain is "tolerable," the nurse will want to perform a more detailed assessment to determine pain location, quality, severity, timing, radiation, precipitating events, and relieving factors. The nurse would also want to perform a follow-up assessment on the client's lower extremities based on the client's report that one leg is swollen (Choice D). Unilateral edema has several causes, and the nurse must perform a focused assessment to evaluate potential conditions. None of the other client comments require a follow-up assessment. The nurse may want to respond to the other comments and reinforce teaching, but a focused assessment is not required.

CJ Cognitive Skill

Recognize Cues

Reference

Williams, 2018, pp. 385–387, 442, 594–599

Thinking Exercise 4-2

Answers

Client Finding	Arterial Thrombus	DVT
Capillary refill = more than 3 seconds	X	
Dull ache or heaviness in the left calf		X
Peripheral pulses are difficult to palpate because of pitting edema		X
Left extremity is pale when elevated on pillows	X	
Decreased mobility	X	X

Rationales

An arterial thrombus (clot) is formed from plaque in an artery that becomes lodged in a vessel and blocks blood flow distal to the occlusion. This blockage occurs in an artery, and therefore blood flow to body tissues is impaired. Symptoms include acute pain; loss of sensory and motor function; absent distal pulse; capillary refill of more than 3 seconds; and pallor, mottling, and cool skin, especially when the extremity is elevated. DVT describes a clot becoming lodged in a deep vein. Venous clots decrease blood flow from the extremities back to the heart. Symptoms of DVT include pain described as a dull ache or heaviness; unilateral pitting edema, which may inhibit the nurse from palpating a pulse; and decreased mobility secondary to pain and edema.

CJ Cognitive Skill

Analyze Cues

Reference

Linton & Matteson, 2020, pp. 661–671

Thinking Exercise 4-3

Answers

The client is ***most likely*** experiencing <u>deep vein thrombosis</u>. The nurse would provide care to prevent <u>pulmonary embolism</u>, which is a potentially life-threatening complication. Together these two health problems are referred to as <u>venous thromboembolism</u>.

Rationales

The client is experiencing dull pain in the calf and unilateral pitting edema. These are symptoms of a deep vein thrombosis (DVT). The client has risk factors for DVT that include recent surgery under general anesthesia, obesity, and bedrest for several days. A client with a DVT in a lower extremity is at risk for activity intolerance secondary to pain and edema; impaired peripheral tissue oxygenation, which results in altered skin pigmentation and ulcerative wounds; and pulmonary embolism, a potentially life-threatening condition caused by the venous clot breaking free and lodging in the pulmonary vasculature. The term *venous thromboembolism* refers to both deep vein thrombosis and pulmonary embolism.

CJ Cognitive Skill

Prioritize Hypothesis

Reference

Linton & Matteson, 2020, pp. 497–499; 670–672

Thinking Exercise 4-4

Answers

Nursing Action	Indicated	Contraindicated	Non-Essential
Apply sequential compression device to unaffected lower extremity.	X		
Instruct the client to gradually increase activity and to stop any activity temporarily if pain occurs.	X		
Administer supplemental oxygen via a nonrebreather mask.			X

Nursing Action	Indicated	Contraindicated	Non-Essential
Use ice packs to decrease leg swelling and pain.		X	
Administer prescribed anticoagulant therapy.	X		
Place client's legs in a dependent position when sitting in a chair.		X	

Rationales

For clients who have a moderate to high risk for a deep vein thrombosis (DVT), sequential compression devices should be administered to both lower extremities as a preventive measure. When a client has a positive diagnosis for a DVT, the leg with the clot should not be massaged or have a cold application, nor should a sequential compression device be used, because of the risk of dislodging the thrombus. The client's legs should not be placed in a dependent position, but instead should be elevated when in bed or chair to improve venous return. The client may be on bedrest initially, but inactivity increases the client's risk for additional venous thrombosis. Activity should begin slowly and increase gradually over several weeks. The nurse would teach the client to stop an activity if pain occurs; once pain subsides, the activity may continue. There is no need to administer supplemental oxygen for DVT.

CJ Cognitive Skill

Generate Solutions

Reference

Linton & Matteson, 2020, pp. 661–675

Thinking Exercise 4-5

Answers

B, C, F, G

Rationales

The hand-off report focuses on changes in the client's status, actions taken, and treatments or tests scheduled. The client's change in status, specifically sudden onset of dyspnea, hypoxia, and chest pain, is most likely related to a pulmonary embolism. The registered nurse needs to know the client's current respiratory assessment findings and what has been done to support the client's respiratory status. This would include current oxygen saturation level, percentage of oxygen being administered, respiratory pattern, and auscultated lung sounds (Choices B and C). Intravenous heparin is commonly prescribed for a pulmonary embolism. Prior to starting heparin, the client will need intravenous access and baseline serum coagulation levels. The status of these necessities would be shared during hand-off report (Choices F and G). As-needed or PRN medications would also be reported, but scheduled medications would not. Assessments of the client's colostomy, intake and output, and immunization status are not essential to report during this transition of care.

CJ Cognitive Skill

Take Action

Reference

Linton & Matteson, 2020, pp. 497–499, 661–675

Thinking Exercise 4-6

Answers

Client Statement	Effective	Ineffective	Unrelated
"I will elevate my legs when sitting to improve circulation."	X		
"I will use an elevated desk to stand at work instead of sitting."		X	
"I will eat a healthy diet with green leafy vegetables every other day."		X	
"I will contact my primary health care provider if I have chest pain or shortness of breath."	X		
"I will drink plenty of water each day."	X		

Rationales

The client is taught to elevate affected extremities to promote circulation and venous return, and to contact the primary health care provider with complications including chest pain and shortness of breath. Prolonged standing, crossing of legs, and massaging or rubbing affected extremities should be avoided. Clients taking warfarin are taught to maintain the same amount of dietary vitamin K each day. Eating a green leafy vegetable every other day may decrease the therapeutic effect of warfarin. The client should be instructed not to make any changes in the diet. Poor fluid intake can cause blood clotting from venous stasis and increased serum osmolality. Therefore drinking plenty of fluids is important for the nurse to reinforce.

CJ Cognitive Skill

Evaluate Outcomes

Reference

Linton & Matteson, 2020, pp. 661–675

Thinking Exercise 4-7

Answers

Nurse's Response	Client Question	Appropriate Nurse's Response for Each Client Question
1 "When the clot in your leg dislodges and moves to your lung it is called a pulmonary embolism. Smoking increases the risk of this complication."	"The night nurse said I needed to stop smoking. What does smoking have to do with my swollen leg?"	5 "Nicotine causes your blood vessels to constrict or narrow, which makes it easier for blood clots to become stuck in the vein."
2 "Increasing your activity slowly may decease your fear. Let's start with getting out of bed and then a short walk later today."	"What can I do to decrease the swelling in my leg?"	6 "Wearing compression stockings as well as elevating your legs when in bed and the chair will help."
3 "Swelling will decrease when the clot is gone, and the medication you are on will dissolve the clot."	"I read on the internet that the clot can go to my lungs if I move my leg. Is that true?"	2 "Increasing your activity slowly may decease your fear. Let's start with getting out of bed and then a short walk later today."

Nurse's Response	Client Question	Appropriate Nurse's Response for Each Client Question
4 "You have many risk factors for a DVT, including smoking."		
5 "Nicotine causes your blood vessels to constrict or narrow, which makes it easier for blood clots to become stuck in the vein."		
6 "Wearing compression stockings as well as elevating your legs when in bed and the chair will help."		
7 "If you have pain when you flex your foot, you should stay in bed."		

Rationales

Nicotine causes vasoconstriction, which increases the client's risk for a thrombus occlusion. The nurse would take this moment to explain to the client the effects of nicotine on the cardiovascular system instead of simply stating that it is one of many risk factors (Response 5). The nurse would teach the client to elevate his legs and how to appropriately apply and wear compression stockings (Response 6). The client is most likely prescribed an anticoagulant medication, not a thrombolytic. Research shows that ambulation does not increase the risk for pulmonary embolus and therefore the client should be encouraged to walk. Increasing activity slowly will decrease the client's anxiety and fear about dislodging the clot. Explaining what a pulmonary embolism is and providing false information about pain on dorsiflexion of the foot will create more fear and do not address the client's concern (Response 2).

CJ Cognitive Skill

Take Action

Reference

Linton & Matteson, 2020, pp. 661–675

CHAPTER 5 Gas Exchange

Answers With Rationales for Thinking Exercises

Exemplar 5A. Asthma (Pediatric Nursing: School-Age Child)

Thinking Exercise 5A-1

Answers

B, C, D, E, F, H

Rationales

The nurse's assessments would focus on signs and symptoms that support potential conditions associated with dyspnea in a child. Dyspnea is commonly associated with an acute respiratory infection; therefore the client's temperature would be assessed as a potential cue for an infectious condition (Option B). Chest trauma, foreign body aspiration, and respiratory disorders such as asthma and acute rhinitis are also common causes of acute dyspnea in children. Inspection of chest symmetry and movement would provide the nurse with information related to the client's breathing pattern and any thoracic abnormalities (Option E). Auscultation of the lungs bilaterally and in a systematic manner would help the nurse identify sounds of abnormal respirations associated with many cardiac and pulmonary disorders (Option F). An examination of the head and neck provides the nurse with essential information related to nasal patency, air hunger (flaring of the nares), tissue oxygenation (cyanotic lips, nose, and gums), and tracheal deviation (Option H). Finally, the nurse would obtain vital signs including heart rate, respiratory rate, and oxygen saturation (Options C and D). These data will be used to determine the severity of the situation and provide a baseline for evaluation of improvement or further decompensation. Height and weight and palpation for abdominal tenderness or masses do not have any relevance to the client's current condition.

CJ Cognitive Skill

Recognize Cues

Reference

Linton & Matteson, 2020, pp. 442–446

Thinking Exercise 5A-2

Answers

The nurse recognizes that the assessment findings could be caused by several medical disorders. Cystic fibrosis is a hereditary disorder characterized by dysfunction of the exocrine glands. Common signs and symptoms are thick, tenacious mucus, progressive dyspnea, activity intolerance, and weight loss. Respiratory syncytial virus is a common respiratory infection that causes bronchiolitis in young children. Symptoms frequently include rhinitis, coughing, and wheezing. Asthma is a potentially reversible, chronic obstructive airway disorder characterized by bronchoconstriction and airway inflammation. Manifestations during an exacerbation usually include dyspnea, anxiety, and audible expiratory wheezes.

Rationales

Cystic fibrosis is a hereditary disorder in which the client experiences thick, tenacious mucus; progressive dyspnea; activity intolerance; and weight loss. Respiratory syncytial virus (RSV) is a common respiratory infection that causes bronchiolitis in young children, often infants 6 months of age or younger. Premature infants and children who have heart disease or chronic lung disease are particularly at risk for this infection. Symptoms typically include rhinitis, coughing, and wheezing. Asthma is a chronic respiratory disorder that causes bronchoconstriction and airway inflammation. As a result, during a flare-up (exacerbation), the client usually has dyspnea, anxiety (due to dyspnea), and audible expiratory wheezes.

CJ Cognitive Skill

Analyze Cues

Reference

Linton & Matteson, 2020, pp. 502–524

Thinking Exercise 5A-3

Answers

Potential Health Problems	Urgent	Non-Urgent	Irrelevant
Inadequate oxygenation related to air trapping	X		
Airway obstruction related to bronchospasm	X		
Potential for injury related to infection			X
Anxiety related to perceived threat of suffocation		X	
Inadequate nutrition related to dyspnea			X

Rationales

The client's low oxygen saturation level, tachypnea, and dyspnea indicate the client is experiencing inadequate oxygenation. This is an urgent problem. The nurse must implement care immediately to prevent tissue hypoxia, acidosis, and cellular death. Airway obstruction related to bronchospasm is also an urgent problem and must be treated immediately to prevent further inflammation, complete airway obstruction, and respiratory failure. Although the client is experiencing anxiety related to perceived threat of suffocation as manifested by his statement of not being able to breathe and needing assistance to get enough air, this is not an urgent issue. The nurse would prioritize the client's airway, breathing, and oxygenation status before addressing the client's anxiety. While taking steps to improve the client's oxygenation, the nurse can try to reduce anxiety by remaining calm and explaining each intervention as it is implemented. The client's findings do not indicate any concerns related to an infection or inadequate nutrition.

CJ Cognitive Skill

Prioritize Hypotheses

Reference

Linton & Matteson, 2020, pp. 502–508

Thinking Exercise 5A-4

Answers

A, D, E, G

Rationales

The treatment plan for a client with asthma is based on symptoms as well as the peak flow meter readings compared with the client's personal best reading (Option G). A peak flow meter reading greater than 80% of the client's personal best indicates the client is doing well, a reading between 50% and 80% of personal best indicates the client needs interventions to relieve acute symptoms, and a reading less than 50% of personal best is a critical situation requiring immediate emergency medical services. The client's oxygen saturation level indicates inadequate oxygenation or hypoxia, and therefore supplemental oxygen would be administered (Option A). The nurse would continuously monitor the client's symptoms for impending respiratory failure and status asthmaticus, a life-threatening episode of asthma (Option D). Signs of impending respiratory failure include tachypnea, shallow respirations, diaphoresis, reddening skin, tachycardia, cardia dysrhythmias, restlessness, drowsiness, and loss of consciousness. A short-acting $beta_2$-agonist (SABA) inhaler will be administered to relieve acute symptoms (Option E). An inhaled leukotriene modifier provides long-term control of asthma symptoms and would not be used during an acute exacerbation. Identifying allergens and environmental triggers via skin testing may be completed during a follow-up visit with the client, but it is not a priority at this time. Adequate hydration will help thin tenacious secretions, but there is no indication that the client needs intravenous hydration at this time.

CJ Cognitive Skill

Generate Solutions

Reference

Linton & Matteson, 2020, pp. 451–452, 646–648

Thinking Exercise 5A-5

Answers

Specific Nursing Action	Planned Intervention	Appropriate Nursing Action for Each Planned Intervention
1 Supply oxygen at 3 L/min via a facemask.	Position the client to improve the use of accessory muscles.	**4** Support the client in a Fowler or tripod position.
2 Perform chest physiotherapy.	Administer the client's short-acting $beta_2$-agonist bronchodilator.	**7** Ask the client to breathe in slowly and as deeply as possible, then hold the breath for a count of 10 if possible.
3 Place a continuous pulse oximetry probe on the client's finger.	Provide supplemental oxygen to keep saturation >92%.	**3** Place a continuous pulse oximetry probe on the client's finger.
4 Support the client in a Fowler or tripod position.	Evaluate peak expiratory flow rates to determine treatment effectiveness.	**5** Ask the client to blow out as hard and as quickly as possible until all of the air is out of the lungs.
5 Ask the client to blow out as hard and as quickly as possible until all of the air is out of the lungs.		
6 Position the client in modified left lateral recumbent position.		
7 Ask the client to breathe in slowly and as deeply as possible, then hold the breath for a count of 10 if possible.		

Rationales

A high-Fowler position can improve breathing in clients who are experiencing dyspnea by relaxing the abdominal muscles, and a tripod position assists by optimizing the use of accessory muscles in the upper chest. This child would be placed in a comfortable, upright position with feet flat on the floor and shoulders relaxed as much as possible. The child may choose to lean forward and rest elbows or hands on knees in a tripod position. The client's bronchodilator is most likely a metered dose inhaler. The client is old enough to self-administer the inhaler, and therefore the nurse would encourage the client use the inhaler appropriately. Steps to using an inhaler with a spacer are (1) breathe out all the way, (2) place the spacer mouthpiece end in the mouth, (3) press down on the inhaler one time, (4) start breathing in slowly, (5) continue breathing in slowly as deeply as possible, and (6) hold the breath for a count of 10 if possible. Oxygen therapy at 3 L/min is an appropriate initial dose, but the nurse would not use a facemask. The child is most likely anxious secondary to breathlessness, and a mask could increase the client's feelings of suffocation. A nasal cannula would be more appropriate for an 8-year-old child. To titrate the supplemental oxygen, the nurse needs to secure a pulse oximetry probe to the client's finger and monitor the client's oxygen saturation continuously. The nurse would assist the client in obtaining a peak expiratory flow reading before and after administering the bronchodilator to evaluate the effectiveness of the medication. These readings would be compared with each other and with the client's personal best. The client is old enough to use a peak expiratory flow meter with directions from the nurse. The appropriate steps are (1) put the mouthpiece in the mouth, (2) close lips tightly around the mouthpiece, and (3) breathe out in one breath as hard and as quickly as possible.

CJ Cognitive Skill

Take Action

References

Linton & Matteson, 2020, pp. 446–452, 502–508; Williams, 2018, pp. 511–512, 518–523, 533–534, 661–662

Thinking Exercise 5A-6

Answers

- Heart rate = 130 beats/min
- Respirations = 28 breaths/min
- Oxygen saturation = 98% (on supplemental oxygen)
- Reports breathing more easily, less shortness of breath
- Decreased use of respiratory accessory muscles
- Expiratory wheezes heard via auscultation only
- Productive cough with tenacious secretions
- Peak expiratory flow rate = 180 L/min (personal best = 240 L/min)

Rationales

The client's peak expiratory flow rate prior to treatment was 160 L/min, or 65% of the client's personal best. The peak expiratory flow rate after treatment is 180 L/min, 75% of personal best, which indicates the client's condition is improving. Other signs of improvement include an increase in the client's oxygen saturation level, decreased use of respiratory accessory muscles, and the client's report of breathing more easily. The client's expiratory wheezes were originally audible (could hear without a stethoscope) and now can be heard only on auscultation. This is also a sign of improvement. The client continues to have a productive cough with tenacious secretions and is experiencing tachycardia and tachypnea. These symptoms must be continuously monitored, and additional interventions may be needed.

CJ Cognitive Skill

Evaluate Outcomes

Reference

Linton & Matteson, 2020, pp. 502–508

Thinking Exercise 5A-7

Answers

Medication	Dose, Frequency, Route	Drug Class	Indication
Albuterol	1–2 aerosol metered doses inhaled every 4–6 hr as needed	**Beta-adrenergic agonist**	Relaxes smooth muscles in the bronchial tree to relieve bronchial constriction
Montelukast	5-mg chewable tablet orally once a day	Leukotriene inhibitor	**Prevents bronchospasm**
Diphenhydramine	25-mg tablet orally every 6 hr as needed	**Antihistamine**	Blocks histamine and dries respiratory secretions
Guaifenesin	1 teaspoon orally every 4 hr as needed	Expectorant	**Thins respiratory secretions for easier expectoration**

Rationales

Albuterol is a bronchodilator that belongs to a class of drugs known as beta-adrenergic agonists. This medication is a short-acting beta agonist (SABA) and is used as a "rescue" inhaler. Montelukast belongs to a class of drugs known as leukotriene inhibitors. By blocking the leukotriene receptors in the lungs, the drug decreases the body's inflammatory response and relaxes smooth muscles to prevent bronchospasm. Diphenhydramine is an antihistamine medication that blocks the body's inflammatory response to an allergic stimulus and minimizes or relieves rhinitis symptoms associated with allergies. Guaifenesin is an expectorant. This medication thins respiratory secretions for easier expectoration or the ejection of phlegm or mucus from the throat and lungs by coughing.

CJ Cognitive Skill

Analyze Cues

Reference

Linton & Matteson, 2020, pp. 453–457

Exemplar 5B. Chronic Obstructive Pulmonary Disease (Medical-Surgical Nursing: Middle-Age Adult)

Thinking Exercise 5B-1

Answers

B, C, E

Rationales

Because of the client's history of COPD, symptoms related to this chronic illness such as a cough for many years and losing weight over the past 6 months are not of immediate concern. The client's desire to smoke and history of multiple hospitalizations need to be explored, but they are also not of immediate concern. Alternatively, dyspnea while resting and a heaviness in the chest are of immediate concern. Clients with COPD often have dyspnea with exertion, but this should subside with rest. A client having trouble breathing while sitting indicates an acute exacerbation or an adjunct pulmonary disorder (Choice B). Heaviness in the chest may be associated with a pulmonary complication, but it may also be related to a cardiac event. The nurse must follow up regarding this symptom immediately (Choice C). In addition, the client's report of difficulty concentrating is very concerning and could indicate inadequate oxygenation to the brain (Choice E).

CJ Cognitive Skill

Recognize Cues

Reference

Linton & Matteson, 2020, pp. 508–510

Thinking Exercise 5B-2

Answers

Client Findings	Inadequate Oxygenation	Cor Pulmonale	Pulmonary Infection
Chest tightness/discomfort	X		X
Difficulty concentrating	X		X
Cyanotic lips	X	X	
Dyspnea	X	X	X
Dependent edema		X	

Rationales

Inadequate oxygenation as a complication of COPD relates to alveolar destruction, bronchospasm, and air trapping. Inadequate oxygenation can interfere with cardiac and brain function when these organs do not receive enough oxygen, resulting in low tissue oxygen levels (hypoxia). The most common symptoms of hypoxia are shortness of breath or dyspnea; confusion or difficulty concentrating; changes in skin color, ranging from blue to cherry red; and chest tightness or discomfort. Cor pulmonale, also known as right-sided heart failure, most commonly occurs as a complication of high blood pressure in the pulmonary arteries (pulmonary hypertension). Pulmonary vascular remodeling secondary to COPD causes an increase in pulmonary artery pressure. Symptoms of cor pulmonale include dyspnea, cyanosis, and peripheral edema. Clients with COPD are at high risk of pulmonary infections because they generally have poor nutrition and have difficulty clearing secretions from the lungs. Stasis secretions may contain bacteria, viruses, dust, and other pollutants that cause an infection. Clients with COPD also have damaged lung tissue, frequently from cigarette smoke, which increases the risk of infection. Symptoms of pulmonary infection are chest pain or discomfort, dyspnea, productive cough, and confusion or delirium.

CJ Cognitive Skill

Analyze Cues

Reference

Linton & Matteson, 2020, pp. 487–489, 508–515

Thinking Exercise 5B-3

Answers

The nurse recognizes that the client is experiencing an exacerbation of COPD with several complications. The ***priority*** client condition is <u>impaired gas exchange</u>. The nurse would intervene immediately to prevent hypoxia, <u>hypercapnia</u>, and <u>respiratory acidosis</u>.

Rationales

Although the client has several problems, impaired gas exchange (affecting airway and breathing) is the priority. The exchange of oxygen and carbon dioxide in the lungs is impaired because of airway obstruction caused by bronchospasm and increased quantity and viscosity of sputum; alveoli destruction secondary to air trapping; and alveolar-capillary membrane changes resulting from bullae and blebs. This ventilation-perfusion mismatch results in hypoxemia (decreased Pao_2), hypercapnia (increased $Paco_2$), and respiratory acidosis.

CJ Cognitive Skill

Prioritize Hypotheses

Reference

Linton & Matteson, 2020, pp. 508–515

Thinking Exercise 5B-4

Answers

Nursing Action	Indicated	Contraindicated	Non-Essential
Slowly increase the oxygen flow rate by 1 liter every 15 minutes until oxygen saturation reaches 90%.	X		
Teach the client that smoking caused his chronic lung disease and that he must quit or he will die.		X	
Type and cross-match for blood products.			X
Help the client to a comfortable high-Fowler position in bed or supported at the bedside.	X		
Schedule treatments, meals, and physical activity so that the client has time to rest.	X		
Administer salmeterol 1 inhalation as needed 15 minutes prior to meals and physical activity.		X	
Place the client on a 1200-mL fluid restriction.		X	

Rationales

The client is hypoxic and needs supplemental oxygen. Increasing the oxygen flow rate slowly will assist the nurse in determining the appropriate amount of oxygen to provide without causing oxygen-induced hypoventilation. To promote full expansion of the lungs and promote use of respiratory accessory muscles, the nurse would place the client in a high-Fowler position. Smoking cessation is essential in the management of COPD. The client may experience severe dyspnea with any exertion, including eating, bathing, and participating in diagnostic tests or treatments. The nurse would attempt to schedule activities so that the client has time to recover and rest. A short-acting $beta_2$-adrenergic agent may be administered prior to a meal or activity to minimize airway resistance and the work of breathing. Salmeterol is a long-acting $beta_2$-adrenergic agent and would not be used as a rescue inhaler. The nurse should discourage smoking in a nonjudgmental manner to maintain a therapeutic relationship. Most clients know that smoking can cause respiratory disease, have attempted to quit smoking, and are unable to overcome the addiction. The nurse should ask the client about his experiences with quitting and provide information about smoking-cessation programs that may be helpful. The client would be encouraged to drink 2500 to 3000 mL of fluid daily to loosen tenacious secretions and promote expectoration. There is no indication that the client requires a blood transfusion, and therefore a type and cross-match is non-essential.

CJ Cognitive Skill

Generate Solutions

Reference

Linton & Matteson, 2020, pp. 508–517

Thinking Exercise 5B-5

Answers

B, C, E, G

Rationales

To adequately titrate supplemental oxygen, the nurse would initiate continuous pulse oximetry to monitor the client's pulse blood oxygen saturation (Choice B). Fluticasone, a corticosteroid, is commonly used to reduce acute airway inflammation. Long-term use of inhaled corticosteroids is not recommended because of their many adverse effects, which include fluid and electrolyte disturbances, increased risk of infection, elevated blood glucose, osteoporosis, and suppression of the adrenal cortex. The nurse would assist the client in rinsing his mouth after administration of inhaled fluticasone to prevent an oral *Candida* infection (Choice E). A registered dietitian nutritionist would be consulted to evaluate the client's nutritional needs and provide recommendations for appropriate high-caloric and high-protein supplements (Choice C). Assistive personnel should use the same scale every morning before breakfast to weigh the client to ensure accurate weight values (Choice G). The other nursing actions are appropriate for this client, but they do not directly relate to the primary health care provider's orders.

CJ Cognitive Skill

Take Action

Reference

Linton & Matteson, 2020, pp. 508–517

Thinking Exercise 5B-6

Answers

Client Finding	Improved	No Change	Declined
Respirations = 34 breaths/min			X
Dependent pitting edema bilaterally		X	
Oxygen saturation = 91% (on room air [RA])	X		
Bilateral wheezes and crackles			X
Oral mucosa and lips pinkish-red	X		

Rationales

Implementation of supplemental oxygen has improved the client's oxygen saturation as demonstrated by an increase in the client's pulse oximetry reading to the desired range of 90% to 92% and improved coloration of the client's lips and oral mucosa from cyanotic to pink. The client's tachypnea has worsened from 28 to 34 breaths/min, and crackles can now be heard in his lung fields. These findings indicate a decline in status and possibly an increase in pulmonary congestion. There is no change in the client's pitting edema in the dependent lower extremities.

CJ Cognitive Skill

Evaluate Outcomes

Reference

Linton & Matteson, 2020, pp. 508–517

Thinking Exercise 5B-7

Answers

A, D, E, F, G

Rationales

The nurse would reinforce teaching on minimizing exposure to irritants, preventing infections, properly taking medications, and improving overall health through nutrition and exercise. The nurse appropriately engages the client in identifying irritants and developing an avoidance plan together (Choice A). The client would be encouraged to obtain vaccines to prevent infection and increase fluid intake to thin tenacious respiratory secretions (Choices D and F). The nurse would reinforce medication teaching and the correct use of prescribed metered-dose inhalers (Choice E). Rescue inhalers are used when the client experiences increased symptoms, but the inhalant should not be repeated every 15 minutes. Most short-acting beta-agonists are prescribed for 1 to 2 sprays every 4 to 6 hours. Taking them more frequently will increase side effects, including tachycardia, headache, and restlessness. The client would be encouraged to exercise, but fitness programs must be designed with periods of activity and rest. The client should not attempt exercise when experiencing an exacerbation of symptoms. The nurse would teach the client that using a several pillows or sleeping in a recliner helps to make breathing easier (Choice G).

CJ Cognitive Skill

Take Action

Reference

Linton & Matteson, 2020, pp. 508–517

Thinking Exercise 5B-8

Answers

Assessment Finding	Improved	Not Changed	Declined
Pao_2 = 75 mm Hg	X		
Stuporous			X
Lung fields clear throughout	X		
$Paco_2$ = 65 mm Hg			X
BP = 145/66 mm Hg		X	

Rationales

The client's vital signs and arterial blood gas (ABG) results indicate that the client is experiencing hypoxia and hypercapnia resulting in respiratory acidosis. Bi-level positive airway pressure (BiPAP) therapy provides noninvasive ventilation support through the use of two levels of pressure, one for inhalation and another for exhalation. BiPAP assists the client by reducing the effort involved in breathing, increasing the volume of each breath, reducing $Paco_2$ levels, and correcting acid-base imbalance. The client's $Paco_2$ level increased, which is a sign of decline. A short-acting $beta_2$-adrenergic agonist is ordered to relax smooth muscles of the airways. Albuterol, a quick-relief bronchodilator, is anticipated to eliminate wheezing caused by airway constriction. The client's lung fields are clear throughout, which is an indication of improvement. Supplemental oxygen is prescribed for this client, with oxygen delivery starting at a low level and increasing slowly based on client symptoms. The client's Pao_2 level has increased, indicating improvement. Hypoxia and hypercapnia are most likely the cause of this client's mental status. Lethargy is consistent with severe drowsiness, but the client can be aroused by moderate stimuli. Stupor means that only vigorous and repeated stimuli will arouse the client. This is a sign that the client is declining. Changes in the client's blood pressure are very minimal, and therefore there is no significant change.

CJ Cognitive Skill

Evaluate Outcomes

Reference

Linton & Matteson, 2020, pp. 508–517

CHAPTER 6 Elimination

Answers With Rationales for Thinking Exercises

Exemplar 6A. Benign Prostatic Hyperplasia/Transurethral Resection of the Prostate (Medical-Surgical Nursing: Older Adult)

Thinking Exercise 6A-1

Answers

Assessment Finding	Assessment Finding That Requires Immediate Follow-Up
Urinary frequency	X
Diabetes mellitus type 2	
Hypertension	
Weak urinary stream	X
Nocturia 2–3 times	X
Postvoid dribbling	X
COPD	

Rationales

The client's main concern is focused on his new-onset urinary symptoms and are therefore of immediate concern to the nurse. His history of other medical conditions is not of immediate concern because they may be controlled or stable.

CJ Cognitive Skill

Recognize Cues

Reference

Linton & Matteson, 2020, p. 1064

Thinking Exercise 6A-2

Answers

A, C, D, G

Rationales

Benign prostatic hypertrophy (BPH) can cause urethral obstruction, causing urinary retention (Choices A and G). Prolonged urinary retention can cause urinary stasis, which can affect the kidneys and cause postrenal chronic kidney disease (Choice D). Urinary retention can also lead to a urinary tract infection (Choice C). Although concentrated urine could contribute to urolithiasis (urinary tract stones), clients who have BPH do not necessarily have concentrated urine. Bladder cancer, polycystic kidney, and atonic bladder are also not typical complications of BPH.

CJ Cognitive Skill

Analyze Cues

Reference

Linton & Matteson, 2020, pp. 1064–1066

Thinking Exercise 6A-3

Answers

The nurse determines, based on the client's urinary symptoms and his prescribed drug regimen, that he ***most likely*** has <u>benign prostatic hyperplasia</u>. If drug therapy is not effective, the client may need to have a partial or total <u>prostatectomy</u>.

Rationales

The client is an older male, which puts him at high risk for benign prostatic hyperplasia (BPH), a common physiologic change of aging. Drug therapy is the first line of treatment. If the client does not respond to this therapy, the client may need to have a partial or total removal of his prostate gland, known as a prostatectomy.

CJ Cognitive Skill

Prioritize Hypotheses

Reference

Linton & Matteson, 2020, pp. 1064–1066

Thinking Exercise 6A-4

Answers

Health Teaching	Indicated	Contraindicated	Non-Essential
"Increase your daily intake of caffeine to help prevent urinary retention."		X	
"Monitor your blood pressure frequently because one of your drugs may cause it to decrease."	X		
"Perform Kegel exercises every day to help manage incontinence."			X
"Avoid alcoholic beverages to help prevent urgency and dribbling."	X		
"Strain your urine with every voiding to remove any stones."			X
"Report burning when you void or cloudy urine to your primary health care provider."	X		

Rationales

Caffeine should be avoided by any client who has urinary problems because it is a diuretic and can cause urge incontinence. Therefore caffeinated beverages should not be increased. Alcohol should also be avoided to prevent increased urgency and dribbling. Kegel exercises are not appropriate for clients who have stress incontinence. Straining the urine is not needed because the client does not have urolithiasis. Because tamsulosin can cause postural hypotension, the client could become dizzy and fall. Therefore the client should monitor his blood pressure to make sure it does not become too low. If hypotension or symptoms associated with urinary tract infection occur, the client should contact the primary health care provider.

CJ Cognitive Skill

Generate Solutions

Reference

Linton & Matteson, 2020, pp. 219, 1064–1066

Thinking Exercise 6A-5

Answers

A, B, D, E, F, G, H

Rationales

For a TURP, the surgeon excises the excess prostatic growth to alleviate urethral obstruction and prevent urinary retention. There is no external incision or surgical dressing for this procedure, but it causes bleeding and pain. Therefore the typical postoperative care includes managing continuous bladder irrigation (CBI) to minimize bleeding and clotting (Choice A). CBI requires a three-way urinary catheter that is tightly taped to keep the balloon in place to compress blood vessels; this tape should not be removed (Choice B). The nurse monitors for clots, bleeding, and infection and encourages fluids in order to dilute and increase urinary output (Choices E, F, and H). The nurse also assesses postoperative pain caused by bladder spasms and administers pain medication as needed (Choice D). The client's sexual ability should not be affected after tissue healing occurs (Choice G).

CJ Cognitive Skill

Take Action

Reference

Linton & Matteson, 2020, pp. 1066–1069

Thinking Exercise 6A-6

Answers

Nurses' Notes

Client states that he is feeling much better and has only occasional bladder spasms. Is voiding less frequently in larger amounts, has no feeling of urgency, and typically has nocturia 2–3 times. Has not tried to have intercourse since surgery but is hoping to try after this visit. Vital signs include: temperature = 98°F (36.7°C), pulse = 78 beats/min, respirations = 18 breaths/min, blood pressure = 154/90 mm Hg. Oxygen saturation = 96%. No adventitious breath sounds. Bowel sounds present × 4. -- *J. L. Miller, LPN*

Rationales

The client is feeling better and does not have urinary symptoms except for nocturia. His vital signs, including oxygen saturation, are stable, indicating no infection. However, his blood pressure is elevated and should be evaluated. Breath sounds and bowel sounds are normal.

CJ Cognitive Skill

Evaluate Outcomes

Reference

Linton & Matteson, 2020, pp. 1066–1069

Thinking Exercise 6A-7

Answers

The nurse calculates that the client's total fluid intake for the 8 hours since he was transferred from the PACU is <u>1480</u> mL and his total urine output for the 8-hour period is <u>720</u> mL.

Rationales

Although some agencies require that bladder irrigation solution be counted as intake, actual fluid intake includes fluids that are taken in via the oral, feeding tube, and intravenous routes. Therefore 1000 mL of IV fluids added to the amounts of water (360 mL) and apple juice (120 mL) = 1480 mL. To calculate the actual urine output, the nurse would need to subtract the amount of the irrigant from the total drainage in the bag: 1600 mL drainage bag output − 880 mL irrigation solution = 720 mL actual urine output.

CJ Cognitive Skill

Take Action

Reference

Linton & Matteson, 2020, pp. 1066–1069

Thinking Exercise 6A-8

Answers

A, B, C, D, E, F, G

Rationales

All of the nurse's statements are correct and should be included in the teaching. Symptoms including acute pain or urinary changes should be reported to his surgeon (Choices A and F). The client should increase his fluid intake and avoid caffeinated beverages (Choices C and D). The nurse reminds the client that although his sexual function should not be impaired, he may experience retrograde ejaculation (Choice E). Before taking any over-the-counter (OTC) drug, the client should check with the surgeon because some OTC drugs can cause urinary retention or diuresis (Choice B). The client should also know that he may need additional treatment or surgery if the prostate enlarges again (Choice G).

CJ Cognitive Skill

Take Action

Reference

Linton & Matteson, 2020, pp. 1066–1069

Exemplar 6B. Ulcerative Colitis/Colostomy (Medical-Surgical Nursing: Middle-Age Adult)

Thinking Exercise 6B-1

Answers

A 38-year-old female client visits her primary health care provider with report of anorexia, increasing diarrhea, moderate to severe abdominal cramping, and blood in her stool. She was diagnosed as having ulcerative colitis 2 years ago. Her current assessment findings include:

- Temperature = 99.8°F (37.7°C)
- Heart rate = 92 beats/min
- Respirations = 20 breaths/min
- BP = 110/58 mm Hg
- Oxygen saturation = 95% (on room air [RA])
- Pain = 6/10

Rationales

All of the highlighted signs and symptoms indicate that the client is experiencing an exacerbation of her ulcerative colitis (UC). She has anorexia, bloody diarrhea with cramping, an elevated body temperature, tachycardia, and moderate pain.

CJ Cognitive Skill

Recognize Cues

Reference

Linton & Matteson, 2020, pp. 755–757

Thinking Exercise 6B-2

Answers

Based on the client data, the nurse recognizes that the client is currently at risk for complications of ulcerative colitis, especially <u>fluid and electrolyte imbalance</u> and <u>inadequate nutrition</u>.

Rationales

The client has increasing diarrhea, which causes a loss of water and potassium. She also has anorexia, which can lead to inadequate nutrition. Eventually she may develop anemia due to bleeding and poor appetite.

CJ Cognitive Skill

Analyze Cues

Reference

Linton & Matteson, 2020, pp. 755–757

Thinking Exercise 6B-3

Answers

The nurse determines that the ***priority*** for care for this client is hydration and ensuring that she has adequate pain management.

Rationales

The nurse's priority is to promote hydration to prevent fluid and electrolyte imbalances, especially dehydration and hypokalemia. The client also needs to have adequate pain management. She has no problem with oxygenation or body temperature. The nurse collaborates with the interprofessional health care team to manage pain, including the administration of drug therapy.

CJ Cognitive Skill

Prioritize Hypotheses

Reference

Linton & Matteson, 2020, pp. 755–757

Thinking Exercise 6B-4

Answers

Nursing Action	Indicated	Contraindicated	Non-Essential
Contact the wound, ostomy, continence nurse (WOCN) about the surgery to determine ostomy placement.	X		
Include any family members or significant others in the teaching as the client requests.	X		
Reinforce teaching about the need to deep breathe and use the incentive spirometer every 1–2 hours.	X		
Remind the client that he will not be allowed to eat or drink anything until the ostomy begins to work.		X	
Reinforce teaching about the purpose of sequential compression/pneumatic devices after surgery.	X		

Rationales

All of these actions would be indicated except for withholding food and fluids from the client until the ostomy begins to function. Because the client is going to have surgery, she needs health teaching about the use of incentive spirometry, deep breathing, and sequential compression devices to help prevent postoperative complications. The WOCN is usually the nurse who marks the client's abdomen for proper ostomy placement before surgery and follows the client postoperatively.

CJ Cognitive Skill

Generate Solutions

Reference

Linton & Matteson, 2020, pp. 310–312

Thinking Exercise 6B-5

Answers

A, E, F, G

Rationales

The client had abdominal surgery with creation of an ascending colostomy for colorectal cancer this morning. The nurse would be sure to help the client to get out of bed and into the chair the same evening, frequently check vital signs and the surgical dressing for bleeding and intactness, and remind the client to use her incentive spirometer every 1 to 2 hours to prevent respiratory complications (Choices A, E, F, and G). It is too soon to change the ostomy pouch and unlikely that the ostomy would be irrigated at any point. Checking for bowel sounds is an appropriate nursing action, but that assessment is not needed every hour.

CJ Cognitive Skill

Take Action

Reference

Linton & Matteson, 2020, pp. 310–312

Thinking Exercise 6B-6

Answers

Client Data	Progressing	Not Progressing
Vital signs stable and without fever	X	
Is unable to do ostomy care including pouch changes		X
Stoma is reddish without surrounding redness	X	
States she can never have sex with her husband again		X
Ostomy draining mostly liquid stool	X	

Rationales

The client's vital signs are stable, which indicates that she does not have an infection. Her ostomy is draining mostly liquid stool, which is normal for an ascending colostomy. The stoma is reddish, showing that it has adequate blood supply. However, she does not want to or is unable to do ostomy care and thinks that she will not be able to have sex with her husband as a result of having the ostomy.

CJ Cognitive Skill

Evaluate Outcomes

Reference

Linton & Matteson, 2020, pp. 310–312

Thinking Exercise 6B-7

Answers

Potential Health Teaching	Appropriate Health Teaching for the Sulfasalazine
"This drug is an antibiotic that is often given to clients who have an acute episode of inflammatory bowel disease."	X
"You will need to take this drug for your entire life."	
"You shouldn't take this drug if you are allergic to sulfa or sulfa medications."	X
"This drug should decrease your trips to the bathroom so you can feel a little more confident."	X
"Be sure to drink lots of fluids to dilute your urine while on this drug."	X

Rationales

Sulfasalazine is a sulfa-based antibiotic that is used to manage inflammation and infection in clients with a variety of diseases. For clients with chronic inflammatory bowel disease such as Crohn's and ulcerative colitis (UC), the drug is given only when there is a disease flare-up, or acute exacerbation. It is not given for life as treatment for UC. When inflammation is decreased, the client's symptoms improve. Because the drug may cause kidney damage, the nurse would teach the client to drink at least 1500 mL of fluid each day.

CJ Cognitive Skill

Take Action

Reference

Linton & Matteson, 2020, p. 854

Thinking Exercise 6B-8

Answers

A, B, D, E

Rationales

Clients with chronic inflammatory bowel disease such as ulcerative colitis (UC) also have a number of associated systemic health problems, including arthritis, hemorrhage, and liver disease (Choice A). They are also at risk for bleeding (hemorrhage) and anemia (Choices B and D). Local complications can include obstruction, abscesses, and fistulas (Choice E). UC can cause dehydration and hypokalemia from diarrhea, rather than fluid overload and hyperkalemia. Polycythemia vera is a disease affecting red blood cells.

CJ Cognitive Skill

Analyze Cues

Reference

Linton & Matteson, 2020, p. 755

Exemplar 6C. Urinary Incontinence (Medical-Surgical Nursing: Older Adult; Young Adult)

Thinking Exercise 6C-1

Answers

The nurse admits a 70-year-old obese female client who had a stroke a week ago to the rehabilitation unit in a skilled facility. The client has right-sided weakness and a history of diabetes mellitus, hypertension, and early dementia. She is able to communicate in short sentences but has trouble understanding what staff or family is saying. The transfer form states that the client needs help with all ADLs and she is incontinent of both bowel and bladder. The nurse contacts Rehabilitation Therapy for initial evaluation.

Rationales

The nurse is concerned that the client's one-sided weakness, early dementia, ADL dependence, and incontinence place her at risk for falling. She may not be able to express her needs because of aphasia that resulted from the stroke. A history of diabetes mellitus and hypertension likely contributed to her stroke, but they are not of immediate concern to the nurse at this time.

CJ Cognitive Skill

Recognize Cues

Reference

Linton & Matteson, 2020, pp. 402–420

Thinking Exercise 6C-2

Answers

Potential Complications	Risk to Client
Constipation	X
Neurovascular compromise	
Pulmonary edema	
Skin breakdown	X
Contractures	X
Deep vein thrombosis	X

Rationales

The client had a stroke, which causes impaired mobility. As a result the client is at risk for constipation, skin breakdown (especially in the presence of incontinence), contractures, and deep vein thrombosis. Pulmonary edema and neurovascular compromise are not typical stroke complications.

CJ Cognitive Skill

Analyze Cues

Reference

Linton & Matteson, 2020, pp. 402–420

Thinking Exercise 6C-3

Answers

The nurse analyzes the assessment data and determines that the client ***most likely*** has urge or functional urinary incontinence, which are both common in clients who experience a stroke. Other risk factors that place the client at risk for urinary incontinence include older age, impaired mobility, and diabetes mellitus.

Rationales

The client has one or two types of urinary incontinence that are common in clients who have a stroke. The client has an immediate urge to void and cannot easily prevent voiding. Because of her one-sided weakness, she is unable to get to the toilet at this time, causing functional incontinence. In addition to stroke, other risk factors for incontinence include being older (bladder muscle becomes weaker); diabetes mellitus, which can cause polyuria; and impaired mobility due to inability to ambulate.

CJ Cognitive Skill

Analyze Cues

Reference

Linton & Matteson, 2020, pp. 222, 402–420

Thinking Exercise 6C-4

Answers

Nursing Action	Indicated	Contraindicated	Non-Essential
Consult with the wound, ostomy, continence nurse (WOCN) to help plan the client's care.	X		
Place the client on a toileting schedule of every 1–2 hours while awake.	X		
Do not offer caffeinated beverages to the client.	X		
Teach the client how to do daily Kegel exercises.			X
Administer oxybutynin to relax the bladder and prevent spasms.		X	
Insert an indwelling urinary catheter to prevent skin breakdown.		X	

Rationales

The client continues to have urinary incontinence and may benefit from consultation with the WOCN. The client should be toileted every 1 to 2 hours and should not be offered any caffeinated beverages. Kegel exercises are not essential because they are most effective for clients who have stress incontinence. Oxybutynin works to relax the bladder and should not be given to older adults owing to side effects such as drowsiness and dry mouth. An indwelling urinary catheter could cause a catheter-related urinary tract infection (CAUTI).

CJ Cognitive Skill

Generate Solutions

Reference

Linton & Matteson, 2020, pp. 222–228

Thinking Exercise 6C-5

Answers

B, D, G, H

Rationales

The client has complications of urinary incontinence including skin breakdown and a yeast infection. The nurse would remind the assistive personnel (AP) to toilet the client every 1 to 2 hours, after meals, and when she first awakens to help keep her dry (Choices D, G, and H). In addition, the client needs treatment for the yeast infection, such as a topical antifungal cream (Choice B). This infection can be very painful, especially when the client's skin is gently washed and dried. The client should not stay in bed, to prevent problems of immobility. When the client is in bed, she should not wear a brief, which creates a dark moist environment for growth of yeast. Fluid restriction or an indwelling urinary catheter would likely cause a urinary tract infection.

CJ Cognitive Skill

Take Action

Reference

Linton & Matteson, 2020, pp. 222–228

Thinking Exercise 6C-6

Answers

Assessment Finding	Effective	Ineffective	Unrelated
Has regular continent bowel movements every 1–2 days.	X		
Is beginning to communicate her need to go to the toilet.	X		
Walks independently with a roller walker and stand-by supervision.	X		
Performs most ADLs independently.	X		
Experienced a fall last night while in the bathroom.		X	
Has symptoms of seasonal allergies.			X
Buttock and perineal skin intact and only slightly pink.	X		
Wears briefs during the day in case of incontinence episode.	X		

Rationales

The client's rehabilitation has been very successful, as evidenced by her ability to ambulate independently, improved communication, ADL independence, and healed skin. However, she recently experienced a fall, which is the most common predictor of future falls. Her seasonal allergy symptoms are not related to her primary health problem.

CJ Cognitive Skill

Evaluate Outcomes

Reference

Linton & Matteson, 2020, pp. 222–228

Thinking Exercise 6C-7

Answers

A, B, C, D, E, F, G

Rationales

All of these statements are correct regarding the function and side effects of bethanechol. This drug is given to clients who have a spastic or reflex bladder to stimulate voiding within an hour of administration (Choice B). If the client is unable to empty his bladder, urine is retained and the client is at risk for a urinary tract infection, which manifests as cloudy, foul-smelling urine (Choices A and G). Common side effects include sweating and flushing, but adverse reactions such as dizziness and tachycardia may occur (Choices C, E, and F). Clients who have asthma or a history of heart disease should therefore not take this medication (Choice D).

CJ Cognitive Skill

Take Action

Reference

Linton & Matteson, 2020, p. 219

Thinking Exercise 6C-8

Answers

A, B, D

Rationales

The quadriplegic client who had a spinal cord injury usually has a spastic or reflex bowel and bladder. There is no muscle control, so he would be unable to do Kegel exercises to strengthen pelvic muscles. After intestinal stimulation with a rectal suppository or oral laxative based on the client's usual bowel schedule, the client can usually empty his rectum (Choices A and B). Scheduling these medications around the client's usual bowel elimination pattern is most effective. The client usually does not require regular manual disimpaction or a mineral oil "cocktail," but this procedure may be needed if the client becomes constipated. An enema may also be needed. Adequate fluid intake (not restriction) and a high-fiber diet can help prevent constipation (Choice D).

CJ Cognitive Skill

Take Action

Reference

Linton & Matteson, 2020, pp. 230–232

CHAPTER 7 Nutrition

Answers With Rationales for Thinking Exercises

Exemplar 7A. Cholecystitis/Cholecystectomy (Medical-Surgical Nursing: Young Adult; Middle-Age Adult)

Thinking Exercise 7A-1

Answers

A 30-year-old female client is brought to the local emergency department by her partner with report of intermittent nausea, vomiting, and diarrhea for the past 3 days; weakness; and abdominal pain that ranges from moderate to severe. Her partner states that the client has had these symptoms since they ate at a new Italian restaurant 3 nights ago. She also has been complaining to her partner about having achiness in many of her joints (arthralgias). The client's medical history includes Crohn's disease, psoriasis, and gastroesophageal reflux disease (GERD), for which she takes multiple medications. Her current vital signs include:

- Temperature = 100.4°F (38°C)
- Apical pulse = 94 beats/min
- Respirations = 22 breaths/min
- Blood pressure = 98/50 mm Hg

An abdominal ultrasound shows cholelithiasis and cholecystitis.

Rationales

The client has had intermittent loss of fluids through vomiting and diarrhea, which puts her at risk for fluid and electrolyte imbalance. Her elevated temperature, tachycardia, and hypotension indicate that she is already dehydrated. Her respirations are slightly increased, but this could be due to the stress and anxiety of her illness. The abdominal ultrasound shows that she has cholecystitis and cholelithiasis, which likely is causing her abdominal pain. All of these signs and symptoms need to be managed at this time. The client's medical history is not of concern at this time.

CJ Cognitive Skill

Recognize Cues

Reference

Linton & Matteson, 2020, p. 778

Thinking Exercise 7A-2

Answers

Assessment Finding	Cholelithiasis/Cholecystitis	Crohn's Disease	Dehydration
Nausea and vomiting	X		
Diarrhea		X	
Abdominal pain	X	X	
Weakness	X	X	X
Arthralgias		X	

Continued

Assessment Finding	Cholelithiasis/Cholecystitis	Crohn's Disease	Dehydration
Tachycardia		X	X
Fever	X	X	X
Hypotension			X

Rationales

The client has a history of Crohn's disease, which may be controlled or have flare-ups (exacerbations). When episodes of this chronic inflammatory bowel disease (IBD) occur, the client usually has diarrhea, abdominal pain, and weakness due to loss of potassium (hypokalemia). Fever may also result from the presence of inflammation. Arthralgias (joint stiffness and discomfort) and other non-GI symptoms may occur in clients with chronic IBD. Clients who have cholecystitis may also report abdominal pain, nausea and vomiting, weakness (from vomiting), and possibly fever due to inflammation. Dehydration is caused by lack of body fluid volume, which decreases blood pressure and increases body temperature. As a compensatory action, the heart rate increases to circulate more quickly to provide oxygen and nutrients to body tissues.

CJ Cognitive Skill

Analyze Cues

Reference

Linton & Matteson, 2020, pp. 91, 755, 778

Thinking Exercise 7A-3

Answers

The nurse recognizes that the ***priority*** need for the client's care includes managing her abdominal pain, dehydration, and possible electrolyte imbalance. Nursing care for the client would include administration of an analgesic and an antiemetic medication.

Rationales

The priority care for this client is to manage dehydration and electrolyte imbalances and administer an antiemetic drug to prevent additional episodes of nausea and vomiting, which will prevent additional fluid and electrolyte losses. In addition, the nurse would promote comfort by administering an analgesic and positioning the client in a sitting position to help relax abdominal muscles.

CJ Cognitive Skill

Prioritize Hypotheses

Reference

Linton & Matteson, 2020, pp. 778–779

Thinking Exercise 7A-4

Answers

A, C, D, E, F, G, H

Rationales

A laparoscopic approach for the removal of the gallbladder (cholecystectomy) requires several small incisions through which the laparoscope is inserted to perform the procedure (Choice A). This surgery is performed under general anesthesia, which for some clients causes postoperative nausea and vomiting (Choice C). She will not need opioid analgesia delivered by a PCA pump. The client will need someone to drive her home because she may be drowsy from the anesthesia (Choice D). For postoperative care, the client will need to avoid high-fat foods because bile stored in the gallbladder helps to break down fats in the digestive system (Choice E). During her recovery, she will need to avoid lifting heavy objects and monitor the incisions for any signs and symptoms of infection (Choices G and H). Within usually 4 to 6 weeks, the surgeon will follow up with the client to ensure that healing has occurred (Choice F).

CJ Cognitive Skill

Generate Solutions

Reference

Linton & Matteson, 2020, pp. 779–782

Thinking Exercise 7A-5

Answers

Nursing Action	Potential Postoperative Complication	Appropriate Nursing Action for Postoperative Complication
1 Teach the client to monitor for rigid boardlike abdomen.	Surgical wound infection	**3** Teach the client to observe for foul-smelling, purulent drainage.
2 Maintain bilateral sequential compression devices.	Nausea and vomiting	**5** Administer an antiemetic medication.
3 Teach the client to observe for foul-smelling, purulent drainage.	Peritonitis	**1** Teach the client to monitor for rigid boardlike abdomen.
4 Apply supplemental oxygen at 2 L/min.	Respiratory complications	**6** Teach the client to deep breathe and cough every 2 hours.
5 Administer an antiemetic medication.	Venous thromboembolism	**2** Maintain bilateral sequential compression devices.
6 Teach the client to deep breathe and cough every 2 hours.		
7 Administer an analgesic mediation.		

Rationales

Postoperative complications are not common after a laparoscopic cholecystectomy but can occur. Because the client is typically discharged on the day of surgery, the nurse teaches the client and family to observe for complications that can occur later, such as surgical wound infection and peritonitis (Actions 1 and 3). Venous thromboembolism can also occur several days after surgery but can be prevented by having the client wear sequential compression devices (Action 2). Because nausea and vomiting can occur as a result of anesthesia, the nurse would administer an antiemetic medication (Action 5). Respiratory complications occur most often in obese clients, who may stay in the hospital overnight after surgery. Deep breathing and the use of incentive spirometry can help prevent these complications (Action 6).

CJ Cognitive Skill

Take Action

Reference

Linton & Matteson, 2020, pp. 284–295, 779–782

Thinking Exercise 7A-6

Answers

Assessment Finding	Effective	Ineffective	Unrelated
Abdominal incisions are closed and healed.	X		
No infection noted in abdominal incisions.	X		
States she has had several episodes of epigastric pain due to food intake.		X	
Breath sounds clear in all lung fields.	X		
Has had increasing problems with constipation since surgery.			X
Bowel sounds present in all four quadrants.	X		
Has red rash on both arms.			X
Has not had any signs or symptoms of deep venous thrombosis.	X		

Rationales

Even though the client had a cholecystectomy, she continues to have episodes of epigastric pain after she eats. Therefore the collaborative interventions for her care are not completely effective. Having constipation and a skin rash are not related to her care that was provided over the past month. However, she has no infection or other postoperative complications and her incisions are closed and healed. These findings indicate that her care was effective in meeting the expected outcomes.

CJ Cognitive Skill

Evaluate Outcomes

Reference

Linton & Matteson, 2020, pp. 284–295, 779–782

Thinking Exercise 7A-7

Answers

The nurse recognizes that the ***priority*** for the client's care is to implement actions that will help prevent postoperative <u>respiratory complications</u> and <u>deep vein thrombosis</u>.

Rationales

This client had a traditional open surgical approach, indicating a high abdominal incision that may affect her ability to take deep breaths or use the incentive spirometer without discomfort. Clients who have this type of operation tend to have shallow breathing, which can lead to atelectasis or pneumonia. They are also at high risk for venous thromboembolism—either deep vein thrombosis or, less commonly, pulmonary embolism.

CJ Cognitive Skill

Prioritize Hypotheses

Reference

Linton & Matteson, 2020, pp. 284–295, 779–782

Thinking Exercise 7A-8

Answers

B, C, D, F, G, I

Rationales

The use of T-tubes is not common today owing to the more common laparoscopic approach for removing the gallbladder. However, for some clients who have had repeated abdominal operations and/or have biliary obstruction, the traditional open approach is used for exploration. To prevent bile buildup during the initial healing time, the client may have a T-tube drainage system that drains by gravity and requires that the drainage bag be kept below the level of the abdomen (Choice D). A J-P drain is used to remove excess fluid near the surgical site. The amount and characteristics of the drainage from both tubes should be measured and documented every shift (Choice C). The NGT drainage should also be measured every shift (Choice F). To help prevent postoperative complications, the nurse would maintain sequential compression devices, teach the client how to do leg ankle exercises to promote venous return, and monitor the surgical dressing for bleeding or other drainage (Choices B, G, and I). While the client has the NGT, she would be NPO. The client should be sitting in a semi-Fowler position and use incentive spirometry every 2 hours to prevent respiratory complications.

CJ Cognitive Skill

Take Action

Reference

Linton & Matteson, 2020, pp. 284–295, 779–782

Exemplar 7B. Peptic Ulcer Disease (Medical-Surgical Nursing: Middle-Age Adult)

Thinking Exercise 7B-1

Answers

A 56-year-old male client visits the urgent care center for report of recent episodes of "stomach burning and pressure." He states that he had similar problems about 3 months ago, but antacids took care of it. However, for the past 2 weeks he has experienced intense upper abdominal pain and burning about 2 to 3 hours after most meals. He continues to take antacids but has noticed that eating more food also helps relieve the burning sensation. His medical history includes hypertension that is controlled with amlodipine, and multiple orthopedic injuries as a result of participation in high school and college athletics. For chronic pain that resulted from these injuries, the client alternates between taking acetaminophen and ibuprofen every day.

Rationales

The nurse would be concerned about the client's acute abdominal pain, especially as it is related to the client's food intake. The client's chronic pain requires daily over-the-counter medications, including ibuprofen, which can be very irritating to the lining of the stomach.

CJ Cognitive Skill

Recognize Cues

Reference

Linton & Matteson, 2020, p. 733

Thinking Exercise 7B-2

Answers

The nurse recognizes that the client's signs and symptoms are associated with <u>**peptic ulcer disease**</u>. Common complications of this health problem include <u>**hemorrhage,**</u> <u>**perforation,**</u> and <u>**obstruction**</u>.

Rationales

The client's signs and symptoms indicate that he has gastric irritation and most likely a duodenal ulcer, also known as peptic ulcer disease (PUD). If the ulcer erodes deep into the mucosal lining of the duodenum, bleeding or obstruction from inflammation may occur. In some cases the ulcer progresses through the duodenal wall, causing bowel perforation. Perforation would allow intestinal contents to leak into the peritoneal space, leading to peritonitis.

CJ Cognitive Skill

Analyze Cues

Reference

Linton & Matteson, 2020, pp. 733–734

Thinking Exercise 7B-3

Answers

B, C, D

Rationales

The client has been placed on drug therapy for possible peptic ulcer disease to manage his symptoms. Most gastric and duodenal ulcers are caused by *H. pylori* infection. Therefore the client would be tested for this bacterium during an EGD (not a colonoscopy) (Choices B and C). If the ulcer is causing bleeding, the client may be anemic, which would be evaluated with a hemoglobin and hematocrit laboratory test (Choice D). The client is not having problems with his liver or pancreas, and therefore tests such as amylase, lipase, albumin, and INR are not necessary.

CJ Cognitive Skill

Prioritize Hypotheses

Reference

Linton & Matteson, 2020, pp. 733–734

Thinking Exercise 7B-4

Answers

Health Teaching	Indicated	Contraindicated	Non-Essential
"Take your medications exactly as directed by your primary health care provider."	X		
"You may have small amounts of alcohol, but avoid smoking and other tobacco products."		X	

Health Teaching	Indicated	Contraindicated	Non-Essential
"Be aware that bismuth may turn your stool darker."	X		
"Take omeprazole at dinner time with food."		X	
"Avoid drugs that can irritate your GI system, especially aspirin, ibuprofen, and other NSAIDs."	X		
"Avoid high-protein foods, which are difficult to digest."			X

Rationales

The client with peptic ulcer disease should not have any alcohol or tobacco products, which could irritate the mucosal lining of the digestive tract and stimulate acid secretions. Omeprazole can be taken with or without food but is best taken first thing in the morning. Foods that the client should avoid are spicy foods, which stimulate gastric secretions. High-protein foods do not need to be avoided.

CJ Cognitive Skill

Generate Solutions

Reference

Linton & Matteson, 2020, pp. 733–735

Thinking Exercise 7B-5

Answers

A, B, E, F, G, H

Rationales

All of these choices are correct, except that there is no dye or other contrast medium that is used in an EGD, and allergies to shellfish or iodine do not need to be considered. An EGD is performed while the client is under moderate sedation rather than general anesthesia.

CJ Cognitive Skill

Take Action

Reference

Linton & Matteson, 2020, p. 705

Thinking Exercise 7B-6

Answers

Nurses' Notes

7/22/21 1400 Client states that he is feeling much better and has only occasional epigastric burning. Vital signs include: temperature = 98°F (36.7°C), pulse = 78 beats/min, respirations = 18 breaths/min, blood pressure = 158/88 mm Hg. Oxygen saturation = 97%. No adventitious breath sounds. Bowel sounds present in all 4 quadrants. States that the arthritis in his knees has recently worsened, but he has gained 14 lb (6.4 kg) in the past few months. ------------ *L.D. Santos, LPN*

Rationales

The client's signs and symptoms have improved, and most of his assessment data are within usual limits, except for his blood pressure, which is elevated. He has gained weight, which is causing more knee pain, but these changes are not related to his peptic ulcer disease.

CJ Cognitive Skill

Evaluate Outcomes

Reference

Linton & Matteson, 2020, pp. 733–735

Thinking Exercise 7B-7

Answers

A, B, C, D, E, G

Rationales

The client is experiencing upper GI bleeding, which requires resting the GI tract by using a nasogastric tube connected to continuous low suction and placing the client on NPO status (Choices A and B). The nurse would monitor the client's vital signs frequently to determine if too much blood loss is leading to hypovolemia and possibly hypovolemic shock (Choice C). Lab tests would include a complete blood cell count to determine if the client is anemic (Choice D). To replace fluids and possibly blood, the client would need IV access (Choice E), but antibiotic therapy would likely not be needed. Placing the client in a sitting position would prevent aspiration from vomiting (Choice G).

CJ Cognitive Skill

Take Action

Reference

Linton & Matteson, 2020, pp. 734–737

Thinking Exercise 7B-8

Answers

History and Physical | **Nurses' Notes** | **Vital Signs** | **Laboratory Results**

- Pain = 9/10
- Temperature = 101.4°F (38.6°C)
- Pulse = 102 beats/min
- Respirations = 28 breaths/min
- Blood pressure = 110/62 mm Hg
- Oxygen saturation = 95% (on room air [RA])
- Abdomen tender, particularly in the right and left upper quadrants

Rationales

The client has severe pain, fever, tachycardia, and tachypnea, all of which are not within usual normal limits. The nurse would be concerned that the client may have a perforation or obstruction caused by peptic ulcer disease.

CJ Cognitive Skill

Recognize Cues

Reference

Linton & Matteson, 2020, pp. 734–737

CHAPTER 8 Mobility

Answers With Rationales for Thinking Exercises

Exemplar 8A. Sports Injury (Pediatric Nursing: School-Age Child)

Thinking Exercise 8A-1

Answers

Client Finding	Requires Immediate Follow-Up
Abrasion on left leg	X
Painful right knee	X
Respirations = 22 breaths/min	
Swollen right knee	X
History of muscular dystrophy (MD)	

Rationales

The child has an acute right knee injury that manifests with pain and swelling. In addition, he has an abrasion on his left leg that could get infected if not treated. His vital signs are within normal/usual limits for his age. His history of muscular dystrophy (MD) could have contributed to his injury but does not affect his immediate care.

CJ Cognitive Skill

Recognize Cues

Reference

Leifer, 2019, pp. 572–573

Thinking Exercise 8A-2

Answers

The nurse recognizes that the child may have fallen due to <u>muscle weakness</u>, which is common in children who have muscular dystrophy. His knee swelling and pain are probably the result of <u>ligament damage</u>.

Rationales

The child with MD typically has muscle weakness, which could have contributed to his fall and subsequent injury. The only symptoms he has are knee swelling and pain rather than changes in alignment, so he likely does not have a fracture. An x-ray would rule out bone involvement. He also does not likely have arthritis because of his young age, although some types of arthritis can occur in his age-group.

CJ Cognitive Skill

Analyze Cues

Reference

Leifer, 2019, pp. 572–573, 581–582

Thinking Exercise 8A-3

Answers

B, C, F

Rationales

The ***priority*** for management of sports injuries require management with RICE (rest, ice, compression, and elevation) to decrease swelling and pain (Choices B, C, and F). Heat or warm compresses would increase blood flow and therefore increase swelling and pain. The child does not need a strong analgesic for pain, nor does he need a cast. After the initial symptoms subside and he begins to heal, a physical therapist may be appropriate, but not at this time.

CJ Cognitive Skill

Prioritize Hypotheses

Reference

Leifer, 2019, pp. 572–573

Thinking Exercise 8A-4

Answers

Nursing Action	Indicated	Contraindicated	Non-Essential
Perform frequent neurovascular checks ("circ checks") of the client's right foot.	X		
Place the client in a high-Fowler bed position.			X
Monitor the surgical dressing for drainage or blood.	X		
Take frequent vital signs until the client is fully awake.	X		
Determine the client's level of consciousness (LOC).	X		
Do not elevate the client's surgical leg to promote perfusion.		X	

Rationales

The child had arthroscopic surgery and would have a surgical dressing that the nurse would monitor for drainage or blood. The dressing and edema from surgery may affect arterial blood flow to the affected foot, and therefore the nurse would perform frequent circulation checks to ensure adequate circulation. Checking the client's LOC and vital signs is common practice for any client who has had surgery. The child's surgical leg will need to be elevated to help reduce swelling, so preventing elevation would be contraindicated. It is not necessary to place the child in a high-Fowler or sitting position.

CJ Cognitive Skill

Generate Solutions

References

Leifer, 2019, p. 577; Linton & Matteson, 2020, pp. 848, 851

Thinking Exercise 8A-5

Answers

The nurse's ***most appropriate*** action at this time is to notify the registered nurse in charge and continue monitoring the client's circulation status.

Rationales

Increased pain, sensory changes, and a weaker pedal pulse are indicators of possible impairment in arterial blood flow. Therefore, after notifying the registered nurse, the nurse would continue to monitor circulation to determine if it worsens.

CJ Cognitive Skill

Take Action

References

Leifer, 2019, p. 577; Linton & Matteson, 2020, pp. 848, 851

Thinking Exercise 8A-6

Answers

Client Finding	Effective	Ineffective	Unrelated
Arthroscopic incisions are closed and healed	X		
No infection noted in arthroscopic incisions	X		
States he has been feeling more weak and tired when he plays sports			X
Says that his right knee feels much better since his surgery	X		
Has increasing problems with constipation since surgery			X
Mother says that she still notices a limp in his right leg at times		X	
States he has problems sleeping since he had his surgery			X
Is getting better grades in school this term			X

Rationales

Healed incisions that are not infected are desired postoperative outcomes. The surgery appears successful because the child states he has less pain in his right knee. However, he still has a limp, which may be due to reluctance of the child to bear complete weight on the injured leg or due to incomplete soft tissue (ligament) healing. The other findings are not related to the child's surgery.

CJ Cognitive Skill

Evaluate Outcomes

References

Leifer, 2019, p. 577; Linton & Matteson, 2020, pp. 848, 851

Thinking Exercise 8A-7

Answers

An 8-year-old girl fell from a scooter onto an asphalt neighborhood road. When her grandfather went outside to check on her, he found her crying and holding her left ankle. When he helped her to a standing position, the child could not bear weight on it. On admission to the emergency department, the nurse notes that the child's left ankle is swollen and beginning to discolor. She is crying and says that it hurts when she tries to walk on it. She also states that her right wrist hurts. Both knees are scraped and bruised with dirt and pieces of stone in the wounds.

Rationales

The child injured her left ankle as a result of falling off a scooter, as manifested by inability to bear weight on the affected leg and a swollen, painful, and discolored ankle. She also has abrasions on both knees, which disrupted skin integrity and could get infected. In addition, she states that her right wrist is painful.

CJ Cognitive Skill

Recognize Cues

Reference

Leifer, 2019, pp. 572–573

Thinking Exercise 8A-8

Answers

B, C, D, G

Rationales

The child had surgery to repair badly torn right ankle ligaments. He has a leg splint that is held in place with a compression bandage. This immobilization device and inflammation from surgery can cause decreased perfusion (arterial blood flow) to the surgical foot and toes. Therefore the nurse would carefully monitor neurovascular status (circulation) (Choice B). To decrease edema formation, the nurse would elevate the surgical leg on pillows and monitor the child's pain (Choices C and D). As for all postoperative clients, the client would remain NPO until he is fully awake and oriented (Choice G). The client would likely not be allowed to bear weight on the surgical leg for several weeks, so he would need to use a swing-through gait when walking with crutches rather than a three-point gait. He will not need heparin for this same-day surgery. The child's mother can stay with him during recovery from surgery.

CJ Cognitive Skill

Take Action

References

Leifer, 2019, pp. 572–573; Linton & Matteson, 2020, pp. 888–889

Exemplar 8B. Fractured Arm/Cast Care (Pediatric Nursing: Preschool-Age Child)

Thinking Exercise 8B-1

Answers

A 4-year-old girl was riding her bicycle on the sidewalk in front of her house when she hit uneven concrete and lost her balance. Although she was wearing a helmet, elbow pads, and knee pads, she injured her left lower arm when she was projected over the bicycle handlebars. Her mother took her to the pediatric urgent care center for evaluation. On admission the nurse noted that the client had a large bruise and swelling on the radial side of her left lower arm. Her mother told the nurse that she does not want her daughter to have any "shots" because she does not believe in immunizations.

Rationales

The child injured her left lower arm when she was projected over the bicycle handlebars. As a result, she has a large bruise and swelling. Although she is 4 years old, she has not had any immunizations, which puts her at risk for common childhood diseases.

CJ Cognitive Skill

Recognize Cues

Reference

Leifer, 2019, pp. 577–580, 749

Thinking Exercise 8B-2

Answers

The nurse recognizes that the child will need a distraction during the treatment of her fracture, such as <u>playing a learning game on a personal electronic device,</u> because this play activity is appropriate for her developmental age.

Rationales

The preschool child begins to play learning games using a personal handheld device such as an iPad. She can likely do that with one hand to help distract her during fracture reduction. The recommended screen time for a child her age is 1 hour a day. A 500-piece puzzle is more than a preschool child would be able to assemble. Modeling clay or slime would take additional ingredients and would need two hands to complete.

CJ Cognitive Skill

Analyze Cues

Reference

Leifer, 2019, pp. 433–434

Thinking Exercise 8B-3

Answers

The ***priority*** for nursing care of the child at this time is to provide <u>discharge teaching</u> and manage the child's <u>pain</u>.

Rationales

The nurse prepares to provide discharge teaching for the child's mother because the child's fracture was managed and immobilized with a cast. The nurse would also collect data about the child's pain by using an appropriate pain scale to determine the need for intervention.

CJ Cognitive Skill

Prioritize Hypotheses

Reference

Leifer, 2019, pp. 577–580, 749

Thinking Exercise 8B-4

Answers

Discharge Teaching	Indicated	Contraindicated	Non-Essential
"It's OK if your daughter's cast gets wet."	X		
"Remind your daughter to keep her arm down by her side most of the time."		X	
"To help with healing, offer your daughter foods high in protein."	X		
"Let your daughter play whenever she wants."			X
"Check every day to determine if your daughter's cast is too tight or too loose."	X		
"Report changes in your daughter's left hand and fingers such as color changes, temperature changes, and increased pain."	X		
"I'd like to review why your daughter needs her preschool vaccines."	X		

Rationales

The nurse would reinforce discharge teaching related to the child's fracture and cast. Unlike a plaster cast, she has a synthetic cast, which can get wet. The nurse would remind the child's mother that she should check if the cast becomes too tight or too loose, and to report any changes that indicate that the circulation is impaired. Initially the affected arm should be elevated (and not down by her side) to decrease or prevent swelling. Foods high in protein and vitamin C promote healing and should be encouraged. The nurse would also remind the child's mother about the importance of getting her immunized before she starts kindergarten.

CJ Cognitive Skill

Generate Solutions

Reference

Leifer, 2019, pp. 577–580

Thinking Exercise 8B-5

Answers

A, C, D, E, F, G

Rationales

The nurse would show the child the cast cutter to demonstrate that it will not cut her skin while the cast is being removed (Choice A). She will not need an analgesic during this procedure. The skin under the cast may be dry and flaky and require frequent applications of lotion after washing with mild soap and water (Choices C, D, and E). After she returns home, the child would be able to return to previous activities (Choices F and G).

CJ Cognitive Skill

Take Action

Reference

Leifer, 2019, pp. 577–580

Thinking Exercise 8B-6

Answers

Client Finding	Progressing Well	Not Progressing Well
Skin on both arms healthy, hydrated, and warm	X	
Lower left arm slightly smaller than lower right arm		X
Has returned to riding her scooter and bicycle with training wheels	X	
Is very inquisitive and excited to start kindergarten next month	X	
Tells the nurse she looks forward to getting an allowance to help with daily chores	X	
Has gained 5 lb (2.3 kg) and 2 inches (5.1 cm) since her 4-year-old annual visit	X	
Has not received any recommended preschool immunizations		X

Rationales

All of these findings show that the child is progressing well after her injury, with the exception that her previously fractured arm is slightly smaller than her left arm. This change may be due to mild muscle atrophy from disuse. However, it is possible that if the child is right-handed, she may have a larger right lower arm due to arm dominance. The child has not received recommended preschool immunizations, which places her at risk for disease and transmission of disease to other children.

CJ Cognitive Skill

Evaluate Outcomes

Reference

Leifer, 2019, pp. 433–434, 577–580

Thinking Exercise 8B-7

Answers

The nurse recognizes that the client is at risk for several complications of his fracture or fracture management, especially compartment syndrome and osteomyelitis.

Rationales

The child had an open, compound fracture, which results in swelling from edema or blood accumulation. Although not common, compartment syndrome occurs when swelling compresses the compartments within the tissues of the lower arm, causing an acute decrease in perfusion or arterial blood flow. This is a potentially limb-threatening complication. Osteomyelitis can occur because the open fracture disrupted the skin and underlying tissues, allowing microbes to enter, causing a wound and possibly bone infection.

CJ Cognitive Skill

Analyze Cues

Reference

Leifer, 2019, pp. 577–580

Thinking Exercise 8B-8

Answers

A 4-year-old girl was a rear seat passenger in her sister's car when she had a motor vehicle accident. After examination by first responders, both sisters were taken to the emergency department for evaluation. The nurse prepares to assess the child, who is crying and asking for her mother. On examination, the nurse notes old bruising on her chest and an old scar on her right upper thigh. She also notes swelling of her right upper arm. X-ray results reveal three old rib fractures and a new right condylar fracture above the elbow.

Rationales

The child has a new arm fracture that needs to be managed, but she also has older injuries. The old scar, bruising, and previous fractures could indicate child abuse and needs to be investigated.

CJ Cognitive Skill

Recognize Cues

Reference

Leifer, 2019, pp. 577–580, 587–590

CHAPTER 9 Metabolism

Answers With Rationales for Thinking Exercises

Exemplar 9A. Diabetes Mellitus (Medical-Surgical Nursing: Middle-Age Adult)

Thinking Exercise 9A-1

Answers

- Oriented × 3, follows all commands
- Reports blurry vision
- Lung fields clear throughout
- Bowel sounds present in all quadrants
- Reports nausea and abdominal discomfort
- Left large toe amputation
- Right lateral lower extremity ulcer with red edges and purulent exudate
- Reports not sleeping well the night before due to needing to urinate every 2 hours

Rationales

The client reports nocturia, or the need to urinate several times during the night. Nocturia in a client with diabetes is usually associated with acute hyperglycemia, can lead to dehydration, and must be followed up by the nurse to ensure adequate hydration. A client with a high blood glucose level may also experience blurred vision, nausea, abdominal pain, and headaches. The nurse would follow up on these findings to determine if they are associated with hyperglycemia or another disorder. Additionally, the nurse would complete a more thorough assessment of the client's right lower extremity ulcer. The presence of purulent exudate indicates an infection, which must be treated quickly to prevent a blood infection called sepsis. Toe amputations occurred over the past 2 years and are not an acute concern requiring follow-up. The other findings are within normal or usual limits.

CJ Cognitive Skill

Recognize Cues

References

Linton & Matteson, 2020, pp. 620–627, 967–972; Williams, 2018, pp. 765–766

Thinking Exercise 9A-2

Answers

Client Findings	Hyperglycemia	Dehydration	Infection
Polyuria	X		
Nausea	X		
Tachycardia		X	X
Nonhealing wound	X		X
Polyphagia	X		

Rationales

Several findings are consistent with acute hyperglycemia. Polydipsia, polyuria, and polyphagia are classic symptoms associated with hyperglycemia. Polyphagia is the term used for excessive hunger. Although there is a large amount of glucose in the body, the cells are unable to use it. Starving cells relay messages that tell the body to consume more food. Polyuria is excessive urination and occurs as the body attempts to excrete excessive glucose. A client with a high blood glucose level may also experience nausea and abdominal pain secondary to gastroparesis.

Symptoms of dehydration are tachycardia, hypotension, poor skin turgor, and dry oral mucosa. The client's wound is not healing properly owing to infection, as manifested by purulent drainage and an elevated white blood cell count. An infection can cause hyperglycemia due to the body's response to increased physiologic stress, and bacteria thrive in the presence of elevated blood glucose. Wound healing and infections are also a complication of diabetes mellitus and result from inadequate blood supply to wound sites. Symptoms of a blood infection (sepsis) are fever, tachycardia, tachypnea, confusion, and decreased urine output.

CJ Cognitive Skill

Analyze Cues

Reference

Linton & Matteson, 2020, pp. 91–92, 967–990

Thinking Exercise 9A-3

Answers

Client Health Problems	Top Two Priority Client Health Problems
Fluid volume deficit related to hyperglycemia	X
Lack of knowledge of dietary management for diabetes mellitus	
Ineffective therapeutic glucose management	X
Impaired skin integrity related to neurologic and circulatory changes	
Infection related to nonintact skin secondary to diabetic ulcers	

Rationales

Prioritizing client needs requires the nurse to evaluate the seriousness of physiologic conditions, risks and benefits of interventions, and client safety. The client's hyperglycemia is the underlying condition leading to other client problems including dehydration, infection, and skin ulcers. Ongoing ineffective management of the client's glucose can result in further complications and life-threatening conditions. Glucose management is therefore a top priority. Dehydration or fluid volume deficit is also a top priority because further depletion of intravascular fluids can result in decreased cardiac output and inadequate perfusion of vital organs. Severe dehydration is a life-threatening condition. Impaired skin integrity and infection are not currently emergent and should be addressed after fluid and glycemic maintenance is established. Knowledge deficits are essential to address and promote the client's self-management of diabetes mellitus. At this time the client's physiologic needs are a greater priority than needs for education.

CJ Cognitive Skill

Prioritize Hypotheses

Reference

Linton & Matteson, 2020, pp. 967–990

Thinking Exercise 9A-4

Answers

The desired outcomes for the client are that she will have blood glucose maintained within 70 and 130 mg/dL (3.9 and 7.2 mmol/L) and pulse and blood pressure within usual limits. To meet these outcomes, the nurse collaborates with the health care team.

Rationales

The client's priority problems are (1) ineffective therapeutic glucose management, and (2) fluid volume deficit related to hyperglycemia. Desired outcomes for ineffective therapeutic glucose management focus on returning the client's blood glucose level to normal limits, 70 to 130 mg/dL (3.9 to 7.2 mmol/L), and maintaining normal blood glucose levels via nursing interventions and client's self-care measures. The best outcome for fluid volume deficit is the establishment of normal extracellular fluid volume. Extracellular volume is most effectively evaluated through blood pressure and heart rate.

CJ Cognitive Skill

Generate Solutions

Reference

Linton & Matteson, 2020, pp. 967–990

Thinking Exercise 9A-5

Answers

Nursing Action	Indicated	Contraindicated	Non-Essential
Obtain the client's current blood glucose level.	X		
Initiate oxygen therapy per nasal cannula.			X
Administer subcutaneous insulin per the sliding scale.		X	
Help the client to drink 120 mL of fruit juice.	X		
Notify the primary health care provider.	X		
Administer 1 mg intramuscular glucagon.			X
Reassess the glucose level 15 minutes after treatment is administered.	X		

Rationales

The nurse's assessment indicates that the client is experiencing a hypoglycemic episode. Symptoms of hypoglycemia include confusion, irritability, blurred or double vision, headache, tachycardia and palpitations, and cool, clammy skin. The nurse would perform a point-of-care test to determine the client's current blood glucose level. Management of a hypoglycemic episode is based on blood glucose level and client symptoms. Because this client can follow simple commands, the nurse would administer 10 to 15 g of oral carbohydrates. A half-cup or 120 mL of fruit juice is indicated and appropriate for the treatment of this client's hypoglycemic episode. The nurse would also continue to monitor the client, reassess the glucose level in 15 minutes, and notify the primary health care provider. As the client's glucose level improves, the nurse will provide the client with a small snack of carbohydrates and protein. The nurse would not administer insulin to this client who is already hypoglycemic, as this would further decrease the blood glucose level. Intramuscular glucagon is not indicated for mild or moderate hypoglycemia. It is used to treat severe hypoglycemia when a client is unable to swallow and no intravenous access is present. Oxygen is not indicated at this time, as it has no impact on the client's symptoms associated with hypoglycemia.

CJ Cognitive Skill

Take Action

Reference

Linton & Matteson, 2020, pp. 990–993

Thinking Exercise 9A-6

Answers

B, E, F

Rationales

This client must be taught to manage blood glucose levels and minimize the risk for further injury. The nurse would reinforce teaching related to proper foot care and maintenance of skin ulcers. Behaviors demonstrating that the client understands how to prevent foot injury include cleansing and inspecting feet daily, wearing clean socks and properly fitting shoes, avoiding walking in bare feet even inside the home, trimming toenails properly, and reporting nonhealing breaks in the skin of the feet to the primary health care provider (Choice B). Management of sick days would be reinforced, including checking blood glucose levels every 4 hours, eating regular meals, drinking adequate fluids, and taking medications as prescribed (Choice E). Clients are taught that exercise can improve blood glucose control, reduce cardiovascular risks, contribute to weight loss, and improve well-being. The nurse would reinforce that both aerobic exercise and resistance training are appropriate types of exercise for this client (Choice F).

CJ Cognitive Skill

Evaluate Outcomes

Reference

Linton & Matteson, 2020, pp. 967–990

Thinking Exercise 9A-7

Answers

Client's Medication List	Appropriate Action or Indication for Each Medication on Client's List
Metformin 500 mg orally twice daily	**8** Decreases glucose production by the liver and increases tissue response to insulin
Exenatide 5 mcg subcutaneous injection twice daily before breakfast and dinner	**2** Stimulates insulin release, suppresses glucagon release, and reduces appetite
Gabapentin 300 mg orally once daily before bed	**5** Relieves neuropathic pain
Glipizide 10 mg orally once daily with breakfast	**6** Promotes insulin secretion by the pancreas
Lisinopril 10 mg orally once daily	**7** Decreases blood pressure and helps prevent kidney disease

Rationales

Metformin, glipizide, and exenatide are all antidiabetic medications used to treat diabetes mellitus type 2. Glipizide helps the pancreas to secrete more insulin. Metformin decreases the production of glucose by the liver and increases the uptake of glucose in tissues. Exenatide belongs to a class of drugs called incretin mimetics and has many actions including stimulating the release of insulin, suppressing glucagon release, and reducing appetite. Gabapentin is an antiepileptic drug (AED) that is also used to treat nerve pain associated with diabetic neuropathy or shingles. Lisinopril belongs to a class of drugs known as angiotensin-converting enzyme (ACE) inhibitors, and is used to treat high blood pressure and heart failure. In clients who have diabetes, it helps to prevent kidney disease from progressing by reducing the amount of protein that goes unfiltered by the kidneys and spills into the urine.

CJ Cognitive Skill

Analyze Cues

Reference

Linton & Matteson, 2020, pp. 967–993

Thinking Exercise 9A-8

Answers

A, B, D, E

Rationales

Hypoglycemia, a common complication of diabetes mellitus, is caused by too much insulin or not enough food. Timing insulin administration with food consumption would assist in the prevention of hypoglycemic episodes (Choice A). The nurse must understand the onset and peak of insulin preparations so that food may be provided at the appropriate times. The nurse must also teach the client to recognize early signs of hypoglycemia so that interventions can be implemented quickly (Choice D). Other complications associated with diabetes mellitus are generally related to microvascular and macrovascular changes. Nephropathy, neuropathy, and retinopathy result from microvascular changes. Macrovascular changes cause coronary artery disease, cerebral vascular disease, and peripheral vascular disease. To prevent injury secondary to visual disturbances caused by retinopathy, the nurse ensures that the room has proper lighting so that the client can safety move around the unfamiliar space including ambulating to the bathroom (Choice B). Peripheral neuropathy impairs sensation in peripheral nerves, especially the feet. Wearing properly fitting shoes minimizes the risk of tissue injury due to abrasions or rubbing that may occur but cannot be felt (Choice E).

CJ Cognitive Skill

Take Action

Reference

Linton & Matteson, 2020, pp. 967–993

Exemplar 9B. Hypothyroidism (Medical-Surgical Nursing: Middle-Age Adult)

Thinking Exercise 9B-1

Answers

B, C, E, F, H

Rationales

The client's actual body temperature is lower than what is considered normal body temperature, but it is not low enough to be considered hypothermia. There are many conditions that manifest with a lower than normal body temperature and cause a client to feel cold. The client is also experiencing bradycardia and recently underwent surgery for a total hip arthroplasty. The nurse would ask questions that provide data on a variety of conditions associated with these symptoms, including questions related to oxygenation, perfusion, metabolic rate, and inflammation. Asking about changes in her mental status and energy level focuses on perfusion, oxygenation, and metabolic rate (Choices B and E). Questions focused on changes in muscles and joints provide the nurse with data related to inflammation and myopathies (Choice C). Asking about shortness of breath assists the nurse in evaluating cardiac and respiratory conditions including infection, heart failure, and pulmonary embolism (Choice F). Weight changes may be related to metabolism, fluid retention or loss, and mental health issues (Choice H).

CJ Cognitive Skill

Recognize Cues

Reference

Linton & Matteson, 2020, pp. 544–545, 646–649, 956–961

Thinking Exercise 9B-2

Answers

Client Findings	Anemia	Hypothyroidism	Heart Failure
Fatigue	X	X	X
Generalized edema		X	X
Frequent headaches	X	X	
Weight gain		X	X
Numbness in extremities	X	X	

Rationales

The client's symptoms are related to several conditions including anemia, hypothyroidism, and heart failure. All three conditions result in fatigue and activity intolerance: anemia due to a lack of oxygen transportation to organs, hypothyroidism due to decreased metabolic rate, and heart failure due to decreased cardiac output and oxygen perfusion. Clients who have anemia or hypothyroidism experience frequent headaches and numbness in extremities. Headaches due to inadequate thyroid hormones are most commonly migraines, and headaches associated with anemia are due to inadequate oxygen perfusion to the brain. Numbness in extremities is also related to inadequate oxygen perfusion in clients with anemia and is related to peripheral neuropathy in clients with hypothyroidism. Generalized edema and weight gain are both manifestations of hypothyroidism and heart failure. Edema and weight gain in a client with heart failure are related to fluid retention. In a client with hypothyroidism, weight gain is related to a decreased metabolic rate, and edema is related to possible myxedema and is generally present on the face, hands, and feet.

CJ Cognitive Skill

Analyze Cues

Reference

Linton & Matteson, 2020, pp. 544–545, 646–649, 956–961

Thinking Exercise 9B-3

Answers

The client is diagnosed with hypothyroidism. The top three ***priority*** problems for this client are activity intolerance related to <u>fatigue</u>, weight gain related to <u>decreased metabolic rate</u>, and potential impaired skin integrity related to <u>dry skin</u> and <u>decreased mobility</u>.

Rationales

Decreased metabolic rates associated with hypothyroidism lead to fatigue and lethargy, which can interfere with clients' ability to tolerate activities and complete ADLs. Weight gain is also related to a decreased metabolic rate. Clients frequently gain weight even with decreased intake of food. Clients with hypothyroidism also have dry, pale, and cool skin. The client is at risk of skin tears and wounds due to the dryness of the skin and is at risk of pressure injuries due to decreased mobility.

CJ Cognitive Skill

Prioritize Hypotheses

Reference

Linton & Matteson, 2020, pp. 544–545, 956–961

Thinking Exercise 9B-4

Answers

Nursing Action	Indicated	Contraindicated	Non-Essential
Teach the client about hormone replacement therapy.	X		
Encourage the client to integrate periods of rest during ADLs.	X		
Assist the client in bathing twice a day to decrease skin drying.		X	
Consult a registered dietitian nutritionist for diet and food option recommendations.	X		
Wear a cloth mask when outside the home to minimize risk of infection transmission.			X

Rationales

Medical treatment for hypothyroidism is the administration of oral thyroid replacement hormones. The client needs to be taught when to take the hormones, when to expect a therapeutic response, and when to report side effects or adverse reactions to the primary health care provider. The client is experiencing activity intolerance related to fatigue. Rest periods during ADLs will enable the client to conserve energy and complete more activities. Impaired skin integrity frequently occurs in clients with hypothyroidism because of dry skin and inactivity. The client would be taught to assess skin daily, use soap-free and non-drying products to bathe, avoid daily tub baths and showers, and change positions at least every 2 hours. The client's decreased metabolic rate may cause increased weight and nutritional deficits. Consulting a registered dietitian nutritionist will help the client to make food choices for gradual weight loss while meeting nutritional needs. Hypothyroidism is not an infectious condition.

CJ Cognitive Skill

Generate Solutions

Reference

Linton & Matteson, 2020, pp. 956–961

Thinking Exercise 9B-5

Answers

Client Questions	Appropriate Nurse's Response for Each Client Question
"Will hormone replacement therapy help me lose weight?"	**4** "Your weight should normalize as your hormone levels are corrected."
"Why did the registered dietarian nutritionist recommend a high-fiber diet with fresh fruits and raw vegetables?"	**1** "Hypothyroidism can cause constipation. Increasing your fluid and fiber intake may minimize this issue."
I feel like my brain isn't functioning correctly. Why am I having trouble thinking?"	**5** "Mental slowness is a symptom of hypothyroidism and should improve with treatment."
"What is the best time for me to take the prescribed levothyroxine dose?"	**3** "Thirty to 60 minutes before breakfast is the best time to take your medication."

Rationales

The nurse provides accurate and therapeutic responses to the client's questions. Most of the symptoms associated with hypothyroidism will be resolved once hormone levels have been corrected. This includes weight gain and neurologic impairments. Constipation is a common manifestation of hypothyroidism. Eating a high-fiber diet with fresh fruits and raw vegetables, along with increased fluid intake and increased activity, will help the client manage bowel issues. Levothyroxine should be administered at the same time each day and on an empty stomach. Taking this hormone replacement 30 to 60 minutes before breakfast each morning is recommended to maximize the drug's effectiveness.

CJ Cognitive Skill

Take Action

Reference

Linton & Matteson, 2020, pp. 956–961

Thinking Exercise 9B-6

Answers

- Vital signs:
  - Temperature = 98.6°F (37°C)
  - Heart rate (HR) = 66 beats/min
  - Blood pressure (BP) = 124/32 mm Hg
  - Respirations = 12 breaths/min
- Alert and oriented × 3
- Client reports feeling fatigue after completing ADLs
- Respirations equal and unlabored
- Lung fields clear throughout
- Client denies pain or stiffness
- Skin cool, dry, and without generalized edema
- Client reports numbness and tingling in extremities
- No change in weight in past 3 weeks
- Thyroid tests
  - Free T_4 = 0.8 ng/dL (10.4 pmol/L)
  - TSH = 4.6 mIU/L

Rationales

The client's free T_4 has increased and is at the low range of normal (0.8 to 2.8 ng/dL). The client's TSH level remains elevated (normal range is 0.4 to 4.0 mU/L). Elevated TSH indicates that the thyroid continues to underproduce thyroid hormones and needs further stimulation. Symptoms associated with hypothyroidism will resolved once hormone levels have been corrected. Treatment with oral thyroid replacement therapy usually takes 6 weeks to correct hormone levels, but clients will begin to see improvement within 2 to 3 weeks. Increased body temperature and heart rate are positive signs that the client's metabolic rate is increasing. Although the client continues to feel fatigue after completing ADLs, this is an improvement from her previous state of lethargy. The client's denial of pain indicates she is no longer experiencing headaches or joint discomfort. A lack of generalized edema is also an indication that the client is improving.

CJ Cognitive Skill

Evaluate Outcomes

Reference

Linton & Matteson, 2020, pp. 956–961

Thinking Exercise 9B-7

Answers

C, E, G

Rationales

Myxedema coma is a life-threatening complication of hypothyroidism and can be triggered by infection, trauma, or exposure to cold. Symptoms of myxedema coma are hypothermia (Choice C), decreased respiratory rate (Choice E), depressed mental function, and decreased level of consciousness (Choice G). Blood glucose levels and cardiac output decrease if interventions are not implemented early. Death can occur from cardiac or respiratory failure. The other client findings are complications of hypothyroidism, but they are not life-threatening and do not need to be reported immediately.

CJ Cognitive Skill

Recognize Cues

Reference

Linton & Matteson, 2020, pp. 956–961

CHAPTER 10 Cellular Regulation: Breast Cancer *(Medical-Surgical Nursing: Middle-Age Adult)*

Answers With Rationales for Thinking Exercises

Thinking Exercise 10-1

Answers

A, C, E, F

Rationales

The risk factors for this client include alcohol use, nulliparity, a strong family history of breast cancer (*BRCA2* positive), and being a female (Choices A, C, E, and F). Being over 50 years of age and having a late menopause are other risk factors for breast cancer, but these factors do not apply to this client.

CJ Cognitive Skill

Recognize Cues

Reference

Linton & Matteson, 2020, p. 1033

Thinking Exercise 10-2

Answers

Based on the stage of the client's cancer, the nurse recognizes that she may select breast-conserving treatment, which includes **lumpectomy** and **external beam radiation**.

Rationales

Breast-conserving treatment avoids removal of one or both breasts. Many women who have early-stage cancer have success with removal of the cancerous lesion (lumpectomy) followed by weeks of external beam radiation. Breast construction is usually done if the breast is removed (mastectomy). Chemotherapy is usually combined with mastectomy surgery to ensure that the cancer cells are destroyed. Internal radiation requires the radiation source to be inserted into a body cavity or in body tissues.

CJ Cognitive Skill

Analyze Cues

Reference

Linton & Matteson, 2020, pp. 1034–1035

Thinking Exercise 10-3

Answers

The nurse recognizes that the ***priority*** for coordinated care of the client's cancer is to <u>prevent metastasis</u>. The nurse's role prior to the client's treatment would be to <u>reinforce client teaching</u>.

Rationales

Any client who has cancer is at risk of its spread, or metastasis. Therefore the priority for coordinated client care is to prevent metastasis. The role of the nurse is to reinforce health teaching about the treatment that the client selects to meet this priority goal.

CJ Cognitive Skill

Prioritize Hypotheses

Reference

Linton & Matteson, 2020, pp. 1034–1035

Thinking Exercise 10-4

Answers

Client Teaching	Appropriate for Client	Not Appropriate for Client
1 "You will have an ink marking to outline the area that will be irradiated."	X	
2 "You will be hospitalized while receiving your radiation therapy."		X
3 "You may wash the ink marking off of your skin once radiation therapy begins."		X
4 "The irradiated skin will likely become irritated after about a week of radiation therapy."	X	
5 "Your radiation treatments may make you very tired."	X	
6 "Your family members will need to stay at least 6 feet from you on days when you have radiation."		X

Rationales

The client will have external beam radiation treatments that would be targeted to her breasts to destroy any remaining cancer cells. Prior to beginning these treatments, the radiation therapy staff mark the area on the skin to direct the radiation beam for each treatment. This marking should not be removed in any way until radiation therapy is completed. The effects of external radiation therapy do not affect other people in any way because it is delivered externally and does not require client hospitalization. *Internal* radiation therapy may require protection for other individuals who encounter the client and may require a hospital stay. Any type of radiation therapy can cause fatigue; external beam therapy often causes skin irritation.

CJ Cognitive Skill

Generate Solutions

Reference

Linton & Matteson, 2020, pp. 110–113

Thinking Exercise 10-5

Answers

A, B, C, D, E, G

Rationales

These chemotherapeutic agents can cause liver toxicity. The nurse monitors the client's liver enzyme levels for increases and teaches the client (and family) to observe for signs and symptoms that indicate liver damage, including jaundice, icterus, and abdominal edema (ascites) (Choices A and B). For clients receiving any type of chemotherapy, the nurse would reinforce teaching about common side effects such as fatigue and loss of hair (alopecia) (Choices D and G). Clients receiving chemotherapy are given antiemetics to help prevent nausea and vomiting (Choice C). The nurse would remind clients to avoid people with infections, especially crowds, because chemotherapeutic agents often cause bone marrow suppression resulting in decreased white blood cells (Choice E). In most cases, these manifestations are temporary while the client is receiving chemotherapy. The client's response to drug therapy is not known at this time.

CJ Cognitive Skill

Take Action

Reference

Linton & Matteson, 2020, pp. 113–114

Thinking Exercise 10-6

Answers

History and Physical	Nurses' Notes	Vital Signs	Laboratory Results

8/4/21 1015 Today the client states she is feeling much better; her last chemotherapy was completed 4 weeks ago. Vital signs: Temperature, 98°F (36.7°C); pulse, 76 beats/min and regular; respirations, 20 breaths/min; blood pressure, 118/74 mm Hg; oxygen saturation, 95%. Yesterday's lab work shows RBCs, WBCs, and platelets increased almost to normal ranges. Has lost 22 lb (10 kg) since beginning chemotherapy and still does not have a good appetite. States that her husband of 2 years has filed for divorce because he "can't handle her health issues." She is looking forward to having her follow-up testing to determine if her tumor has decreased in size. ------------------------------------P. Brown, LVN

Rationales

The client's vital signs are within usual parameters, which indicates that the client does not have any major complications of chemotherapy or cancer complications. She states she is feeling better, which is supported by her RBCs, WBCs, and platelets returning to almost normal ranges. Chemotherapy can cause bone marrow suppression resulting in decreased blood cell counts. However, she is not progressing well related to her appetite, which is poor and has resulted in significant loss of weight.

CJ Cognitive Skill

Evaluate Outcomes

Reference

Linton & Matteson, 2020, pp. 113–114

Thinking Exercise 10-7

Answers

Nursing Action	Indicated	Contraindicated	Non-Essential
Apply oxygen therapy at 2 L/min.			X
Monitor the amount and color of the J-P drainage.	X		
Remind the staff to avoid taking blood pressures or drawing blood in the affected arm.	X		
Keep the client's head of the bed flat at all times.		X	
Elevate the affected arm on a pillow.	X		
Observe the surgical dressing for bleeding.	X		
Keep the client in bed for at least 48 hours.		X	
Begin to reinforce client teaching about how to perform postmastectomy exercises.	X		

Rationales

Clients who have a radical mastectomy also have nearby lymph nodes removed, which places them at high risk for lymphedema. Therefore the nurse reminds the staff to avoid invasive procedures and taking blood pressure in the surgical or affected arm and keeps the arm elevated on a pillow to prevent lymphedema. Postmastectomy exercises increase mobility and help minimize arm swelling. The client should get out of bed the day of surgery and maintain a semi-Fowler or Fowler position (not flat) to help prevent edema and decrease respiratory effort. Oxygen therapy is not necessary unless the client has a chronic respiratory problem. For any postoperative client, the nurse would observe the surgical dressing for bleeding and monitor the amount and characteristics of drainage from any drain or other tube.

CJ Cognitive Skill

Generate Solutions

Reference

Linton & Matteson, 2020, pp. 280–282, 284–296, 1036–1037

Thinking Exercise 10-8

Answers

Assessment Finding	Effective	Ineffective	Unrelated
Incisions show no sign of infection.	X		
Reports an inability to straighten her left elbow.		X	
Mastectomy and reconstruction incisions are healed without redness or drainage.	X		
Left arm is very swollen and much larger than the right arm.		X	
Reports frequent heart palpitations when she drinks caffeinated beverages.			X

Rationales

The client assessment findings demonstrate that she is progressing well and that treatment interventions were effective. However, her left surgical arm is swollen, preventing her from straightening her elbow. Her report of heart palpitations is a new problem that is not related to her breast cancer or surgery.

CJ Cognitive Skill

Evaluate Outcomes

Reference

Linton & Matteson, 2020, pp. 1036–1037

CHAPTER 11 Infection

Answers With Rationales for Thinking Exercises

Exemplar 11A. Pneumonia (Medical-Surgical Nursing: Middle-Age Adult)

Thinking Exercise 11A-1

Answers

B, C, D, F, G, H

Rationales

The nurse would be concerned about the client's respiratory signs and symptoms including expectorating thick mucus when coughing, achiness in her chest, tachypnea, and a low oxygen saturation of below 95% (Choices D, F, G, and H). The client also has tachycardia and hypotension, which are indicative of possible dehydration (Choices B and C). Her fever likely caused her to be dehydrated and possibly anorexic. However, having a decreased appetite is not as concerning to the nurse at this time. Clients who have infections with fever often have anorexia.

CJ Cognitive Skill

Recognize Cues

Reference

Linton & Matteson, 2020, pp. 91, 489

Thinking Exercise 11A-2

Answers

The nurse recognizes that the client's assessment findings suggest that the client ***most likely*** has **pneumonia**. Based on her current vital signs, she also seems be **dehydrated**.

Rationales

The client has the typical assessment findings that are associated with a respiratory infection such as community-acquired pneumonia, rather than asthma or another respiratory illness. Her vital signs are typical of dehydration and include fever, tachycardia, and hypotension. Inadequate fluid volume can cause a decreased blood pressure. The heart attempts to compensate for lack of blood volume by increasing its work to get the oxygenated blood to vital body organs and tissues.

CJ Cognitive Skill

Analyze Cues

Reference

Linton & Matteson, 2020, pp. 91, 489

Thinking Exercise 11A-3

Answers

The ***priority*** for the client's care in the hospital will be to treat her **infection** and increase her **oxygenation**. She will also require **IV fluids** to manage **dehydration**.

Rationales

The client will require antibiotic therapy and respiratory support to increase her oxygenation. She will also need additional oral fluids and IV therapy to provide fluids and an access for IV antibiotic therapy.

CJ Cognitive Skill

Prioritize Hypotheses

Reference

Linton & Matteson, 2020, pp. 91, 489

Thinking Exercise 11A-4

Answers

Primary Health Care Provider Order	Indicated	Contraindicated	Non-Essential
Obtain a sputum specimen for culture and sensitivity and chest x-ray stat.	X		
Start supplemental oxygen therapy via nasal cannula.	X		
Refer the client to physical therapy to help manage her fatigue.			X
Provide access for IV fluid and antibiotic therapy.	X		
Place the client in a lateral position to prevent aspiration of secretions.		X	

Rationales

The primary health care provider will need to confirm the pneumonia diagnosis and determine the pathogen that is causing the client's infection. A sputum analysis can provide information about the type of pneumonia the client has, and a chest x-ray helps confirm the diagnosis. The client will need supplemental oxygen, antibiotic therapy, and IV fluids to start managing her infection. At this time she is not ready for physical therapy to help her increase endurance because of fatigue until the infection begins to resolve. She should be in a sitting position (rather than a lateral position) at all times while in bed to prevent secretion aspiration and promote thoracic expansion.

CJ Cognitive Skill

Generate Solutions

Reference

Linton & Matteson, 2020, pp. 489–492

Thinking Exercise 11A-5

Answers

A, C, D, F, G, H, I, J

Rationales

Because the client previously had a successful nebulizer treatment for her respiratory distress, the nurse would request that the respiratory therapist administer another treatment (Choice A). Increasing the oxygen level would improve oxygenation, and giving an antitussive would help decrease her coughing episodes (Choices C and D). The client needs to maintain a sitting or high-Fowler position to increase thoracic expansion and facilitate breathing, and also needs to increase fluids to thin secretions (Choices G and H). The nurse would take vital signs and listen to breath sounds to compare these findings with previous results (Choices F and I). All of the client's findings and nursing actions would need to be documented (Choice J).

CJ Cognitive Skill

Take Action

Reference

Linton & Matteson, 2020, pp. 489–492

Thinking Exercise 11A-6

Answers

History and Physical	Nurses' Notes	Vital Signs	Laboratory Results

12/3/21 1015 Client states that she has only 2–3 coughing spells a day and has not coughed up any mucus since yesterday. VS: T = 99° F (37.2° C), P = 84, R = 22, B/P = 118/70, oxygen saturation = 95% (on room air). Continues to report extreme fatigue and anorexia. Understands that she needs to continue taking her antibiotic until the prescription is completed. Also able to demonstrate use of inhaler for home use to improve breathing. --- *S. Myers, LPN*

Rationales

The client's coughing episodes have decreased and her cough is not productive now. Additionally, her vital signs have improved, indicating that the infection is resolving and she is well hydrated. Her oxygen saturation is improving without supplemental oxygen.

CJ Cognitive Skill

Evaluate Outcomes

Reference

Linton & Matteson, 2020, pp. 489–492

Thinking Exercise 11A-7

Answers

Nursing Action	Indicated	Contraindicated	Non-Essential
Remind assistive personnel to keep the client NPO.	X		
Maintain the client in a position with the head of the bed at 10 degrees or higher.		X	
Be sure that suction equipment is on hand and working.			X
Consult with the speech-language pathologist (SLP) to perform a swallowing study.	X		
Mix liquid beverages with a thickening agent to prevent choking.		X	

Rationales

Even though the client had a mild stroke, he should remain NPO until the SLP performs a swallowing study and documents the results. No fluids or food should be offered to the client, so beverages with a thickening agent should not be offered. While NPO, the client should not need to be suctioned unless he has a problem later with managing his secretions.

CJ Cognitive Skill

Generate Solutions

Reference

Linton & Matteson, 2020, pp. 404, 489–492

Thinking Exercise 11A-8

Answers

The nurse suspects that the client ***most likely*** has COVID-19, which is a highly transmissible respiratory infection, and is at high risk for decreasing oxygenation. If the client is confirmed to have this health problem by means of a point-of-care test, she would probably be discharged or transferred to her home.

Rationales

The client who is young (under 60) without comorbidities would be expected to be asymptomatic or have mild symptoms if she had COVID-19, which is a coronavirus that causes varied clinical manifestations across populations. At this time her symptoms are mild, and she can be discharged to home. The nurse would teach the client to go to the emergency department if her condition worsens, especially if she has increasing respiratory problems.

CJ Cognitive Skill

Prioritize Hypotheses

Reference

Ignatavicius et al., 2021, p. 569

Exemplar 11B. Respiratory Syncytial Virus (Pediatric Nursing: Toddler)

Thinking Exercise 11B-1

Answers

A 16-month old female toddler is brought to the emergency department (ED) by her parents. Her mother tells the nurse that the toddler started having a "runny" nose and cough 2 days ago. This morning, she had a "little" fever, was very fussy, and seemed to have a couple of pauses in her breathing. Current vital signs include: axillary temperature, 100°F (37.8° C); apical pulse, 102 beats/min; respirations, 34 breaths/min; blood pressure, 76/50 mm Hg; oxygen saturation, 88%. The nurse auscultates occasional low-pitched wheezes in both lungs. The child is admitted to the acute care pediatric unit.

Rationales

The nurse is concerned about the client's increased respirations and the mother's report that the toddler had pauses in breathing. The child has a low oxygen saturation level and occasional low-pitched wheezes in her lungs. These assessment findings are concerning because they can worsen and place the child at high risk for respiratory failure.

CJ Cognitive Skill

Recognize Cues

Reference

Leifer, 2019, pp. 600–601

Thinking Exercise 11B-2

Answers

Client Finding	Asthma	RSV
Low-grade fever		X
Fussiness	X	X
Low oxygen saturation	X	X
Wheezing	X	X
Cough	X	X

Rationales

The main difference between assessment findings associated with asthma versus RSV is the fever that occurs with RSV. Treatment for these two diseases is also different.

CJ Cognitive Skill

Analyze Cues

Reference

Leifer, 2019, pp. 600–601

Thinking Exercise 11B-3

Answers

A, B, C, G

Rationales

The priority for a child who has RSV is to maintain a patent airway and prevent worsening respiratory problems that could result in respiratory failure (Choices A and G). Management of the child would also include preventing infection transmission and promoting hydration while she has a fever (Choices B and C).

CJ Cognitive Skill

Prioritize Hypotheses

Reference

Leifer, 2019, pp. 600–601

Thinking Exercise 11B-4

Answers

Nursing Action	Acute Respiratory Distress	Dehydration
Weigh the child every day and report weight loss.		X
Suction the child if thick secretions are present.	X	
Maintain the oxygen saturation at a minimum of 90% to 95%.	X	
Provide oral hydration fluids, such as Pedialyte.		X
Report high-pitched wheezing to the registered nurse immediately.	X	
Document accurate intake and urinary output.		X
Report tachypnea to the registered nurse immediately.	X	

Rationales

Interventions for preventing or managing dehydration would be to provide additional fluids, measure and document intake and output, and weigh the child at the same time on the same scale every day. Weight is the most reliable indicator of fluid gain or loss. To improve the child's respiratory effort and prevent acute distress, the nurse would administer supplemental oxygen and monitor for high-pitched wheezing. If needed, the nurse would also suction the child to remove secretions that may be hindering breathing.

CJ Cognitive Skill

Generate Solutions

Reference

Leifer, 2019, pp. 600–601, 673–674

Thinking Exercise 11B-5

Answers

A, B, C, F

Rationales

RSV is not an airborne pathogen but is spread by droplet and contact with surfaces or objects that have been contaminated. These surfaces and objects are disinfected to minimize infection transmission (Choice F). In addition to handwashing, contact precautions and wearing a mask provide protection for RSV transmission (Choices A, B, and C).

CJ Cognitive Skill

Take Action

Reference

Leifer, 2019, pp. 600–601

Thinking Exercise 11B-6

Answers

Assessment Finding	Effective	Ineffective	Unrelated
Has occasional low-pitched wheezing		X	
Temperature = 99°F (37.2°C)	X		
Oxygen saturation = 96% (on room air [RA])	X		
Respirations = 26 breaths/min	X		
Weight = 23 lb (10.4 kg)			X
Urine output = 18 mL/hr	X		
Diarrheal stools due to teething			X
No cough or rhinorrhea	X		

Rationales

The toddler's respiratory status has improved except that she still has a few auscultated wheezes. Her weight and diarrheal stools are not related to her RSV recovery.

CJ Cognitive Skill

Evaluate Outcomes

Reference

Leifer, 2019, pp. 600–601

Thinking Exercise 11B-7

Answers

The nurse recognizes that the infant is at high risk for RSV because he has **a history of congenital heart defect**. The medication that is given to help prevent RSV infection in high-risk infants is a monoclonal antibody called **palivizumab**, which is typically given once a month from November through March.

Rationales

Infants who have poor immune function, are premature, and/or have significant congenital heart disease are at high risk for RSV infection. Therefore they are candidates for palivizumab, which is given monthly at the beginning of the RSV season from November through March.

CJ Cognitive Skill

Analyze Cues

Reference

Leifer, 2019, pp. 600–601

CHAPTER 12 Mood and Affect: Depression/Suicide Risk *(Mental Health Nursing: Older Adult)*

Answers With Rationales for Thinking Exercises

Thinking Exercise 12-1

Answers

- Oriented to person, place, and time
- Sitting in chair with slumped posture
- Avoids eye contact with nursing staff
- Reports feeling hopeless on most days over the past 3 weeks
- Heart rate (HR) = 72 beats/min
- Respirations = 14 breaths/min
- Lung fields clear throughout all lobes
- Moves all extremities with moderate strength
- Refuses to participate in ADLs or take meals in the dining hall
- Reports thinking about death frequently but denies thoughts of hurting herself

Rationales

The nurse recognizes that several client findings indicate an abnormal emotional and/or behavioral response to the current situation. These findings include slumped posture, poor eye contact, and withdrawal from ADLs. The nurse must follow up with these observations to determine underlying physical and mental causes. The client's report of hopelessness over the past 3 weeks alerts the nurse to a prolonged period of symptoms, which must be further assessed. Follow-up assessments would focus on current emotions and perceptions related to the loss of health, pain and other underlying conditions, changes in appetite and sleep patterns, and support systems and coping skills.

CJ Cognitive Skill

Recognize Cues

Reference

Morrison-Valfre, 2017, pp. 203–209; 237–240

Thinking Exercise 12-2

Answers

	Anxiety	Delirium	Depression
Impaired cognition	X	X	X
Reduced appetite			X
Agitation	X	X	X
Sleep disturbances	X	X	X
Activity avoidance	X		X

Rationales

All three disorders impair cognition. Anxiety is an emotional response to a real or imagined threat or stressor. During severe anxiety the client may experience impaired memory, attention, and concentration. Delirium is a rapid change in consciousness that is associated with an underlying physical condition. Disorganized thinking, decreased attention span, and fluctuating levels of consciousness occur with delirium. Depression is a mood disorder that involves emotional, physical, intellectual, social, and spiritual problems. Clients experiencing major depression experience difficulty concentrating and making decisions. Depression is also associated with a reduced appetite with weight loss. Anxiety and delirium do not usually result in a reduced appetite. The emotional state of clients with all three disorders fluctuates. Clients may feel sad, uneasy, fearful, irritable, and agitated.

Sleep cycle disruptions are commonly present in all three disorders. Sleep deprivation is a risk factor for anxiety, and insomnia is a manifestation. Clients with delirium often have reversed sleep cycles, with emotional nights filled with hallucinations and delusion, and lethargic days during which the client sleeps continuously. Client experiencing major depression may experience insomnia or other sleep disturbances. Although clients with delirium may have difficulty participating in ADLs because of cognitive changes, these clients do not withdraw from social encounters or avoid activities. Alternatively, both anxiety and depression are associated with emotional distress that interferes with everyday life and avoidance of situations.

CJ Cognitive Skill

Analyze Cues

Reference

Morrison-Valfre, 2017, pp. 192–193, 203–209, 237–240

Thinking Exercise 12-3

Answers

Based on the client's feelings of hopelessness for more than 2 weeks, as well as insomnia, poor concentration, and reduced appetite with weight loss, the nurse determines that the client is ***most likely*** experiencing <u>major depressive episode</u>. The nurse's ***priority*** is to closely monitor the client for <u>suicidal thoughts</u> to prevent client injury.

Rationales

Mild depression is short-lived and is usually triggered by a life event or situation outside the client's control. Major depressive episode is the term used when symptoms of depression are more severe and last more than 2 weeks. Classic manifestations of major depression are persistent sadness and feelings of hopelessness, reduced appetite with weight loss, insomnia, excessive fatigue, and difficulty concentrating. Major depressive disorder is the term used to describe multiple episodes of major depression over at least a 2-year period. Suicidal thoughts are frequently associated with major depressive episodes and are viewed by the client as the only way to cope with the physical, mental, and emotional misery. The nurse must identify suicidal thoughts early to ensure the client remains safe and free of harm.

CJ Cognitive Skill

Prioritize Hypotheses

Reference

Morrison-Valfre, 2017, pp. 237–234

Thinking Exercise 12-4

Answers

Nursing Action	Indicated	Contraindicated	Non-Essential
Teach the client meditation and relaxation techniques.	X		
Encourage frequent oral care.			X
Isolate the client from other rehabilitation clients.		X	
Remind the client that it may take several weeks for antidepressant drugs to begin working.	X		
Monitor the client for increasing blood pressure.	X		
Obtain consent for electroconvulsive therapy (ECT).		X	

Rationales

The client is prescribed venlafaxine, a serotonin norepinephrine reuptake inhibitor (SNRI) antidepressant drug. Therapeutic effects may take 2 to 3 weeks to occur, and therefore the client would be reminded that the drug takes time to work and would be encouraged to continue taking the medication. Venlafaxine can cause hypertension, and therefore the nurse would monitor for increasing blood pressure, especially diastolic blood pressure. The client would be expected to perform the usual oral care rather than more frequent care, which is not essential for the client's care.

Nonpharmacologic treatments for depression include exercise, group therapy, and use of meditation and relaxation techniques. The client would be encouraged to participate in activities instead of being isolated. In most settings, ECT is used only in clients with severe, long-lasting depression after other therapies and medications have failed. The client's depressive episode does not qualify for ECT. In addition, the client is recovering from a myocardial infarction, and therefore the treatment would be contraindicated.

CJ Cognitive Skill

Generate Solutions

Reference

Morrison-Valfre, 2017, pp. 68–72, 244–249

Thinking Exercise 12-5

Answers

A, D, E, F, G

Rationales

Standard evidence-based suicide prevention precautions include protecting the client from self-harm, removing dangerous items from the environment, and observing the client closely (Choices A and E). Establishing rapport with the client is essential. Encouragement and advocacy from a nurse may help a suicidal client to develop more effective strategies for coping and living (Choice G). Although the client may be experiencing many emotions, the client may agree to establish a "no self-harm contract" (a promise not to engage in self-destructive behaviors) with the care provider (Choice D). Constant observation is needed even when a client agrees to a no self-harm contract. Asking a client about the suicide plan does not put ideas in the client's head. Instead it provides the nurse with a better assessment of the client's level of suicidal behavior. The nurse must determine if the client has a detailed plan to hurt herself (Choice F).

CJ Cognitive Skill

Take Action

Reference

Morrison-Valfre, 2017, pp. 314–324

Thinking Exercise 12-6

Answers

Client Statements	Is Progressing	Is Not Progressing
"I am looking forward to seeing my grandchildren this afternoon."	X	
"Everything seems to run together in my mind. I don't know if it is day or night."		X
"I need to take a nap after working so hard in physical therapy."	X	
"I feel comfortable sharing my hopes and fears in group therapy."	X	
"My clothes are not soiled. I can continue wearing them for several more days."		X

Rationales

Clients with major depression experience feelings of despair in every thought and activity. The client's anticipation of visiting grandchildren and ability to work hard in physical therapy do not indicate despair or hopelessness. Instead, these statements present a client who is engaged with others, is participating in activities to improve her health, and has plans for the future. The client's ability to fully participate in group therapy is also a sign of progression. Sharing hopes and fears demonstrates that the client is becoming more self-aware of her feelings and is open to exploring with a group of people ways to effectively cope. Additional manifestations of major depression are confusion, inability to concentrate, loss of interest and motivation, and poor personal hygiene. Although the client's clothing may not be soiled, wearing the same clothes every day and a lack of interest in her personal appearance indicates that the client is not progressing. The client's statements that "everything seems to run together in my mind" and "I don't know if it is day or night" indicate that the client is not fully oriented and is not thinking accurately. A lack of interest in the outside world and mental confusion are not signs of progression; these are classic signs of depression.

CJ Cognitive Skill

Evaluate Outcomes

Reference

Morrison-Valfre, 2017, pp. 237–249

Thinking Exercise 12-7

Answers

A, C, E, F, G

Rationales

Screening for suicidal thoughts is an essential role of the nurse. A series of questions must be asked to bring out expressions of suicidal thoughts if present. Asking direct questions will not encourage the client to take any suicidal actions. Instead, these questions give the client permission to discuss feelings and attitudes. Questions would focus on the client's thoughts about hurting himself or ending his life (Choices A and C), any plans to attempt suicide (Choice E), and concerns about suicide (Choice F). Finally, the nurse will ask if a "no self-harm contract" would be accepted by the client (Choice G). The other choices focus on assessing a client for symptoms of depression and anxiety. They are not specific to assess a client's potential for suicide.

CJ Cognitive Skill

Take Action

Reference

Morrison-Valfre, 2017, pp. 314–324

CHAPTER 13 Stress and Coping

Answers With Rationales for Thinking Exercises

Exemplar 13A. Generalized Anxiety Disorder/Loss (Mental Health Nursing: Older Adult)

Thinking Exercise 13A-1

Answers

Client Finding	Client Finding That Requires Follow-up by the Nurse
Client's heart rate	
Shape and size of client's chest	
Spouse's behavior	X
Client's sputum color and consistency	
Use of oxygen by the client	
Client's dyspnea	X
Spouse's response to the nurse	X
Client's orientation level	

Rationales

The client's level of orientation correlates with the diagnosis for Alzheimer disease. The client is alert and talkative, which indicates a positive mood and affect, and no need for follow-up. The client's respiratory status correlates with the diagnosis of COPD. There is no need for the nurse to follow up with the chest and sputum assessments. The client has an oxygen saturation level of 92%, which is appropriate for a client with COPD; therefore there is no concern with the use of 4 L of oxygen via nasal cannula. Dyspnea, especially with exertion, is a common symptom of COPD, but a client who becomes short of breath during a basic conversation may be experiencing progression of the disease or a respiratory infection. The nurse would want to follow up on this assessment finding. The spouse appears to be fretting and experiences difficulty concentrating. She also responds, "I've got this," which suggests issues with control. Her behavior and responses must be followed up on as they could be related to issues with the spouse and/or the client. The client's heart rate is within the normal range.

CJ Cognitive Skill

Recognize Cues

Reference

Morrison-Valfre, 2017, pp. 203–213

Thinking Exercise 13A-2

Answers

To further analyze the situation, the nurse would **establish rapport** and ask the client's spouse to **talk about her feelings**.

Rationales

Behaviors of the wife indicate the presence of anxiety. Older adults frequently deny their anxiety, and therefore the nurse must establish a relationship and environment that allows the client to comfortably express how she is feeling. After establishing rapport with the client's wife, the nurse would simply ask the client to explain her anxious feelings. Older adults usually appreciate the interest of concerned health care providers.

CJ Cognitive Skill

Analyze Cues

References

Williams, 2018, pp. 212–213; Morrison-Valfre, 2017, p. 209

Thinking Exercise 13A-3

Answers

Potential Health Problems	Probable	Remote	Improbable
Ineffective coping	X		
Paranoia			X
Anxiety disorder	X		
Social isolation		X	
Avoidant personality disorder			X

Rationales

The wife is most likely experiencing an anxiety disorder and ineffective coping. She states that she frequently experiences anxiety, a vague uneasy feeling experienced in response to real or imagined stress, but feeling anxious is not the same as an anxiety disorder. Other assessment findings that suggest an anxiety disorder include difficulty concentrating, insomnia, fretting, and chronic worrying about everyday events. The wife's coping abilities are also overwhelmed and she loses emotional control, which are symptoms of an anxiety disorder. Ineffective coping is exhibited by the wife's decreased use of social support and available resources and difficulty attending to daily activities.

Social isolation occurs when a client experiences a general lack of interest and withdrawal from others or is absent of meaningful interactions with others. The wife has stopped going to church, but her friends visit once a week. She may be experiencing social isolation, but it is not the most likely explanation for the situation. The wife is not exhibiting delusions or behaviors marked by suspiciousness, and therefore a diagnosis of paranoia is improbable. Although the wife is afraid to leave her husband, it is unlikely that she is experiencing avoidant personality disorder. The client is concerned about being a burden to her friends and family; she is not afraid of rejection or humiliation.

CJ Cognitive Skill

Prioritize Hypotheses

Reference

Morrison-Valfre, 2017, pp. 171–175, 203–213, 353–360, 364–371

Thinking Exercise 13A-4

Answers

Based on the nurse's suspected diagnosis, the nurse would plan interventions to meet desired client outcomes. The desired outcomes for older adults with anxiety disorders are to **develop effective coping mechanisms** and **experience fewer episodes of anxiety**.

Rationales

Older adults must cope with several anxiety-causing life changes, including loss of health, self-determination, and control. Therefore the focus on nursing care for an older adult with anxiety is to help the client identify methods to reduce anxiety and cope with daily uncertainties. Coping strategies previously used by the client may no longer work, and new coping mechanisms may need to be developed as the adult ages. In addition, the nurse would expect the client to experience fewer episodes of anxiety after implementation of various interventions.

CJ Cognitive Skill

Generate Solutions

References

Williams, 2018, pp. 212–213; Morrison-Valfre, 2017, pp. 209

Thinking Exercise 13A-5

Answers

B, C, E, F, H

Rationales

Therapeutic interventions for anxiety disorders usually involve a combination of mental health therapies and drug therapy. For older adults, antianxiety medications, especially benzodiazepines, frequently cause side effects that place the client at risk for injury. Therefore drug therapy for anxiety disorders in older adults should be implemented carefully. A focus on mental health therapies is safer and often more effective for older adults. The most effective way to cope with anxiety is to recognize anxiety symptoms early and implement preventive coping mechanisms. The nurse would teach the wife to recognize signs of anxiety within herself and explore a variety of coping strategies to prevent or minimize anxieties (Choices C and F). The nurse may also teach relaxation techniques and encourage the wife to share feelings of anxiety, fear, and stress (Choices E and H). Discussing feelings of anxiety may be difficult for older adults, so the nurse will need to establish a safe environment for group sessions. Cognitive-behavioral therapy is also useful in the treatment of older adults. This therapy helps clients intellectually understand the ineffective behaviors used to cope with anxiety and replace them with more successful behaviors (Choice B).

CJ Cognitive Skill

Take Action

References

Williams, 2018, pp. 212–213; Morrison-Valfre, 2017, pp. 209–216

Thinking Exercise 13A-6

Answers

Client statements	Is Progressing	Is Not Progressing
"I pay a certified nursing assistant to care for my husband on Sunday mornings so that I can attend church."	X	
"I participate in group therapy with others who have spouses with Alzheimer disease."	X	
"I complete housework in the middle of the night when I cannot sleep."		X
"I don't want to burden others, so I stopped allowing friends and family to visit."		X
"I encourage my husband to do as much for himself as he can."	X	

Rationales

Expected outcomes for this client were to use coping strategies to reduce anxiety and experience fewer anxiety episodes. Anxiety occurs as a results of a perceived threat to one's self. Going to church and participating in group therapy are signs that the wife is accepting of the situation and not threatened by changes in her life and her husband's illness. These statements also indicate that she is more comfortable leaving her husband with others and is open to discussing her fears and concerns with a group of peers. In addition, allowing her husband to do as much as he can for himself is a reflection on the wife's ability to manage feelings of worry that led to her fretting. Sleep disturbances are a sign of anxiety, and therefore the client's comment that she does not sleep through the night is an indication that she is not progressing. Similarly, not allowing visitors at the house demonstrates her projection of anxiety and ineffective coping.

CJ Cognitive Skill

Evaluate Outcomes

Reference

Morrison-Valfre, 2017, pp. 209–216

Thinking Exercise 13A-7

Answers

A, C, D, H

Rationales

The nurse would be alert for symptoms of grief associated with the recent death of the client's spouse. Grieving is different for everyone and depends on an individual's coping abilities. Unhealthy or ineffective grief reactions may lead to anxiety or depressive disorders. For this client, the nurse would identify the client's lack of energy, disinterest in daily activities, and refusal to engage with anyone as signs of loss or grief (Choices A and C). The client is oriented and therefore her statement about calling her husband would alert the nurse to the possibility of unresolved or complicated grieving and continued denial of the loss (Choice D). Feelings of despair and worthlessness are additional signs of ineffective grief (Choice H). The nurse will want to evaluate the client for suicidal thoughts based on these client statements. The client's other comments display effective coping and a lack of signs associated with depression and anxiety.

CJ Cognitive Skill

Recognize Cues

Reference

Morrison-Valfre, 2017, pp. 226–230

Thinking Exercise 13A-8

Answers

Nursing Actions	Indicated	Contraindicated	Non-Essential
Allow the client to make choices whenever possible.	X		
Ensure the same nurse is assigned to provide the client's bed bath each day.		X	
Explain the reasons when changes in the client's plan of care occur.	X		
Respect the client's right to refuse care and activities.	X		
Coordinate with the kitchen to provide the client's favorite foods.			X

Rationales

In institutional settings, it is essential to allow the client opportunities to exert control. The client should be provided options and allowed to make choices whenever possible. The ultimate power is the client's right to refuse care. Health care professionals must respect this right and provide good explanations for important treatments or medications to overcome objections and relieve conflict. Changes in the client's plan of care must also be explained as soon as the change is known. The client is more likely to accept the change when he understands the circumstances of the change and does not think it occurred because the nurse is attempting to assume control of his right to make choices. In addition, the client should be encouraged to do as much as possible for himself, and the environment should be adapted to encourage independence. Performing a daily bed bath strips the client of all independence and power. Providing the client's favorite foods is a nice gesture, but it does not address the client's feelings of loss. In addition, he has diabetes and needs to follow the appropriate diet to control his glucose.

CJ Cognitive Skill

Generate Solutions

Reference

Williams, 2018, pp. 214–216

Exemplar 13B. Substance Use Disorder (Mental Health Nursing: Older Adult)

Thinking Exercise 13B-1

Answers

History and Physical | **Nurses' Notes** | **Vital Signs** | **Laboratory Results**

Health History

Benign prostatic hyperplasia

Hyperlipidemia

Osteoarthritis

Social History

Married with three adult children and several grandchildren

Retired primary school teacher

Denies alcohol use

Medications

Acetaminophen 650 mg orally every 12 hours

Atorvastatin 20 mg orally once daily

Tamsulosin 0.4 mg orally once daily

Rationales

The client states that he drinks whiskey each evening, but the health history documented in the client's medical record indicates that he denies alcohol use. This discrepancy must be followed up on by the nurse. If the client does drink alcohol, then the nurse must evaluate the client's medication list for contraindications and other potential risks. Acetaminophen is metabolized by the liver and so is alcohol. Taking both substances increases the client's risk for liver damage, and over time this risk is cumulative and synergistic in a negative way. Tamsulosin belongs to a class of drugs called alpha-adrenergic blockers. Drinking alcohol with this medication may increase the client's risk for orthostatic hypotension, a common side effect of alpha-adrenergic blockers. The nurse will want to follow up on both of these medications and client symptoms.

CJ Cognitive Skill

Recognize Cues

References

Morrison-Valfre, 2017, pp. 326–340; Linton & Matteson, 2020, pp. 1219–1240

Thinking Exercise 13B-2

Answers

A, B, C, F, H

Rationales

The nurse will want to ask questions to assess the client's alcohol use. The Short Michigan Alcohol Screening Test–Geriatric Version (SMAST-G) is a screening instrument used to evaluate "at-risk" alcohol use, alcohol abuse, or alcoholism in older adults. The 10-question tool asks yes-or-no questions and assigns one point for each "yes" response. A score of 2 or higher is indicative of an alcohol problem. Choices A, C, and F are questions from the SMAST-G tool. The CAGE assessment, which is an acronym formed from key terms on the questionnaire, is another simple screening tool used to identify potential problems with alcohol. The four question CAGE assessment asks yes-or-no questions to determine if substance use exists. Choice H is a CAGE question. Choice B, although not part of an alcohol screening tool, is essential to ask. If the client takes alcohol to help him sleep, he may take other substances. Over-the-counter and recreational drugs may interact with current prescriptions and/or alcohol and place the client at risk for injury. The other questions do not address the client's statement about using alcohol to help him sleep.

CJ Cognitive Skill

Analyze Cues

References

Morrison-Valfre, 2017, pp. 326–340; Linton & Matteson, 2020, pp. 1219–1240

Thinking Exercise 13B-3

Answers

The client's use of alcohol increases his risk for impaired judgment and coordination, which may lead to falls and medication misuse.

Rationales

Older adults usually become intoxicated with less alcohol intake than young and middle-age adults because of decreased muscle mass and water in the body, as well as slower metabolic processes. During intoxication, older clients can experience impaired judgment, coordination, and reaction time. Too much alcohol may also lead to balance problems, falls, and medication misuse, resulting in overdose.

CJ Cognitive Skill

Prioritize Hypotheses

References

Williams, 2018, pp. 233–234; Morrison-Valfre, 2017, pp. 326–340; Linton & Matteson, 2020, pp. 1219–1240

Thinking Exercise 13B-4

Answers

Nursing Action	Indicated	Contraindicated	Non-Essential
Withhold the client's dose of pain medication.		X	
Confront the client about his alcohol use and consequences.	X		
Encourage the client to agree to participate in a treatment program.	X		
Contact adult protective services to report elder abuse.			X
Monitor the client for physiologic changes related to detoxification.	X		

Rationales

Denial is common with clients who have a substance-related problem. Identifying the problem is the first step toward change, and therefore the nurse should confront the client about his alcohol use. Confrontation should be done an environment that is safe for the client, family and friends involved, and any health care staff. A personal commitment by the client to participate in a treatment program significantly increases the likelihood of success. Alcohol withdrawal is a life-threatening condition. The nurse must identify withdrawal signs and promptly intervene to halt the progression of symptoms. Nurses must ensure that the client has appropriate pain management and postoperative care. Withholding the client's medication would be unethical and could cause physiologic and psychological issues related to pain. There is no need to contact adult protective services for this client.

CJ Cognitive Skill

Generate Solutions

References

Morrison-Valfre, 2017, pp. 326–340; Linton & Matteson, 2020, pp. 1219–1240

Thinking Exercise 13B-5

Answers

B, E, F, H

Rationales

Symptoms of alcohol withdrawal can quickly advance to life-threatening delirium tremors. The nurse must effectively communicate the client's current withdrawal symptoms so that the receiving nurse is prepared to promptly intervene and decrease the potential for seizures or a hypertensive emergency. The nurse would report current vital signs (Choice B) because the client's heart rate, blood pressure, and temperature can be used as predictors for stages of withdrawal. These values may increase to extreme levels during withdrawal. Anxiety is an early sign of withdrawal and is usually followed by irritability and agitation. The nurse would present the client's current mood and behavior (Choice F), as well as orientation assessment (Choice H). As withdrawal stages progress, the client's level of orientation will decline, leading to confusion, disorientation, and hallucinations. Finally, the nurse will need to report any actions taken or medications administered to treat symptoms (Choice E). Lorazepam and chlordiazepoxide are most commonly used to prevent severe consequences of withdrawal symptoms. The other options are not essential information to share with the registered nurse at this time.

CJ Cognitive Skill

Take Action

References

Morrison-Valfre, 2017, pp. 326–340; Linton & Matteson, 2020, pp. 1219–1240

Thinking Exercise 13B-6

Answers

Client Finding	Effective	Ineffective	Unrelated
"I will be prescribed methadone to help me overcome my addiction."		X	
"It is my choice to participate in the alcohol treatment program."	X		
"Treatment may consist of individual, group, and family therapy."	X		
"I can't join Alcoholics Anonymous (AA) until after I complete the treatment program."		X	
"Eating a low-fat, high-protein diet will assist my recovery from alcoholism."			X
"Decreasing my alcohol intake to only one glass a day is a positive step."		X	

Rationales

Participation in alcohol treatment programs is usually voluntary. Family and friends may encourage a client to participate in an inpatient or outpatient program, but the client's desire to participate improves therapy outcomes. Alcohol treatment programs consist of drug education; individual, group, and family therapy; recreational and occupational therapy; milieu therapy; diagnosis and treatment of addiction; and an introduction to community resources for clients with alcohol addictions. Clients may join Alcoholics Anonymous (AA) when desired. There is no need to complete a treatment program before participating in AA. The client should not drink any alcohol. Even one drink for an alcoholic is a relapse. A client entering an alcohol treatment program must understand that any alcohol is prohibited. Methadone is used to treat heroin addiction. The nurse must clarify that that client will not receive methadone for his addiction. No particular diet is needed for alcohol addiction therapy.

CJ Cognitive Skill

Evaluate Outcomes

References

Morrison-Valfre, 2017, pp. 326–340; Linton & Matteson, 2020, pp. 1219–1240

Thinking Exercise 13B-7

Answers

A, C, D, E, G

Rationales

Older adults experience social and physical changes that increase their vulnerability to substance misuse and substance use disorders. Physical risk factors for substance use disorder in older adults are chronic pain, physical disabilities, reduced mobility, chronic illness, and an overall poor health status (Choice C). Older adults who experience transitions in living or care situations, loss of loved ones, and changes in income are also at high risk for substance misuse (Choices A and D). Psychiatric risk factors include an avoidance coping style, history of substance use disorders, previous or current mental illness, and feeling socially isolated (Choices E and G). The other statements are not associated with risk factors of a substance use disorder.

CJ Cognitive Skill

Analyze Cues

References

Morrison-Valfre, 2017, pp. 326–340; Linton & Matteson, 2020, pp. 1219–1240

Exemplar 13C. Elder Abuse/Neglect (Mental Health Nursing: Older Adult)

Thinking Exercise 13C-1

Answers

- Heart rate (HR) = 88 beats/min
- Blood pressure (BP) = 126/65 mm Hg
- Respirations (R) = 14 breaths/min
- Oxygen saturation = 94% (on room air [RA])
- Height = 5 foot 10 inches (1.8 m); weight = 122 lb (55.5 kg)
- Alert and oriented to self and place, confused to time and situation
- Follows simple commands
- Skin is warm and dry
- No skin tears, bruising, or wounds present
- Poor eye contact with son
- Avoids answering direct questions when son is in room

Rationales

The client's height and weight calculate to a body mass index (BMI) that is lower than normal or underweight. The nurse needs to communicate these data related to a state of malnutrition. The client's confusion to time and situation must be reported and further assessed to determine if disorientation is an acute response to hospitalization or a chronic condition. Poor eye contact and avoiding direct questions are radically different responses from the talkative and cooperative client initially assessed. These findings also must be reported to the registered nurse and further evaluated. Other findings are within normal limits and do not need to be reported to the registered nurse.

CJ Cognitive Skill

Recognize Cues

References

Morrison-Valfre, 2017, pp. 300–307; Williams, 2018, pp. 21–26, 209–216

Thinking Exercise 13C-2

Answers

A, B, D, E, G, H

Rationales

Elder abuse and neglect by a family member generally occurs because of increased demands on limited resources and caregiver physical exhaustion or mental fatigue. Intentional abuse occurs when a person deliberately plans to mistreat or harm another person, but not all forms of abuse are intentional. Unintentional abuse or neglect is just as devastating to the older adult and frequently occurs when the caregiver lacks necessary knowledge, resources, and stamina to care for the older family member. Comments related to no sleep or interrupted sleep at night (Choice A), working continuously at the job and at home (Choice B), and becoming frustrated with his father (Choice H) are all signs that the son is struggling to balance the continuous demands of his father's care with work obligations and his personal health. Not having anyone to stay with or check on his father (Choice G) indicates a lack of resources and support for the client's care. Locking the client in his room (Choice E) demonstrates ineffective coping and rationalizing "to keep him from hurting himself." Finally, the client not eating when alone (Choice D) is a sign of self-neglect due to the client's inability or lack of awareness to eat. It is also a sign that the client does not have the resources needed for effective care around the clock.

CJ Cognitive Skill

Analyze Cues

References

Morrison-Valfre, 2017, pp. 300–307; Williams, 2018, pp. 21–26, 209–216

Thinking Exercise 13C-3

Answers

Potential Health Problems	Priority Health Problems
Decreased/impaired nutrition due to possible neglect	X
Delayed growth due to inadequate caregiving	
Knowledge deficit about community support and resources for home care	X
Poor self-esteem due to negative family interactions	X
Acute pain due to physical injuries	

Rationales

The client has physiologic and psychological problems due to unintentional abuse and neglect. The client has decreased/impaired nutrition as manifested by current height and weight values, low BMI, and reports of inadequate food intake. This physical problem is a priority, as fluid and nutritional status impacts basic functions of the body and may contribute to other health problems or conditions. Emotional or psychological abuse, including verbal and nonverbal communications of frustration, displeasure, and disgust, can damage an older adult's self-esteem and even destroy the will to live. Although this problem will need to be addressed over a period of time, the nurse may prioritize the client's mental and emotional status to promote safety and prevent self-harm. In addition, the client and his son lack resources and support services necessary for the health and well-being of both. The client needs additional assistance during the day when the son is at work, and the son needs support to more effectively cope with stress related to being a family caregiver. Knowledge deficit related to community support and resources for home care is a priority, as without services the abuse may escalate. The client is an older adult and therefore does not have any growth issues. The client also has no signs of physical injuries and denies pain.

CJ Cognitive Skill

Prioritize Hypotheses

References

Morrison-Valfre, 2017, pp. 300–307; Williams, 2018, pp. 21–26, 209–216

Thinking Exercise 13C-4

Answers

The desired outcomes for this client are remaining free from injury, eating adequate nutrients to maintain health, feeling safe and secure at home, and practicing behaviors that promote self-confidence. Desired outcomes for the client's son are to perform the caregiver role with competence and confidence and use strategies and resources to promote stress reduction.

Rationales

The client's plan of care must address both the client and the caregiver. To prevent further abuse and neglect, the client's son needs to feel comfortable with his role as a family care provider and know when and how to meet the physical and psychosocial needs of his father while not neglecting his own health and desires. The son must also use resources and coping strategies to effectively address personal stressors and achieve stress release in a safe manner. Understanding the client's medications and dietary needs is important but not a priority for the client's son at this time. There is no indication that the son is intentionally harming the client. Being a family care provider for an older adult is a difficult role with many responsibilities. An outcome focused on personality deficits does not address any of the client's priority problems.

CJ Cognitive Skill

Generate Solutions

References

Morrison-Valfre, 2017, pp. 300–307; Williams, 2018, pp. 21–26, 209–216

Thinking Exercise 13C-5

Answers

A, C, D, E, G

Rationales

The client is malnourished and may need nutritional supplements. The nurse will consult with a registered dietitian nutritionist (Choice A) to determine appropriate diets and supplements necessary to meet the client's needs. Teaching the client's son coping strategies (Choice C) and connecting the client with a social worker to identify community resources (Choice D) will address the son's knowledge deficit related to support and resources for home care. The nurse will address concerns with the client and son individually. Providing privacy (Choice G), using therapeutic communication techniques, and providing emotional support are essential during these conversations. Finally, the nurse must document findings accurately and objectively (Choice E). Abuse and neglect, whether intentional or unintentional, are not acceptable and may cause the nurse to experience strong emotions. The nurse must remember to document actual findings and actions in the client's chart and not allow personal feelings or biases to be reflected in documentation or care provided. The other actions do not address the current problems or assist in the achievement of desired outcomes.

CJ Cognitive Skill

Take Action

References

Morrison-Valfre, 2017, pp. 300–307; Williams, 2018, pp. 21–26, 209–216

Thinking Exercise 13C-6

Answers

Client Finding	Effective	Ineffective	Unrelated
Client eats 100% of meals and supplements.	X		
Client's son has joined a support group for caregivers of older adults.	X		
Client is oriented to person and place and follows basic commands.			X
Client's son is afraid to use available respite care.		X	
Client states he is interested in going to the senior day care center.	X		

Rationales

Changes in weight and BMI will be slow, but the client's ability to eat and take appropriate supplements on a regular schedule will promote a healthy nutritional status and is a positive outcome. The client's interest in going to a senior day care center also demonstrates that interventions were effective. Interactions with others may improve his nutritional intake during the day when his son is at work and decrease any social isolation he may have when home alone for extended periods. Joining a support group to share feelings and learn new strategies to improve coping skills demonstrates that interventions were effective, but the son's reluctance to use respite care owing to guilt, fear, or other misguided emotions indicates that interventions were not effective. The client's orientation and ability to follow commands have not changed since admission and are not relevant when evaluating desired outcomes.

CJ Cognitive Skill

Evaluate Outcomes

References

Morrison-Valfre, 2017, pp. 300–307; Williams, 2018, pp. 21–26, 209–216

Thinking Exercise 13C-7

Answers

Nursing Action	Indicated	Contraindicated	Non-Essential
Ensure confidentiality when discussing concerns with the client and wife together.		X	
Consult the primary health care provider to evaluate the client's behavior and medication regimen.	X		
Assess the client's range of motion and strength to determine he is physically capable of hitting his wife.			X
Consult the case manager regarding alternatives for the client's discharge plan.	X		
Notify appropriate reporting agencies for suspected elder abuse.	X		

Rationales

Because the wife spoke with the nurse outside the client's room, it appears that she may be hesitant about speaking about abuse in the presence of the client. Interviewing the wife separately from the client provides an opportunity to identify inconsistencies regarding abuse and ensures both the client and the wife are safe. The wife indicates that the client's confusion creates behavioral outbursts and agitation. An evaluation of the client's neurologic status, behavior, and potential causes including medication is essential to determine the root cause. Medications or other therapies may also be available to help control the client's aggressive behavior. Nurses are mandated reporters of elder abuse; therefore the nurse must follow state reporting laws if abuse is suspected. There may be alternative options for discharge that do not require the client to go directly home. The nurse would consult with the case manager to begin evaluating these options. There is no need for the nurse to evaluate the client's ability to physically harm his wife.

CJ Cognitive Skill

Generate Solutions

References

Morrison-Valfre, 2017, pp. 300–307; Williams, 2018, pp. 21–26, 209–216

CHAPTER 14 Reproduction

Answers With Rationales for Thinking Exercises

Exemplar 14A. Uterine Leiomyoma/Hysterectomy (Medical-Surgical Nursing: Middle-Age Adult)

Thinking Exercise 14A-1

Answers

Client Finding in PACU	Client Finding on Surgical Unit	Client Finding Requiring Immediate Follow-up
Temperature = 99°F (37.2°C)	Temperature = 99°F (37.2°C)	
Apical pulse = 84 beats/min; strong and regular	Apical pulse = 100 beats/min; fairly strong and regular	**X**
Respirations = 20 breaths/min	Respirations = 18 breaths/min	
Blood pressure = 122/78 mm Hg	Blood pressure = 102/54 mm Hg	**X**
Oxygen saturation = 95% (on room air [RA])	Oxygen saturation = 95% (on room air [RA])	
Abdominal surgical dressing dry and intact	Abdominal surgical dressing dry and intact	
Mild abdominal distention	Moderate abdominal distention	**X**
Bowel sounds absent × 4	Bowel sounds absent × 4	
Pain level = 7/10	Pain level = 9/10	**X**
No nausea or vomiting	Reports feeling "a little nauseated"	
IV of D5/RL infusing at 80 mL/hr	IV of D5/RL infusing at 80 mL/hr	

Rationales

The client experienced several assessment finding changes when she was admitted from the PACU to the surgical unit, including an increased pulse, decreased blood pressure, increased pain, and increased abdominal distention. These assessment changes are significant and need immediate follow-up by the nurse.

CJ Cognitive Skill

Recognize Cues

Reference

Linton & Matteson, 2020, pp. 91, 1025–1028

Thinking Exercise 14A-2

Answers

When interpreting the admission assessment data, the nurse recognizes that the client is ***most likely*** experiencing <u>internal bleeding</u> as evidenced by a(n) <u>decreased blood pressure</u>, <u>increased apical pulse</u>, and <u>increased pain level</u>.

Rationales

The nurse would observe that there is no overt bleeding, even though the pulse increased and the blood pressure dropped. The client also has increased abdominal pain and distention. Therefore the nurse would suspect internal bleeding as a possible complication of surgery.

CJ Cognitive Skill

Analyze Cues

Reference

Linton & Matteson, 2020, pp. 91, 1025–1028

Thinking Exercise 14A-3

Answers

Based on the changes in the client's condition in the surgical unit, the nurse needs to plan care to meet the ***priority*** goals of preventing hypovolemic shock and managing pain.

Rationales

If the client's bleeding continues or is massive, the client experiences fluid loss, which causes hypovolemia and possibly hypovolemic shock. She is also experiencing a 9/10 pain in her abdomen, which is likely due to the internal bleeding.

CJ Cognitive Skill

Prioritize Hypotheses

Reference

Linton & Matteson, 2020, pp. 91, 1025–1028

Thinking Exercise 14A-4

Answers

Potential Primary Health Care Provider Orders	Anticipated	Contraindicated	Non-Essential
Increase IV rate to 150 mL/hr.	X		
Obtain a complete blood count (CBC) and basic metabolic panel (BMP) stat.	X		
Monitor oral temperature every hour.			X
Give regular insulin per sliding scale.			X
Keep the client in a high-Fowler position.		X	
Maintain NPO status until further orders.	X		

Rationales

As a result of likely hypovolemia, the client would need fluid replacement by increasing the IV rate. The client may need surgery depending on the results of the diagnostic imaging tests, so the nurse would maintain the client's NPO status for the time being. Blood work to determine if the client is anemic or has an electrolyte imbalance would also be needed. Because the client is NPO, she would likely not need insulin at this time. The nurse knows that any client who is hypotensive would benefit from lowering the head of the bed rather than sitting the client up. Therefore a sitting position for this client would be contraindicated. The client's temperature would not need to be taken every hour, but the nurse would take her respiration, pulse, and blood pressure at least every hour until her diagnosis is confirmed.

CJ Cognitive Skill

Generate Solutions

Reference

Linton & Matteson, 2020, pp. 91, 1025–1028

Thinking Exercise 14A-5

Answers

A, B, D, E, F, G, H

Rationales

The nurse teaches the client how to care for herself at home after her surgery, including when to report changes to her surgeon such as signs of incisional infection (Choices A and E) or deep vein thrombosis (Choice G). Because the client had a short-term urinary catheter, the client should also monitor for and report any urinary burning or frequency to the surgeon (Choice B). The client does not have to remain on bedrest for a week but should not overexert, including avoiding heavy lifting (Choice D). She can take a shower if she protects her incision (Choice F). Because she has had a removal on one ovary and on her uterus, she has surgically induced menopause (Choice H).

CJ Cognitive Skill

Take Action

Reference

Linton & Matteson, 2020, pp. 1025–1028

Thinking Exercise 14A-6

Answers

- Temperature = 98.8°F (37.1°C)
- Blood pressure = 166/94 mm Hg
- Oxygen saturation = 95%
- Incision clean, dry, and edges approximated
- Clear yellow urine
- Reports difficulty sleeping and excessive sweating at night
- No abdominal pain

Rationales

The highlighted client findings are all within normal or usual limits and show that the client is progressing well. Her blood pressure, however, is high, and she has a history of hypertension. She is also having sleeping issues and excessive sweating, which are likely the result of her surgically induced menopause.

CJ Cognitive Skill

Evaluate Outcomes

Reference

Linton & Matteson, 2020, pp. 1025–1028

Thinking Exercise 14A-7

Answers

A, B, D, E, F, G, H

Rationales

To prevent postoperative complications, the nurse would teach the client to use the incentive spirometer at least every 2 hours, deep breathe every hour, and exercise her legs and ankles to prevent deep vein thrombosis (DVT) (Choices A, B, and D). The nurse also ensures that the client moves soon after surgery by getting out of bed into a chair to prevent DVT and respiratory complications (Choice F). To help the client know what to expect postoperatively, the nurse explains about her surgical bandages, teaches her about the usual amount of vaginal drainage as a result of the surgical procedure, and reminds her to sit up in bed to relieve tension on abdominal muscles and thus reduce pain (Choices E, G, and H).

CJ Cognitive Skill

Take Action

Reference

Linton & Matteson, 2020, pp. 1025–1028

Exemplar 14B. Peripartum Care (Maternal-Newborn Nursing: Young Adult)

Thinking Exercise 14B-1

Answers

Signs of Pregnancy	Positive Signs of Pregnancy
Morning nausea	
Audible fetal heartbeat	X
Abdominal and breast striae	
Breast tenderness	
Amenorrhea	
Abdominal enlargement	
Ultrasound image of fetus	X

Rationales

Although all of these signs may occur in a pregnant woman, only the evidence of a fetus can confirm pregnancy and be considered a positive sign of pregnancy.

CJ Cognitive Skill

Recognize Cues

Reference

Leifer, 2019, pp. 54–55

Thinking Exercise 14B-2

Answers

The nurse takes the client's blood pressure as a baseline because increased blood pressure during pregnancy may indicate preeclampsia/eclampsia. The nurse also schedules the client for a glucose tolerance test because some pregnant women develop gestational diabetes mellitus during pregnancy, which can lead to diabetes mellitus type 2 later in the woman's life.

Rationales

When a woman is pregnant, she experiences an increase in blood volume, which can cause increased high blood pressure. If this problem is not managed or does not respond to management, she can develop preeclampsia, which can harm the both the mother and the fetus if it progresses to eclampsia. Because of the additional demand of a fetus on the mother, some women develop gestational diabetes mellitus (DM), which can result in DM type 2 later in the woman's life.

CJ Cognitive Skill

Analyze Cues

Reference

Leifer, 2019, pp. 97–100, 102–103

Thinking Exercise 14B-3

Answers

The nurse recognizes that the variable decelerations are ***most likely*** caused by umbilical cord compression and therefore the ***priority*** for client care is repositioning to her left side.

Rationales

During labor contractions, the fetal umbilical cord can become compressed. The nurse repositions the client first on her left side. If this action does not work to increase the fetal heart rate, supplemental oxygen may be administered to the client.

CJ Cognitive Skill

Prioritize Hypotheses

Reference

Leifer, 2019, p. 143

Thinking Exercise 14B-4

Answers

Nursing Action	Indicated	Contraindicated	Non-Essential
Obtain blood for coagulation studies, complete blood count, and blood typing.	X		
Administer an enema.		X	
Ensure that informed consent is obtained.	X		
Shave the perineal area to remove excess hair.			X
Insert an indwelling urinary catheter.	X		
Keep client NPO.	X		

Rationales

The nurse prepares the client for possible surgery to deliver the baby by keeping her NPO and inserting a urinary catheter to prevent bladder injury during the procedure. The nurse ensures that informed consent is obtained by the surgeon and that all of the necessary blood work, including type and crossmatch, is completed.

CJ Cognitive Skill

Generate Solutions

Reference

Leifer, 2019, pp. 189–190

Thinking Exercise 14B-5

Answers

A, B, C, D, E, F, H

Rationales

Postoperative nursing care for the woman having a cesarean section includes the same actions as those for any abdominal surgery, such as documenting urinary output, administering analgesic medication for pain, and monitoring vital signs and the abdominal dressing for drainage and intactness (Choices A, D, E, and H). In addition, because the client had a baby, the nurse would check lochia and the condition of the postpartum uterus (Choices B and C). The client had spinal anesthesia and would be monitored for her ability to move her legs by at least 1 to 2 hours after surgery (Choice F).

CJ Cognitive Skill

Take Action

Reference

Leifer, 2019, p. 191

Thinking Exercise 14B-6

Answers

Nursing Action	Effective	Ineffective	Unrelated
Temperature = 98°F (36.7°C)	X		
Oxygen saturation = 97% (on room air [RA])	X		
Small incisional area in right lower abdominal quadrant reddened and oozing yellow drainage		X	
States that her seasonal allergies are especially annoying this year			X
Has lost 22 lb since delivery	X		
States she feels tired most of the time because the baby is hungry every 2 hours	X		

Rationales

The client's vital signs are within usual limits and she has lost a significant amount of weight since delivery, indicating that she is progressing well and her care was effective. Being tired with a 4-week old infant is expected. However, her abdominal incision should not show signs of infection. Her report of allergies is not related to her postpartum care.

CJ Cognitive Skill

Evaluate Outcomes

Reference

Leifer, 2019, pp. 218–220

Thinking Exercise 14B-7

Answers

Health Teaching Statement by Nurse	Client's Discomfort of Pregnancy	Health Teaching That Client Can Use to Manage Discomfort of Pregnancy
1 "Elevate your legs whenever you can."	Constipation	**3** "Eat food high in fiber."
2 "Avoid gas-forming and greasy foods."	Backache	**4** "Use good body mechanics."
3 "Eat food high in fiber."	Ankle edema	**1** "Elevate your legs whenever you can."
4 "Use good body mechanics."	Fatigue	**6** "Take naps during the day as needed."
5 "Eat ginger several times a day."	Shortness of breath	**8** "Sleep with several pillows at night."
6 "Take naps during the day as needed."		
7 "Increase fluid intake to at least four glasses a day."		
8 "Sleep with several pillows at night."		

Rationales

The client's discomforts are typical of pregnant women but are managed the same way as they would be for women who are not pregnant. For example, ankle edema can decrease if the client elevates her legs and feet frequently. Using good body mechanics can help prevent backaches, and naps will help with fatigue. The fetus, especially in the third semester, can press on the woman's diaphragm, causing shortness of breath. Sitting upright using pillow support can help make breathing easier.

CJ Cognitive Skill

Take Action

Reference

Leifer, 2019, pp. 70–71

Thinking Exercise 14B-8

Answers

A, B, D, E, F, G

Rationales

Teaching the client about fetal monitoring can help alleviate the laboring woman's anxiety. The purpose of this device is to continuously monitor the baby's heart rate, which is expected to change during contractions (Choices A, D, and E). It consists of a transducer and two sensors that are placed on the abdomen to detect the place where the fetal heart rate (FHR) is the strongest (Choice B). FHR is recorded during labor, and the mother's vital signs are monitored (Choices F and G).

CJ Cognitive Skill

Take Action

Reference

Leifer, 2019, pp. 137–143

Exemplar 14C. Newborn Care (Maternal-Newborn Nursing: Newborn)

Thinking Exercise 14C-1

Answers

A, B, D, E, F, G

Rationales

The nurse would expect the highest score of 2 on four of the five aspects of the Apgar scoring system. Babies typically have a pink body with blue extremities at 1 minute after birth for a total Apgar score of 9 instead of 10 (Choice E). Unless the baby is born in a high-altitude area, the cyanosis typically disappears within 5 minutes. The baby's heart rate is over 100, which is normal (Choice A). The baby also has active spontaneous motion, a flexed body position, a strong cry, and a prompt response to stimuli, all of which are normal (Choices B, D, F, and G).

CJ Cognitive Skill

Recognize Cues

Reference

Leifer, 2019, p. 158

Thinking Exercise 14C-2

Answers

Newborn Finding	Apgar Subscore
Heart rate = 98 beats/min	1
Strong spontaneous cry	2
Flexed body posture	2
Prompt response to stimuli such as suction	2
Body pink, extremities blue	1
Total Apgar Score	**8**

Rationales

The Apgar scoring system rates five aspects of newborn assessment, which are each scored as a 0, 1, or 2 (normal). The baby had a heart rate of 98, which is scored as a 1 because the newborn should have a heart rate of over 100 beats/min. Having blue extremities would score a 1 rather than a 2, which is normal.

CJ Cognitive Skill

Analyze Cues

Reference

Leifer, 2019, p. 158

Thinking Exercise 14C-3

Answers

The nurse recognizes that the ***priority*** for the newborn is to support thermoregulation to prevent complications such as <u>hypoglycemia</u> and <u>respiratory distress</u>. To prevent becoming hypothermic, the newborn is kept <u>in a radiant warmer</u> until the newborn's temperature is stabilized.

Rationales

The nurse knows that keeping the baby warm in a radiant warmer is a priority to prevent complications such as hypoglycemia and respiratory distress.

CJ Cognitive Skill

Prioritize Hypotheses

Reference

Leifer, 2019, p. 157

Thinking Exercise 14C-4

Answers

Nursing Action	Indicated	Contraindicated	Non-Essential
Provide the opportunity for the newborn to have skin-to-skin contact with the mother.	X		
Administer vitamin K to the newborn subcutaneously in the abdomen.		X	
Keep the umbilical cord moist and covered.		X	
Prepare the newborn for circumcision.			X
Perform a heel stick on the newborn to test for phenylketonuria (PKU).	X		
Ensure that the mother's and newborn's identification bands match.	X		

Rationales

The nurse provides skin-to-skin contact between mother and baby to promote maternal bonding and ensures that the identification bands match between mother and baby for safety and security. The nurse also keeps the umbilical cord dry (not moist) and performs a heel stick to obtain a blood sample to test for PKU. Vitamin K is administered as an intramuscular (IM) injection rather than a subcutaneous one. The baby is a girl, so circumcision preparation does not apply.

CJ Cognitive Skill

Generate Solutions

Reference

Leifer, 2019, pp. 158–160

Thinking Exercise 14C-5

Answers

Nurse's Response	Client Question	Appropriate Nurse's Response for Each Client Question
1 "Breastfeeding is cheaper than buying milk formula."	"How often should I breastfeed the baby?"	**2** "Feed the baby on a 2- to 3- hour schedule."
2 "Feed the baby on a 2- to 3- hour schedule."	"How do I make sure that the baby is latching onto my breast?"	**3** "Be sure that the baby's mouth covers the entire breast areola."
3 "Be sure that the baby's mouth covers the entire breast areola."	"How do I stop the baby from eating?"	**7** "Put your finger in the corner of the baby's mouth."
4 "Burp the baby halfway through the feeding."	"What is the main advantage of breastfeeding?"	**6** "Breastfeeding helps build a relationship with your baby and the milk is easily digested."
5 "Feed the baby when she cries."		
6 "Breastfeeding helps build a relationship with your baby and the milk is easily digested."		
7 "Put your finger in the corner of the baby's mouth."		

Rationales

Breastfeeding has many advantages including helping to build a mother-baby relationship and providing nutrition that is easy for the baby's GI system to digest. The baby's mouth should cover the entire areola of the breast, and the baby should be fed every 2 to 3 hours on a schedule. To remove the baby from the breast, the mother can put her finger in the corner of the baby's mouth to unlatch.

CJ Cognitive Skill

Take Action

Reference

Leifer, 2019, pp. 231–238

Thinking Exercise 14C-6

Answers

Newborn Finding	Is Progressing	Is Not Progressing
Unable to hold head/chin up		X
Grasp reflex is intact	X	
Focuses on surroundings	X	
Weight = 8 lb (3.6 kg)		X
Holds hands closed most of the time	X	

Rationales

A 4-week-old infant should be able to hold her head/chin up and focus on objects in her environment. Her grasp reflex should still be intact and she should hold her hands closed in a fist most of the time. She should have also gained a little weight, but she has lost weight. It is expected that newly born babies lose a few ounces during the first few days but then should regain that weight and perhaps even more than at birth by 4 weeks.

CJ Cognitive Skill

Evaluate Outcomes

Reference

Leifer, 2019, pp. 285, 394

Thinking Exercise 14C-7

Answers

The nurse recognizes that the newborn ***most likely*** has dehydration due to inadequate fluid intake.

Rationales

The baby is not getting enough fluid from breastfeeding and is likely becoming dehydrated. He is very fussy because he is hungry and needs fluids.

CJ Cognitive Skill

Analyze Cues

Reference

Leifer, 2019, pp. 231–238

Thinking Exercise 14C-8

Answers

A, B, E, F, G

Rationales

Because the baby is hungry and likely dehydrated, the nurse would assess his vital signs, weight (as the most reliable indicator of fluid status), skin turgor, and mucous membranes for dryness (Choices A, B, F, and G). Because the baby wears a diaper, measuring the amount of urinary output is not possible as a sign of dehydration. However, the nurse would ask about the number of diaper changes during the day to determine if the baby is urinating. Newborns are expected to need a minimum of 6 to 8 diaper changes each day; many newborns need more than 10 diaper changes each day .

CJ Cognitive Skill

Take Action

Reference

Leifer, 2019, pp. 231–238

CHAPTER 15 Perfusion

Answers With Rationales for Thinking Exercises

Exemplar 15A. Hypertension (Medical-Surgical Nursing: Older Adult)

Thinking Exercise 15A-1

Answers

- Alert and oriented
- Fidgety and restless
- Reports vision is "foggy around the edges"
- Heart rate (HR) = 88 beats/min
- Blood pressure (BP) = 164/88 mm Hg
- Respirations = 17 breaths/min
- Oxygen saturation = 94% (on room air [RA])
- Reports a headache at the back of her head, rated 6/10
- Respirations equal and unlabored
- Lung fields clear throughout
- Abdomen round and soft
- Bowel sounds present

Rationales

The client's restless behavior may be a sign of anxiety. There are many reasons the client could be feeling anxious, and the nurse must complete a more thorough assessment to determine the cause. Pain must always be assessed completely. Headaches can have a variety of causes including some life-threatening conditions. A headache with an accompanying report of vision changes is especially concerning, and the nurse must urgently follow up on these symptoms. The client's vital signs are within normal limits with the exception of the blood pressure, which is elevated. Because the nurse does not know the client's health history, it is essential for the nurse to follow up on the blood pressure to determine if it is related to acute pain and anxiety or to another primary problem that is causing the client's headache, visual changes, and anxious feelings. The other client findings are all within usual limits.

CJ Cognitive Skill

Recognize Cues

Reference

Linton & Matteson, 2020, pp. 677–690

Thinking Exercise 15A-2

Answers

A, B, E, F, G, H

Rationales

Headache, vision changes, and anxiety are associated with life-threatening conditions including stroke and intracranial hemorrhage. The nurse needs to complete a thorough neurologic assessment to determine if the client has any additional signs of these disorders. The nurse assesses the client's cranial nerves, including pupils for size, shape, and reaction (Choice A) and facial movement for symmetry (Choice E). Because the nurse knows little about the client's health history, the nurse will also ask questions to obtain more information about the client's health status and healthy or risky behaviors. Questions focused on nutrition (Choice F), exercise, sleep (Choice H), and stress will help the nurse to identify health risks. Questions focused on use of nicotine (Choice B), alcohol, and other substances must also be asked. Finally, the nurse will assess for any history of headaches or migraines, because visual changes may accompany migraine headaches (Choice G). Assessing peripheral pulses and recent immunizations will not assist the nurse in analyzing cues and identifying priority client needs.

CJ Cognitive Skill

Analyze Cues

Reference

Linton & Matteson, 2020, pp. 677–690

Thinking Exercise 15A-3

Answers

The client ***most likely*** has previously undiagnosed <u>hypertension</u>. The nurse's ***priority*** is to implement a plan of care to prevent complications, including heart failure, <u>stroke</u>, and <u>kidney disease</u>.

Rationales

The client is not experiencing any other neurologic deficits related to intracranial hemorrhage or a transient ischemic attack. The client also states she has no health or medical issues. The client has many risk factors for hypertension including age, a diet high in fat and sodium, use of nicotine tobacco, unhealthy sleep habits, and daily stress. The client most likely has hypertension that was undiagnosed owing to her lack of annual health checkups. Prolonged hypertension causes thickening of arteriolar walls, which decreases their ability to expand and increases peripheral vascular resistance. The long-term effect of hypertension is decreased blood flow to various organs. The organs that are most sensitive to vascular changes are the heart, kidneys, brain, and eyes. Ineffective management of hypertension increases the client's risk of heart failure, stroke, and chronic kidney disease.

CJ Cognitive Skill

Prioritize Hypotheses

Reference

Linton & Matteson, 2020, pp. 677–690

Thinking Exercise 15A-4

Answers

Nursing Action	Indicated	Contraindicated	Non-Essential
Consult a registered dietitian nutritionist to facilitate a low-fat and low-sodium diet.	X		
Provide client teaching focused on nutrition, exercise, and medication therapy.	X		
Monitor for therapeutic and side effects of antihypertensive medications.	X		
Collaborate with a physical therapist for passive range-of-motion activities when orthostatic hypotension occurs.		X	
Ensure naloxone is on the unit in case of an overdose of antihypertensive medications.			X

Rationales

Hypertension is a chronic disease that requires long-term management. Client education is critical for effective management and must be included in the client's plan of care. The client's immediate concerns and questions should be addressed first, followed by information on diet therapy, exercise, and medications. Goals of diet therapy for a client with hypertension are to maintain ideal body weight and prevent fluid retention. A low-fat and low-sodium diet would be implemented. The client will be started on new medications. The nurse must monitor the client for therapeutic and side effects of drug therapy to ensure that the client's blood pressure is successfully lowered without negative symptoms. The nurse will collaborate with physical therapy and occupational therapy personnel to ensure that the client is safe during all activities. Antihypertensive medications increase the client's risk for orthostatic hypotension, and passive range of motion would not be performed when blood pressure is low. The client should continue fully participating in therapies.

CJ Cognitive Skill

Generate Solutions

Reference

Linton & Matteson, 2020, pp. 677–690

Thinking Exercise 15A-5

Answers

B, D, E, F, H

Rationales

The client is starting hydrochlorothiazide (HCTZ), a diuretic that is a first-line treatment for hypertension. This drug increases urinary output to rid the body of excessive fluid and decrease intravascular volume (Choice E). The nurse would monitor the client's intake and output to ensure fluid balance (Choice H). Electrolytes would also be monitored because the HCTZ causes loss of sodium (desired to help lose excessive fluid) and potassium (not desired and must be replaced). Both HCTZ and amlodipine can cause dizziness and orthostatic blood pressure changes, requiring nurse monitoring (Choice F). Side effects of amlodipine include bradycardia, hypotension, headache, and ankle and foot edema (Choice B). If dependent edema occurs, the nurse would teach the client the need to elevate her lower extremities while sitting (Choice D).

CJ Cognitive Skill

Take Action

Reference

Linton & Matteson, 2020, pp. 677–690

Thinking Exercise 15A-6

Answers

Client Statement	Effective	Ineffective	Unrelated
"I will use the resources provided to begin a smoking cessation program."	X		
"Once my blood pressure is within normal limits, I can stop taking the medication."		X	
"I will add more fruits and vegetables to my diet and eat less fast food."	X		
"Spices, garlic, and onions can add flavor to my food without adding more sodium."	X		
"I will take my pulse for a full minute prior to taking my antihypertensive medications."			X

Rationales

Smoking aggravates hypertension, and therefore clients with hypertension will be encouraged to quit. The nurse will provide the client with information about local resources including the American Heart Association's smoking cessation programs. The nurse will help the client develop healthy eating habits based on a diet moderately low in sodium and low in fat. Eating more fruits and vegetables and low-fat dairy products can help the client to eat the prescribed diet. Seasoning foods with spices, garlic, and onions instead of salt may also assist the client in decreasing sodium intake. Antihypertensive medications should be taken as prescribed and not stopped unless instructed to do so by the primary health care provider. Suddenly stopping these drugs may cause the client's blood pressure to rise rapidly. Although her antihypertensive medications will lower heart rate, there is no need for the client to take her pulse for a full minute before taking the medications.

CJ Cognitive Skill

Evaluate Outcomes

Reference

Linton & Matteson, 2020, pp. 677–690

Thinking Exercise 15A-7

Answers

A, B, D, F, G, H

Rationales

A client taking these prescribed medications may experience several side effects. Orthostatic hypotension, a common side effect, occurs when the vasculature does not constrict quickly enough to adjust the client's blood pressure with position changes, usually from supine to standing. This slow vascular response causes the client to feel lightheaded or dizzy. The nurse would evaluate for symptoms of orthostatic hypotension because they increase the client's risk of falls and injury (Choice A). Many older adults remain sexually active as they age, and therefore the nurse must assess for sexual dysfunction, a side effect of diuretics and beta blockers (Choice B). Ingesting foods high in potassium is recommended to clients prescribed diuretics including hydrochlorothiazide. Assessing what the client eats assists the nurse in determining if the client understands the recommended diet and knows which food items are high in potassium (Choice F). The nurse would also evaluate for signs of palpitations caused by hypokalemia or a side effect of the calcium channel blocker (Choice G). Depression is a side effect of beta blockers and is also a serious concern for older adults. Depression lowers a client's motivation, impairs quality of life, and can lead to suicide. The nurse would assess for signs of depression including feelings of hopelessness (Choice H), changes in sleep and eating patterns, trouble concentrating, and thoughts of suicide (Choice D).

CJ Cognitive Skill

Evaluate Outcomes

Reference

Linton & Matteson, 2020, pp. 677–690

Exemplar 15B. Stroke (Medical-Surgical Nursing: Older Adult)

Thinking Exercise 15B-1

Answers

Client Finding	Priority Client Finding That Requires Follow-Up by the Nurse
Level of consciousness	X
Blood pressure	X
Oxygenation status	
Pain	
Dysarthria	X
Heart rate	

Rationales

The client is experiencing lethargy, disorientation, and slurred speech (dysarthria). These findings indicate a change in the client's neurologic status from shift change 30 minutes earlier. The nurse must recognize that this change in status is not within the expected outcomes for the client and is potentially a life-threatening situation. The client's vital signs are within normal limits with the exception of the client's blood pressure. Normal blood pressure is a systolic pressure less than 120 mm Hg and a diastolic pressure less than 80 mm Hg. The client's blood pressure at 160/92 mm Hg is elevated and must be evaluated further to determine if it is creating the client's situation or is a result of the situation. The client denies pain.

CJ Cognitive Skill

Recognize Cues

Reference

Linton & Matteson, 2020, pp. 401–420

Thinking Exercise 15B-2

Answers

Client Finding	Anemia	Sepsis	Hypoglycemia	Stroke
Lethargy	X		X	X
Slurred speech		X		X
Confusion		X	X	X
Pallor	X		X	

Rationales

The nurse will evaluate potential problems related to acute neurologic changes. Based on the client's history of diabetes mellitus, the nurse will assess for signs of an abnormal blood glucose level, specifically hypoglycemia. Relevant findings for hypoglycemia include mental confusion, lethargy or fatigue, and pallor. The nurse may obtain the client's capillary blood glucose level to further evaluate the client for a potential hypoglycemic episode. The client also has a history of anemia. Client findings relevant to anemia are cool skin, pallor, and lethargy. The nurse may further assess the client for shortness of breath, chest pain, and lightheadedness, as well as morning laboratory results, specifically hemoglobin and hematocrit levels.

The client has several risk factors for a stroke including advanced age, recent surgery, diabetes mellitus, and hypertension (BP = 160/92 mm Hg). Client findings relevant to a stroke are lethargy, slurred speech, and confusion. Assessing for additional unilateral changes including weakness and numbness, as well as aphasia and dysphasia, will assist the nurse in further analyzing the client for a potential stroke. The client's advanced age and history of diabetes mellitus increase the client's risk for a blood infection called sepsis. An acute change in mental status, including confusion, disorientation, and slurred speech, is relevant to sepsis.

CJ Cognitive Skill

Analyze Cues

Reference

Linton & Matteson, 2020, pp. 401–420

Thinking Exercise 15B-3

Answers

The client is ***most likely*** experiencing a stroke. The nurse must intervene immediately to prevent aspiration pneumonia.

Rationales

A stroke is the most likely explanation for the client's current condition. The five most common symptoms of a stroke are (1) sudden confusion or trouble speaking; (2) sudden numbness or weakness of the face, arm, or leg; (3) sudden trouble seeing from one or both eyes; (4) sudden dizziness, trouble walking, or loss of balance or coordination; and (5) sudden severe headache with no known cause. The client is currently experiencing several of these symptoms, including confusion, dysarthria, hemiplegia, and blurred vision. In addition, the client is not anemic (hemoglobin/hematocrit, 12 g/dL/39%) and both her blood glucose level (188 mg/dL) and her white blood cell count (8000/mm^3) are normal. Because the client is having a stroke, she is at risk for aspiration pneumonia and should remain NPO until she has swallowing studies.

CJ Cognitive Skill

Prioritize Hypotheses

Reference

Linton & Matteson, 2020, pp. 401–420

Thinking Exercise 15B-4

Answers

Nursing Action	Potential Complication	Appropriate Nursing Action for Each Potential Complication
1 Explain what is happening, why interventions are implemented, and what can be expected.	Inability to communicate effectively due to dysarthria	**4** Explore communication methods to determine what works best for the client.
2 Provide a note pad for the client to communicate in writing.	Anxiety due to loss of function or fear of disability	**1** Explain what is happening, why interventions are implemented, and what can be expected.
3 Assess family strengths and resources.	Pulmonary infection due to impaired neuromuscular function and mobility	**7** Continuously monitor oxygen saturation levels and breath sounds; suction oral secretions as needed.
4 Explore communication methods to determine what works best for the client.	Potential for falls related to hemiplegia	**6** Frequently remind the client to use the call light if the client needs to use the bathroom.
5 Perform postural drainage and percussion therapy to mobilize bronchial secretions.		
6 Frequently remind the client to use the call light if the client needs to use the bathroom.		
7 Continuously monitor oxygen saturation levels and suction oral secretions as needed.		

Rationales

Dysarthria is the inability to speak clearly as a result of weakened facial muscles. Clients who have dysarthria are difficult to understand, but they understand what is said and have no difficulty putting together thoughts. The nurse would provide several tools and resources to help the client communicate effectively. The client should choose the communication method that works best for her; the nurse should not decide. Anxiety and fear are common during the acute phase of a stroke. The client may not understand what is happening to her or why she is experiencing neuromuscular issues. Acknowledging signs of anxiety and identifying the source will assist the nurse in addressing the client's emotions. Providing information about what is happening, what the health care staff is doing, and what the client can expect will also decrease anxiety.

During the acute phase of a stroke, airway clearance is a high priority. The client is experiencing left-side hemiplegia and drooling from the left side of the mouth. Excessive sputum and an inability to clear secretions effectively increase the client's risk for aspiration, pulmonary infection, and respiratory distress. The nurse will position the client to decrease secretions from pooling in the mouth, perform oral suctioning to remove secretions, and continuously monitor the client's oxygen saturation level and breath sounds. The client, who is experiencing hemiplegia, cognitive changes, and potential sensory impairments, is also at high risk for injury including falls, skin breakdown, and extremity trauma. The client will be on bedrest during the acute phase but may try to get out of bed to go to the bathroom. The nurse would frequently remind the client to use her call light if she wants to get out of bed. The nurse would also position the client to prevent skin breakdown and promote adequate blood flow to all extremities.

CJ Cognitive Skill

Generate Solutions

Reference

Linton & Matteson, 2020, pp. 401–420

Thinking Exercise 15B-5

Answers

A, B, E, F, H

Rationales

The nurse would contact the Rapid Response or Stroke Team immediately (Choice A). A stroke is a medical emergency and should be treated immediately to reduce or prevent permanent disability. Rapid Response and Stroke Teams consist of experts in acute stroke assessment and management. The nurse would also assist in completing the facility's approved stoke scale while awaiting for the Stroke Team to arrive (Choice B). Establishing a baseline assessment with a valid and reliable tool assists in the diagnosis and determination of treatment options. The National Institutes of Health Stroke Scale (NIHSS) assessment is the most frequently used assessment tool and assesses for level of consciousness, orientation, communication deficiencies, visual deficits, sensory impairment, and motor function (Choice H). Finally, the nurse would prepare the client for an imaging examination, most likely a computed tomography perfusion (CTP) scan and/or computed tomography angiography (CTA). Imaging scans are used to definitively diagnose a stroke and must be completed prior to the administration of IV thrombolytic therapy. The nurse would assess for known allergies to contrast media (Choice E) and remove all personal and medical equipment that would not be transported with the client to the radiology department.

The client's change in status requires care to be transferred to a registered nurse. When providing the transition of care report, the nurse must report the time symptoms began (Choice F). The client should remain NPO until a swallow evaluation is completed and on bedrest in a comfortable position. Positioning the client in a flat position increases risk of aspiration.

CJ Cognitive Skill

Take Action

Reference

Linton & Matteson, 2020, pp. 401–420

Thinking Exercise 15B-6

Answers

Client Statement	Effective	Ineffective	Unrelated
"Rehabilitation will teach me new ways to compensate for my loss of function."	X		
"I will remain in the rehabilitation center until I can complete ADLs independently."		X	
"I look forward to having a window in my room at the rehabilitation center."			X
"The purpose of rehabilitation is for me to achieve the highest level of functioning possible with my deficits."	X		
"I am excited to learn how to use personal assistive devices to obtain more independence."	X		
"I will get to know several therapists who will take the place of a nurse during my rehabilitation."		X	

Rationales

General goals of stroke care during the rehabilitation phase are to maximize functional abilities and teach new ways to compensate for losses. The rehabilitation phase is managed by an interdisciplinary team that consists of many health care providers including nurses. Members of rehabilitative teams usually consist of nurses, physicians, physical therapists, occupational therapists, speech and language pathologists, social workers, psychologists, recreational therapists, vocational rehabilitation counselors, and registered nutritional dietitians.

The main focus of stroke rehabilitation is to assist the client in achieving the highest level of functioning possible. A variety of assistive devices and environmental adaptations can foster a return to independence. Clients are usually unable to remain in acute rehabilitation facilities until independence with all ADLs is achieved. Outpatient therapy and family care providers are needed for a client to achieve the highest level of function and remain safe. The nurse would not have taught the client anything about the facility's decor.

CJ Cognitive Skill

Evaluate Outcomes

Reference

Linton & Matteson, 2020, pp. 401–420

Thinking Exercise 15B-7

Answers

Client Finding	Is Progressing	Is **Not** Progressing
Uses picture boards to communicate effectively	X	
Experiences reflexive coughing during meals		X
Voids 600 mL dark amber urine in past 24 hours		X
Requires verbal cues to initiate voluntary movements	X	
Reports feeling hopeful about recovery process	X	

Rationales

Using picture boards or other communication methods to effectively communicate is a positive step for a client who has expressive aphasia (difficulty speaking and writing). The ability to communicate needs and emotions will assist the client in fully participating in rehabilitation activities including speech therapy. Dyspraxia is the partial inability to initiate coordinated voluntary motor acts. Any part of the body with motor function can be affected. Clients can often move spontaneously, but they are unable to move willfully. Health care providers use verbal cues to help clients initiate voluntary responses. The client's ability to respond to these verbal cues and initiate voluntary movements is a sign of progression. Recovering from a stroke can cause many emotions including anxiety and depression. The client's verbalization of hope is a sign that the client is coping effectively with the situation.

Dysphagia or difficulty swallowing is a very serious problem for stroke clients because it increases the risk of malnutrition, dehydration, aspiration, and pneumonia. This client exhibits a reflexive cough during meals. Reflexive coughing acts primarily to protect the airway and clear away aspirated material. This finding indicates that the client is aspirating during meals and therefore is not tolerating the prescribed diet. Dark amber urine and less than 30 mL of urine output each hour are signs of dehydration. This client finding also indicates the client is not progressing and is at risk for serious complications.

CJ Cognitive Skill

Evaluate Outcomes

Reference

Linton & Matteson, 2020, pp. 401–420

Thinking Exercise 15B-8

Answers

A, C, D, H

Rationales

Homonymous hemianopsia is a condition in which a client's loses half of the field of vision. This creates problems for self-care and safety. Clients often need to be reminded to scan the affected visual field, especially when walking and eating. The client will form new observation habits with time, and the son can assist with frequent reminders (Choice A). Clients with impaired sensation are at risk for pressure ulcers and other injuries. The nurse will teach the client and his family to assess affected areas for signs of pressure (Choice C), how to avoid pressure, and what to do if signs of pressure are present. The nurse would also advise not to apply heat or cold to affected areas, as the client will not be able to feel if the application is too hot or too cold (Choice D).

The client should not be lying in bed most of the day. The client needs to be able to access food, water, and bathroom facilities, and a family caregiver or respite care provider needs to be present if the client is unable to access these necessities independently. Resources for respite care, community resources, and support groups should be provided to assist the client and his son in dealing with ongoing disabilities and care responsibilities (Choice H). The client should be encouraged to be as independent as possible, with the environment adapted (raised commode seat, bathtub rails, shower seat, and so on) to promote this independence. Personal assistive devices encourage independence with impaired mobility by helping clients dress, bathe, and eat. An indwelling catheter increases the client's risk of infection and would not be used.

CJ Cognitive Skill

Take Action

Reference

Linton & Matteson, 2020, pp. 401–420

CHAPTER 16 Mobility

Answers With Rationales for Thinking Exercises

Exemplar 16A. Parkinson Disease/Complications of Impaired Mobility (Medical-Surgical Nursing: Older Adult)

Thinking Exercise 16A-1

Answers

- Lives at home with his wife, who cares for him
- Needs assistance with ADLs on days when his rigidity is worse
- Walks short distances in the house using a rollator walker
- Is alert and oriented × 2–3
- Wife states that he sometimes talks to himself and seems scared
- Has resting tremors in both arms and hands, but left hand is worse than the right (client is right-handed)
- Chokes at times when he eats
- Has fallen three times in the past week
- Has a stage 2 sacral pressure injury that is 2 cm × 1 cm without drainage
- Blood pressure (BP) (sitting) = 118/70 mm Hg; BP (standing) = 98/64 mm Hg
- Heart rate = 68 beats/min and regular
- Takes losartan for a 10-year history of hypertension
- Takes a carbidopa/levodopa combination for PD

Rationales

The client is expected to have resting tremors and muscle rigidity, which would require ADL assistance and an ambulatory aid such as a walker. However, he has fallen, chokes at times while eating, and has a stage 2 pressure injury, none of which are expected as a usual manifestation of PD. The difference between his sitting and standing systolic blood pressure is 20 mm Hg, which indicates orthostatic hypotension, which may be a contributing factor to falls because of dizziness or light-headedness. This problem may be the result of drug therapy or another cause and needs to be followed up. His wife states that the client sometimes talks to himself and seems scared, perhaps indicating possible hallucinations that require follow-up.

CJ Cognitive Skill

Recognize Cues

Reference

Linton & Matteson, 2020, pp. 383–386

Thinking Exercise 16A-2

Answers

Client Finding	Parkinson Disease	Orthostatic Hypotension
Needs assistance with ADLs on days when his rigidity is worse	X	
Has resting tremors in both arms and hands, but left hand is worse than the right (client is right-handed)	X	
Has fallen three times in the past week	X	X
Chokes at times when he eats	X	
Blood pressure (BP) (sitting) = 118/70 mm Hg; BP (standing) = 98/64 mm Hg		X
Wife states that he sometimes talks to himself and seems scared	X	

Rationales

The difference between the client's sitting and standing systolic blood pressure is 20 mm Hg, which indicates orthostatic hypotension, which may be a contributing factor to falls as a result of dizziness or light-headedness. He also experiences muscle rigidity, which requires that he use a walker and could contribute to falls. With the exception of the BP readings, all of the client findings are associated with PD.

CJ Cognitive Skill

Analyze Cues

Reference

Linton & Matteson, 2020, pp. 383–386

Thinking Exercise 16A-3

Answers

Based on the client findings, the nurse recognizes that the ***priorities*** for the client's care at this time are ensuring client safety and preventing additional complications of impaired mobility.

Rationales

Given the client's fall history, orthostatic hypotension, and rigidity, the nurse's priorities would be to prevent injury and promote client safety. He already has a stage 2 pressure injury from decreased mobility and would need interventions that help prevent additional complications of impaired mobility.

CJ Cognitive Skill

Prioritize Hypotheses

Reference

Linton & Matteson, 2020, pp. 383–386

Thinking Exercise 16A-4

Answers

Nursing Action	Indicated	Contraindicated	Non-Essential
Refer the client to a registered dietitian nutritionist for food choices that are less likely to cause choking.			X
Refer the wife to hospice care for the client.			X
Remind the client and wife that he should get up slowly from the bed or chair.	X		
Suggest to the wife to keep a diary of the client's hallucinations or other mental and emotional changes.	X		
Teach the client how to care for the sacral pressure injury and report worsening or redness around the wound.	X		
Remind the wife to continue monitoring the client's blood pressure daily.	X		

Rationales

The client does not need hospice care because his disease is not at a late stage. The nurse would refer the client to a speech-language pathologist to evaluate his swallowing ability and determine the food consistency that he needs. A dietitian is not qualified to assess swallowing status. The nurse would teach the client to monitor his blood pressure and remind him to move slowly when changing positions owing to orthostatic hypotension. The nurse would also review how to care for his pressure injury and keep a diary of the client's mental and emotional behaviors, including any additional hallucinations.

CJ Cognitive Skill

Generate Solutions

Reference

Linton & Matteson, 2020, pp. 383–386

Thinking Exercise 16A-5

Answers

A, B, C, D, F, G

Rationales

To help manage the symptoms of the client's disease, the nurse would teach the wife and client to remind him to chew his food slowly and thoroughly before swallowing (Choice A). To prevent complications of decreased mobility, the nurse would also teach the wife and client to take frequent walks, perform active and active-assisted exercises, and drink adequate fluids to prevent constipation (Choices C, D, and G). Teaching to help prevent falls includes wearing firm rubber-soled shoes and stretching and marching in place before ambulating with his walker (Choices B and F).

CJ Cognitive Skill

Take Action

Reference

Linton & Matteson, 2020, pp. 383–386

Thinking Exercise 16A-6

Answers

Client Finding	Is Progressing	Is Not Progressing
Wife states that he has been choking less frequently in the past month on food or liquids.	X	
Blood pressure (BP) (sitting) = 130/76 mm Hg; BP (standing) = 124/72 mm Hg.	X	
Client walks every day inside and outside with his walker.	X	
Client has not fallen within the last 3 months.	X	
Client reports feeling sad and depressed most days.		X
Stage 2 sacral pressure injury is smaller at 1.5 cm × 0.8 cm; no drainage or surrounding redness.	X	

Rationales

The client shows improvement in all swallowing and walking and has not fallen in the last 3 months prior to this visit. His pressure injury is beginning to heal, as evidenced by a smaller size without drainage or redness, and the difference between his sitting and standing blood pressures is decreased. However, the client is experiencing feelings of sadness, which means he may be experiencing clinical depression. Depression could interfere with his desire to continue ambulating and participating in his care.

CJ Cognitive Skill

Evaluate Outcomes

Reference

Linton & Matteson, 2020, pp. 383–386

Thinking Exercise 16A-7

Answers

A, B, C, D, H

Rationales

A client with moderate-stage PD slows in movements and has cogwheel muscle rigidity, slurred speech, lack of facial expression, and gait disturbances that affect balance (Choices A, B, C, D, and H). Although the client usually has hand tremors, they tend to occur when resting. Visual disturbances and lower extremity tingling are not common in PD but commonly occur in clients who have multiple sclerosis.

CJ Cognitive Skill

Recognize Cues

Reference

Linton & Matteson, 2020, pp. 383–386

Exemplar 16B. Osteoarthritis/Total Knee Arthroplasty (Medical-Surgical Nursing: Older Adult)

Thinking Exercise 16B-1

Answers

Client Finding	Client Finding That Requires Follow-up
Knee pain = 7/10 on a 0 to 10 pain rating scale	X
Right knee reddened and swollen	X
Height = 6 ft (1.8 m); weight = 265 lb (111.1 kg)	X
Blood pressure = 154/90 mm Hg	X
Blood glucose = 124 mg/dL (6.9 mmol/L)	
Right quadriceps have less tone than left quadriceps	X

Rationales

All of these client findings are relevant data that are significant when planning care. The client's right knee is red, swollen, and painful. His knees are weight-bearing joints that are bearing excessive weight because of his obesity. The client's blood pressure is well above the normal range and needs to be addressed. His glucose level is only slightly elevated and would be monitored, but does not require follow-up at the moment.

CJ Cognitive Skill

Recognize Cues

Reference

Linton & Matteson, 2020, pp. 857–860

Thinking Exercise 16B-2

Answers

The nurse recognizes that the client's knee pain is ***most likely*** due to <u>osteoarthritis</u> as a result of <u>aging</u>, <u>obesity</u>, and his <u>occupation</u>.

Rationales

Osteoarthritis is a common health problem associated with aging (especially in women) as the joint cartilage degenerates and the joint space narrows. Certain occupations that require manual labor can also worsen or accelerate the disease.

CJ Cognitive Skill

Analyze Cues

Reference

Linton & Matteson, 2020, pp. 857–860

Thinking Exercise 16B-3

Answers

Based on an analysis of the client findings, the nurse recognizes that the ***priority*** health problems for the client at this time are **chronic pain** and **inflammation**.

Rationales

The client's right knee is painful, red, and swollen, which could interfere with his mobility and quality of life. Therefore chronic pain and inflammation are the priority problems.

CJ Cognitive Skill

Prioritize Hypotheses

Reference

Linton & Matteson, 2020, pp. 857–860

Thinking Exercise 16B-4

Answers

Health Teaching	Indicated	Contraindicated	Non-Essential
"Use heat on both knees to help relieve pain and promote healing."		X	
"Use assistive-adaptive devices as needed (e.g., sock aids, shoehorns, dressing sticks, extenders)."			X
"Seek out a weight reduction program to help reduce knee pain and promote general health."	X		
"Take acetaminophen when needed for pain."	X		
"Try to work on finding a new occupation that allows you to sit more."			X
"Follow up with all physical therapy appointments as prescribed."	X		
"Wear good firm shoes to support your knees."	X		

Rationales

The nurse would teach the client to use ice rather than heat for an inflamed joint. The knee is already red and swollen, implying heat due to increased blood flow to the area for healing. He does not need to find a new occupation or use assistive-adaptive devices for ADLs at this point. The nurse would teach the client to manage pain by losing weight, taking acetaminophen as needed, attending physical therapy sessions, and wearing good firm shoes to support his knees when walking.

CJ Cognitive Skill

Generate Solutions

Reference

Linton & Matteson, 2020, pp. 857–860

Thinking Exercise 16B-5

Answers

A, C, D, E, G

Rationales

Before discharge, the nurse would need to teach the client about the need to ambulate with his walker, being careful to bear weight as instructed (Choices A and C). Venous thromboembolism (deep vein thrombosis and pulmonary embolus) is a common complication after total knee and hip arthroplasty. Therefore the client should be taught to continue wearing his antiembolism stockings and notify the surgeon if either calf is swollen, red, and/or painful (Choices D and F). The surgeon should also be notified if the surgical incision becomes reddened and swollen, with or without drainage (Choice G).

CJ Cognitive Skill

Take Action

Reference

Linton & Matteson, 2020, pp. 857–860

Thinking Exercise 16B-6

Answers

Client Finding	Effective	Ineffective	Unrelated
Ambulates several times a day with a cane	X		
Incision healed without redness or drainage	X		
Right knee is slightly swollen and warm at times	X		
Reports new-onset toothache for the past few days			X
Blood pressure = 126/80 mm Hg	X		
Reports no right knee pain but has “a little soreness”	X		

Rationales

All of these client findings demonstrate progress following a total knee arthroplasty. For many clients, the surgical knee is typically swollen, warm, and sore for several months postoperatively because of the complexity of the knee joint and its weight-bearing function. Having a toothache is not related to the client’s surgery.

CJ Cognitive Skill

Evaluate Outcomes

Reference

Linton & Matteson, 2020, pp. 857–860

Thinking Exercise 16B-7

Answers

The nurse reinforces the teaching provided by the physical therapist about how to use a cane, including the need for the client to place the cane **on her right side** when ambulating. To ensure proper cane height, the top of the cane should be at the level of the client's **greater trochanter**.

Rationales

A cane should be used on the strong, unaffected side and advanced when the surgical leg goes forward for extra support. The height of the cane should be at the level of the client's greater trochanter, which is parallel to the wrist of most clients.

CJ Cognitive Skill

Take Action

Reference

Linton & Matteson, 2020, p. 890

Thinking Exercise 16B-8

Answers

History and Physical	Nurses' Notes	Vital Signs	Laboratory Results

10/24/21 Reports severe intermittent pain in most of her hand joints, with right thumb base being the worst at 6/10 when picking up objects. Numerous enlarged bony nodules on most finger joints preventing the client from making a tight fist. Several finger nodules warm to touch. Chronic back pain (cervical and lumbosacral) for over 45 years with report of frequent crepitus when moving neck and shoulders. Minimal joint involvement in lower extremities, except for knees. Able to perform ADLs independently but beginning to have problems with opening containers, jars, and bottles. Job requires working long hours at a computer at home. Takes ibuprofen 800 mg orally every morning, which wears off by dinner time. States that if she takes too much of the drug, she gets nosebleeds. Is hoping to have other choices for decreasing pain and reducing deformity. --R. J. Youseff, LPN

Rationales

The nurse would want to follow up on the client's report of chronic finger joint and back pain, which is likely affecting her quality of life. She is still able to care for herself and perform ADLs, but at some point she might need an adaptive device to help her open containers, jars, and bottles. The nurse would also be concerned about her nosebleeds caused at times by ibuprofen. The client may be at risk for internal bleeding if she is having nosebleeds.

CJ Cognitive Skill

Recognize Cues

Reference

Linton & Matteson, 2020, pp. 857–860

Exemplar 16C. Fractured Hip/Open Reduction, Internal Fixation (Medical-Surgical Nursing: Older Adult)

Thinking Exercise 16C-1

Answers

- Alert but unable to determine orientation due to severe pain
- Crying out and grabbing her right hip
- Right leg shorter than left and externally rotated
- Has history of severe osteoporosis for which she is prescribed risedronate
- Has been walking with a rollator walker or cane when ambulating before her fall
- Heart rate = 92 beats/min
- Respirations = 28 breaths/min
- Blood pressure = 162/90 mm Hg
- Oxygen saturation = 90% (on room air [RA])
- No other apparent injury noted

Rationales

The client fell and sustained an injury with a painful hip, which needs to be addressed as soon as possible. Her blood pressure may be elevated because of acute pain but should be followed up. The oxygen saturation level is below normal, but she does not have any symptoms. However, this abnormality should be followed up and monitored for the potential need for supplemental oxygen.

CJ Cognitive Skill

Recognize Cues

Reference

Linton & Matteson, 2020, pp. 890–895

Thinking Exercise 16C-2

Answers

The nurse analyzes client findings and recognizes that the client ***most likely*** has a <u>fractured hip</u>. This trauma can lead to complications including <u>bleeding</u> and <u>neurovascular impairment</u>.

Rationales

The client has classic symptoms that are consistent with a displaced fractured hip because she has severe pain and her right leg is shortened and externally rotated. Long bones are very vascular, which can result in bleeding if they break. Neurovascular impairment may occur, as bone ends can impinge on blood vessels and nerves that supply the lower leg and foot.

CJ Cognitive Skill

Analyze Cues

Reference

Linton & Matteson, 2020, pp. 890–895

Thinking Exercise 16C-3

Answers

In addition to monitoring for fracture complications, the ***priorities*** of care for the client are to manage pain and assess for delirium.

Rationales

A major priority is to manage the client's pain by reducing and immobilizing the fracture. The nurse would also assess for delirium, or acute confusion, which is a common health problem that occurs in older adults after a hip fracture.

CJ Cognitive Skill

Prioritize Hypotheses

Reference

Linton & Matteson, 2020, pp. 890–895

Thinking Exercise 16C-4

Answers

Nursing Action	Potential Postoperative Complication	Appropriate Nursing Action for Postoperative Complication
1 Turn the client and inspect skin every 1–2 hr.	Atelectasis	**6** Teach the client to use incentive spirometry every 1–2 hr.
2 Maintain bilateral sequential compression devices.	Nausea and vomiting	**5** Administer antiemetic medication.
3 Monitor the incision for redness and drainage.	Delirium	**7** Reorient the client frequently.
4 Apply supplemental oxygen at 2 L/min.	Pressure injury	**1** Turn the client and inspect skin every 1–2 hr.
5 Administer antiemetic medication.	Venous thromboembolism	**2** Maintain bilateral sequential compression devices.
6 Teach the client to use incentive spirometry every 1–2 hr.		
7 Reorient the client frequently.		

Rationales

Atelectasis can occur unless the client's lungs are frequently expanded through deep breathing and the use of incentive spirometry every 1 to 2 hours. Nausea and/or vomiting can be treated with an antiemetic medication; venous thromboembolism (VTE) is prevented with anticoagulant therapy and by wearing sequential compression (pneumatic) devices. Pressure injuries and delirium are common complications in clients who have a surgical hip repair. The nurse would be sure that the client is turned every 1 to 2 hours to prevent pressure injury. Frequent orientation helps reduce the risk of delirium, but acute confusion can occur due to analgesics, surgery, and relocation to the hospital.

CJ Cognitive Skill

Generate Solutions

Reference

Linton & Matteson, 2020, pp. 890–895

Thinking Exercise 16C-5

Answers

A, B, C, E, F

Rationales

The nurse includes the need for the client to continue measures to help prevent venous thromboembolism (VTE), including taking an anticoagulant and wearing compression or antiembolism stockings (Choices A and B). The client should avoid sleeping on her operative hip until healing has occurred, and therefore can sleep on her back or on her unaffected leg with a pillow between her legs to prevent hip dislocation (Choice E). However, the nurse reminds the client and daughter that the client should not stay in any one position too long to prevent skin breakdown (Choice F). Finally, the nurse reminds the daughter and client to contact the surgeon immediately if the incision shows signs of infection (Choice C).

CJ Cognitive Skill

Take Action

Reference

Linton & Matteson, 2020, pp. 890–895

Thinking Exercise 16C-6

Answers

Client Finding	Is Progressing	Is Not Progressing
Temperature = 97.8°F (36.6°C)	X	
Surgical incision healed without redness or drainage	X	
Reports soreness in her incisional area but not severe pain	X	
Walks independently with a cane on her left side	X	
Performs ADLs without assistance	X	
Has no calf pain or redness	X	

Rationales

All of the listed client findings indicate usual or normal assessment findings or improvement after surgery. The client has no evidence of complications, such as pressure injury, infection, or deep vein thrombosis, and she is performing ADLs independently.

CJ Cognitive Skill

Evaluate Outcomes

Reference

Linton & Matteson, 2020, pp. 890–895

Thinking Exercise 16C-7

Answers

C, D, E

Rationales

The nurse would plan interventions to prevent pressure injury while the client is in traction and perform frequent neurovascular assessments to check for circulation impairment (Choices C and E). It is very important for the traction weights to hang freely and for all ropes and pulleys to be intact (Choice D). For Buck's traction (also called skin traction), the total weight should be 5 to 10 lb (2.7 to 4.5 kg). Buck's traction is used less often today for hip fractures, but the nurse may encounter client situations similar to this client's case.

CJ Cognitive Skill

Take Action

Reference

Linton & Matteson, 2020, pp. 890–895

CHAPTER 17 Sensory Perception: Cataracts *(Medical-Surgical Nursing: Older Adult)*

Answers With Rationales for Thinking Exercises

Thinking Exercise 17-1

Answers

Client Finding	Client Finding That Requires Follow-up by the Nurse
History of diabetes mellitus type 2	X
History of hypertension	X
Was treated several years ago for depression after partner died	
Has worn glasses for almost 60 years	
Has new onset of decreased visual acuity	X
Sees floaters and spots at times, especially in her left eye	X
Sees better at night than during the day	X

Rationales

The client has decreased vision and sees abnormal spots and floaters, especially in her left eye. These eye changes may have caused or contributed to her car accident and should be followed up. Her history of diabetes mellitus and hypertension may have been factors in the visual changes because these diseases can cause changes in blood vessels in the retina. Therefore the nurse would explore how the client has been managing these diseases.

CJ Cognitive Skill

Recognize Cues

Reference

Linton & Matteson, 2020, pp. 970, 1175

Thinking Exercise 17-2

Answers

The nurse recognizes that the client ***most likely*** has cataracts, a common problem of the eye associated with aging. The client needs to have an eye examination to accurately diagnose this problem.

Rationales

The visual changes reported by the client are consistent with the typical signs and symptoms caused by cataracts, in which the lens of the eyes become opaque, preventing clear vision. This problem is very common as a physiologic change of aging. The client needs to have a thorough eye examination by a qualified health care professional.

CJ Cognitive Skill

Analyze Cues

Reference

Linton & Matteson, 2020, p. 1175

Thinking Exercise 17-3

Answers

The ***priority*** for the client related to her visual changes is to ensure improvement in her visual acuity.

Rationales

The client is an older adult and is at risk for falling and other injuries related to aging changes, including having impaired vision. Therefore to ensure client safety, the priority is to improve her visual acuity.

CJ Cognitive Skill

Prioritize Hypotheses

Reference

Linton & Matteson, 2020, p. 1175

Thinking Exercise 17-4

Answers

B, C, D, E, G, H

Rationales

The client is scheduled to have her left cataract removed as a same-day ambulatory care procedure. She will likely need to instill many eyedrops into her left eye to prepare for surgery, including an antibacterial drug (Choice B), an anti-inflammatory drug (Choice E), a mydriatic drug to allow better access to her lens, and a cycloplegic drug to decrease movement of the eye and its anatomic parts. All eyedrops should be used at room temperature (Choice C); each type of eyedrop should be administered at least 5 minutes apart from other types (Choice H). The best practice for administering eyedrops includes looking up to the ceiling (not the floor), pulling the lower lid down, and gently closing the eye while moving it around to distribute the drug (Choices D and G).

CJ Cognitive Skill

Generate Solutions

Reference

Linton & Matteson, 2020, pp. 1148–1150

Thinking Exercise 17-5

Answers

A, B, C, D, E, F, G, H

Rationales

All of these actions would be performed by the nurse, including health teaching about any physical restrictions, the wearing of an eye patch, the administration of eyedrops, and the care of the surgical eye (Choices C, D, E, F, and G). In addition, the nurse would assess the client's pain level, review the pain management plan, and remind the client when she should contact the surgeon (Choices A and B). Because the client is a diabetic and surgery is a stressor, the client needs to carefully monitor her blood glucose (Choice H).

CJ Cognitive Skill

Take Action

Reference

Linton & Matteson, 2020, pp. 970, 1176–1177

Thinking Exercise 17-6

Answers

Client Finding	Is Progressing	Is Not Progressing
Temperature = 97.8°F (36.6°C)	X	
Blood pressure = 128/74 mm Hg	X	
No drainage from left eye	X	
Moderate redness in sclera	X	
Reports no severe eye pain	X	
Blood glucose = 195 mg/dL (10.8 mmol/L)		X

Rationales

The client's surgical eye is healing as evidenced by the absence of severe eye pain and drainage. Moderate redness is expected for a number of weeks after surgery owing to the trauma of surgery. The only abnormal finding is that the client's blood glucose is above usual limits, and this should be followed up by her primary health care provider.

CJ Cognitive Skill

Evaluate Outcomes

Reference

Linton & Matteson, 2020, pp. 975, 1176–1177

Thinking Exercise 17-7

Answers

Drug Action	Drug Name	Appropriate Action for Each Prescribed Drug
1 Prevents eye infection	Latanoprost	**5** Increases aqueous humor outflow
2 Constricts pupils of the eye	Timolol	**4** Decreases aqueous humor formation
3 Increases ocular hypertension	Epinephrine	**6** Dilates pupils of the eye
4 Decreases aqueous humor formation		
5 Increases aqueous humor outflow		
6 Dilates pupils of the eye		

CJ Cognitive Skill

Take Action

Reference

Linton & Matteson, 2020, pp. 1179–1180

CHAPTER 18 Infection: Pneumonia *(Medical-Surgical Nursing: Older Adult)*

Answers With Rationales for Thinking Exercises

Thinking Exercise 18-1

Answers

Client Finding	Most Important Client Findings That Require Follow-up by the Nurse
Acute confusion	X
Barrel-shaped chest	
Dark-red sputum	X
Oxygen saturation = 86% (on 2 L/min oxygen via NC)	X
Yellowed fingertips	

Rationales

The client has no history of dementia; therefore new-onset confusion is a change in status and must be followed up because, in older adults, acute confusion is a common change indicating an acute health problem. Chronic cough is a symptom of chronic obstructive pulmonary disease (COPD) and may be dry or productive with pale or yellow sputum. Dark-red sputum is not associated with COPD. The nurse would prioritize this finding and further assess to determine the cause. Clients with chronic lung disease frequently have a lower oxygenation level, usually between 92% and 88%. The client's current oxygen saturation of 86% is too low and must be followed up immediately.

Clients with COPD frequently develop a barrel-shaped chest in the later stages of the disease. This occurs as a result of chronically overinflated alveoli and air trapping. Yellowed fingertips are a common finding in clients who smoke. Nicotine and tar found in cigarettes stains nails and nail beds. In addition, smoking causes vasoconstriction, which can block oxygen to fingertips, resulting in clubbing and yellow-hued fingers. The client's barrel-shaped chest and yellowed fingernails are not a priority.

CJ Cognitive Skill

Recognize Cues

Reference

Linton & Matteson, 2020, pp. 488–492

Thinking Exercise 18-2

Answers

Client Finding	COPD	Pneumonia	Lung Cancer
Productive cough	X	X	X
Dark-red sputum		X	X
Dyspnea	X	X	X
Wheezing	X		
Acute confusion		X	

Rationales

The client has a history of chronic obstructive pulmonary disease (COPD); therefore the nurse would first analyze symptoms to determine whether an exacerbation has occurred. Client findings that correspond with symptoms of a COPD exacerbation are dyspnea, productive cough, and wheezing. The client has several risk factors for pneumonia including smoking, chronic illness, and undernutrition (BMI = 19). Relevant client findings for pneumonia are acute onset of confusion, a productive cough with dark-red sputum, and dyspnea. As a smoker, the client is also at risk for recurrent lung cancer. Lung cancer generally does not cause symptoms until advanced stages. Client findings that are relevant to lung cancer are dark-red or rusty-colored sputum, chronic cough, and dyspnea. Other common symptoms of lung cancer are difficulty swallowing; hoarseness; swelling in face or neck; and shoulder, neck, or chest pain. Wheezing is rare in both pneumonia and lung cancer.

CJ Cognitive Skill

Analyze Cues

Reference

Linton & Matteson, 2020, pp. 488–492, 508–517, 523–525

Thinking Exercise 18-3

Answers

The nurse determines that the client is ***most likely*** experiencing pneumonia as evidenced by his new-onset confusion, lateral chest pain, and fever. The nurse is most concerned with the client's oxygenation and orientation findings.

Rationales

The client has classic symptoms of pneumonia, including new-onset confusion or delirium, fever, shaking chills, stabbing lateral chest pain, and hemoptysis. The client's dyspnea and productive cough may be enhanced at this time, but these are chronic symptoms and not specific enough to differentiate pneumonia. Undernutrition is a risk factor for pneumonia and may be exacerbated by an infection. Wheezing is not usually a symptom of pneumonia.

Prioritizing client concerns requires the nurse to determine which findings are life-threatening, urgent, and nonurgent. The client's oxygenation status is most alarming, and saturation levels at 86% indicate the client is experiencing hypoxemia. The client is also experiencing mental changes due to a lack of oxygen perfusion to the brain. Changes in orientation are very concerning, as they indicate early signs of hypoxia. Persistent hypoxia can cause permanent damage to organs and is life-threatening. Therefore the nurse would be most concerned with the client's life-threatening oxygenation and orientation findings. Fever and pain are urgent issues but not life-threatening at this time. The client's lung sounds consist of wheezes, which are a chronic finding related to his underlying lung disease. Wheezing, caused by airway inflammation and bronchoconstriction, may be treated to help improve ventilation and subsequently oxygenation levels, but wheezing is not a priority concern.

CJ Cognitive Skill

Prioritize Hypotheses

Reference

Linton & Matteson, 2020, pp. 488–492

Thinking Exercise 18-4

Answers

Nursing Action	Client's Priority Problem	Appropriate Nursing Action for Each Priority Client Problem
1 Provide a high-calorie, low-protein diet to promote the immune system.	Inadequate oxygenation	**4** Provide supplemental oxygen to keep saturation levels between 88% and 92%.
2 Assist the client in changing positions every 2 hours to help mobilize secretions.	Airway obstruction	**2** Assist the client in changing positions every 2 hours to help mobilize secretions.
3 Place the client in a supine position to decrease pressure of abdominal organs on the diaphragm.	Inadequate nutrition	**5** Arrange for food options that are attractive and preferred by the client to enhance appetite.
4 Provide supplemental oxygen to keep saturation levels between 88% and 92%.		
5 Arrange for food options that are attractive and preferred by the client to enhance appetite.		

Rationales

The client's current oxygen saturation level is dangerously low and causing neurologic changes. Providing supplemental oxygen is essential. The use of oxygen for a client with chronic lung disease must be monitored closely to maintain effective oxygen levels for physiologic needs without overoxygenating and causing oxygen-induced hypoventilation. Keeping the client's oxygenation level between 92% and 88% is ideal. The client would be placed in a semi-Fowler position or in a reclining chair to promote gas exchange and decrease pressure of abdominal organs on the diaphragm. Accumulation of secretions in the respiratory tract impairs gas exchange. The administration of antimicrobials, decongestants, and expectorants will help the client to remove secretions by coughing. Repositioning the client frequently will also help to loosen and mobilize secretions in the client's lungs.

The client's body mass index (BMI) is low, indicating undernutrition. This is most likely secondary to his chronic lung disease but has a significant impact on the client's ability to fight infection and heal. Good nutrition is essential for a client with pneumonia, and a typical diet usually consists of high protein and high calories. Fatigue and dyspnea may interfere with adequate food intake, and therefore the nurse will attempt to entice an appetite by arranging foods in an attractive and convenient manner, providing foods the client prefers, placing the client in a comfortable position with the head elevated, and assisting with oral care before and after meals.

CJ Cognitive Skill

Generate Solutions

Reference

Linton & Matteson, 2020, pp. 488–492

Thinking Exercise 18-5

Answers

- Ciprofloxacin 400 mg IV every 12 hours
- Blood cultures × 2
- Supplemental oxygen to keep saturations at 88% to 92%
- Nutritional consultation
- Chest physiotherapy
- Sputum culture

Rationales

The nurse's priority action is to assess the client's oxygenation saturation level and titrate supplemental oxygen to maintain a level of 88% to 92%. Appropriate oxygenation levels must be maintained to ensure organ function. Blood and sputum cultures must be completed next. Clients with an infection are generally prescribed a broad-spectrum antibiotic until cultures reveal the actual microorganism causing the infection. Blood and sputum cultures must be completed prior to initiating antibiotic therapy to ensure that the organism is properly identified. After the cultures, the nurse would prioritize the antibiotics and then collaborate with the registered dietitian nutritionist for the nutritional consultation and with the respiratory therapist for the chest physiotherapy.

CJ Cognitive Skill

Take Action

Reference

Linton & Matteson, 2020, pp. 488–492

Thinking Exercise 18-6

Answers

Client Finding	Is Progressing	Is Not Progressing
Oxygen saturation = 93% (on 4 L/min via NC)	X	
Drinks a protein shake between each meal	X	
Dyspnea with activity and at rest		X
Right pleural effusion present on chest x-ray		X
Dry, nonproductive cough	X	

Rationales

The client's priority problems were inadequate oxygenation, airway obstruction, and inadequate nutrition. The desired outcome for oxygenation was a saturation level of 88% to 92%. The client's current oxygen saturation level of 93% on 4 L of oxygen indicates the desired outcome was met. The client may tolerate a decrease in the amount of supplemental oxygen currently being used. The client's cough has returned to the preinfection, chronic cough he most likely experiences with COPD. This is a sign the client is progressing. In addition, the client is tolerating three protein shakes each day, which is a positive sign. These shakes will hopefully improve his nutritional status, but changes in weight and nutrition will take more than 3 days to fully evaluate.

The client is still experiencing dyspnea at rest. Clients with COPD frequently experience dyspnea with activity but not at rest. The client's ongoing shortness of breath is a sign of not progressing and could be related to the right pleural effusion present on the client's chest x-ray. Pleural effusion is the accumulation of fluid between the pleura that surrounds the lungs and the pleura that lines the thoracic cavity. This fluid takes up space in the thoracic cavity, causing shortness of breath. A large amount of fluid can lead to collapse of the lung. Pleural effusion is a complication of pneumonia and a sign of not progressing.

CJ Cognitive Skill

Evaluate Outcomes

Reference

Linton & Matteson, 2020, pp. 488–492

Thinking Exercise 18-7

Answers

Nursing Action	Indicated	Contraindicated	Non-Essential
Ensure suction equipment is available at the bedside.	X		
Encourage the client to tilt her head back when swallowing.		X	
Keep the head of bed elevated during enteral feedings.	X		
Remove choking hazard foods such as hotdogs and grapes.			X
Perform oral hygiene frequently.	X		

Rationales

Aspiration pneumonia is prevented by implementing care to avoid aspiration and treating aspiration promptly. To avoid aspiration, the client will be taught to sit upright with the neck in a neutral position or slightly bent forward during meals. A swallow study will determine the consistency of foods and beverages the client can safely swallow. Thickened fluids are easier to swallow than thin liquids and are often prescribed for clients who are at risk for aspiration. Although hotdogs and grapes are a choking hazard for toddlers, these foods are usually not an issue for adults who can chew. Before each bolus enteral feeding, the nurse will check the tube position per agency policy, measure residuals, and elevate the head of the bed. The client will remain in a position with the head of the bed elevated until 30 minutes after the bolus feeding is finished.

Suction equipment must be readily available in case the client aspirates. If aspiration is suspected, the nurse will suction the client to try to remove the foreign material and place the client in a side-lying position to promote drainage from the airway. Clients who experience swallowing issues or other conditions associated with aspiration pneumonia may aspirate their own secretions, which are full of oral bacteria. When these bacteria are introduced into the warm and highly oxygenated lungs, they can quickly multiply and become a serious infection. Performing frequent oral care helps to control bacteria in the oral cavity and prevent pneumonia.

CJ Cognitive Skill

Generate Solutions

Reference

Linton & Matteson, 2020, pp. 488–492

Thinking Exercise 18-8

Answers

A, B, D, E, H

Rationales

When teaching a client who has pneumonia, the nurse will focus on activity and rest, nutrition and fluids, and antibiotic therapy. Infection may cause fatigue, and therefore the client will be taught to increase activity slowly (Choice A), take periods of rest as needed, and eat smaller meals more frequently if a large meal is too tiring (Choice H). A high-protein diet will help the client to heal, and the nurse should provide examples of food items that are high in protein and low in fat (Choice E). A good cough is essential for removal of secretions. The nurse may teach the client deep-breathing and coughing exercises as well as positioning and splinting techniques to decrease pain during deep breathing and coughing exercises. Adequate fluids will also help mobilize pulmonary secretions for expectoration and would be encouraged as part of the teaching (Choice D). The client needs to complete the entire antibiotic course, even when feeling better, to decrease risk of future resistant infections (Choice B). The client is not required to self-quarantine for 14 days but may want to limit visitors and activities because of fatigue. Nausea and vomiting are common side effects of azithromycin and do not need to be reported.

CJ Cognitive Skill

Take Action

Reference

Linton & Matteson, 2020, pp. 488–492

CHAPTER 19 Cognition

Answers With Rationales for Thinking Exercises

Exemplar 19A. Delirium (Mental Health Nursing: Older Adult)

Thinking Exercise 19A-1

Answers

- Temperature = 97.8°F (36.5°C)
- Heart rate = 82 beats/min
- Blood pressure = 158/88 mm Hg
- Oxygen saturation = 95% (on room air [RA])
- Is alert and oriented × 3
- Is ADL independent and lives alone
- Has knee and hip pain most days from arthritis, which runs in her family
- States she has had a hard time recently controlling her bladder; feels like she has to void all the time
- Has nocturia 2 to 5 times every night, which makes her feel tired during the day
- Tries to drink plenty of water but is thinking she should restrict fluids to help with her bladder problem

Rationales

The client has a history of hypertension, which may not be under control because her current blood pressure is higher than the normal range and requires follow-up. She also has pain due to a family history of osteoarthritis, which may be interfering with her quality of life or possibly the ability to perform ADLs. The client's main concern for the current visit, though, is that she is having problems with urination control, including urgency and nocturia. She wants to restrict her fluid intake to decrease the number of times she gets up or feels urgency, but fluid restriction may actually cause more problems, including dehydration and possible urinary tract infection. Therefore all of the cues about her urinary pattern are relevant for the nurse to follow up.

CJ Cognitive Skill

Recognize Cues

Reference

Linton & Matteson, 2020, pp. 203–204, 207

Thinking Exercise 19A-2

Answers

The nurse recognizes that the client is ***most likely*** experiencing <u>delirium</u> as a result of <u>oxybutynin</u>.

Rationales

The client became acutely confused and had a visual hallucination as a result of a new medication that was prescribed for her urinary pattern changes, oxybutynin. Oxybutynin is an anticholinergic medication used for urge incontinence but can cause major side/adverse effects, especially in older adults. Examples include acute confusion, blurred vision, dry mouth, and constipation. Acute confusional behaviors include delusions, hallucinations, and disorientation.

CJ Cognitive Skill

Analyze Cues

Reference

Linton & Matteson, 2020, pp. 208, 223–224

Thinking Exercise 19A-3

Answers

A, D, G

Rationales

The client is disoriented, is acutely confused, and has difficulty following conversation (Choice G). Therefore she would likely have poor judgment and get out of bed without assistance, making her at risk for falling (Choice A). Safety is always the priority for client care. Given that the client has been taking oxybutynin for urge urinary incontinence for less than 24 hours, she would still likely have that problem (Choice D).

CJ Cognitive Skill

Prioritize Hypotheses

Reference

Linton & Matteson, 2020, pp. 207–208

Thinking Exercise 19A-4

Answers

Nursing Action	Indicated	Contraindicated	Non-Essential
Apply oxygen therapy at 2 L/min.			X
Place a fall alarm on the client's mattress.	X		
Reorient the client frequently.	X		
Withhold oxybutynin until the client's delirium resolves.	X		
Apply a vest restraint to ensure that the client does not try to get out of bed.		X	
Remind assistive personnel to toilet the client every 2 hours.	X		

Rationales

The client is not having any problems with breathing, and therefore applying supplemental oxygen therapy is not needed. The client would not be placed in a vest restraint because it could cause harm to the client and is not in compliance with hospital accreditation standards or best practices.

CJ Cognitive Skill

Generate Solutions

Reference

Linton & Matteson, 2020, pp. 207–208, 223–224

Thinking Exercise 19A-5

Answers

Primary Health Care Provider's Orders	Orders That Are Priority for the Nurse to Implement First
Discontinue oxybutynin for urge incontinence	X
Amlodipine 10 mg orally every morning	
Vital signs every 4 hours	
Continuous pulse oximetry	
Out of bed with assistance to bedside commode	
Toilet every 2 hours	X
Diet as tolerated	
Continuous IV 5%D/0.45%NS at 80 mL/hr	
Fall precautions	X

Rationales

The priority orders for the nurse to implement are focused on keeping the client safe (Fall Precautions) and preventing her from getting out of bed to go to the bathroom for her urge incontinence. Toileting every 1 to 2 hours would help decrease her incontinence. The drug that is most likely causing the client's confusion and disorientation needs to be discontinued to help resolve her delirium. Delirium can be reversed if the cause is identified and removed.

CJ Cognitive Skill

Take Action

Reference

Linton & Matteson, 2020, pp. 207–208, 223–224

Thinking Exercise 19A-6

Answers

Client Finding	Is Progressing	Is <u>Not</u> Progressing
Has not experienced a fall while hospitalized	X	
Able to walk with minimal assistance	X	
Continues to have urge urinary incontinence		X
Is alert and oriented × 2	X	
Has had no hallucinations while hospitalized	X	

Rationales

All of the findings show that the client is improving with the exception of her urge urinary incontinence. She is less confused, has not had a fall during her hospital stay, and is more oriented than she was at admission.

CJ Cognitive Skill

Evaluate Outcomes

Reference

Linton & Matteson, 2020, pp. 207–208

Thinking Exercise 19A-7

Answers

B, C, D, E, F

Rationales

Benzodiazepines, antidepressants (especially tricyclics), antihistamines, and hypnotics all affect the central nervous system (CNS) and can cause acute confusion and other emotional/behavioral symptoms (Choices B, D, E, and F). Most diuretics can cause sodium loss, which is needed for neuronal cell function. When hyponatremia occurs, the client can experience acute confusion and weakness (Choice C). Mydriatrics are ophthalmic drugs that cause pupil dilation, antibiotics are used to treat bacterial infections, and anticoagulants prevent excessive clotting. None of these drugs usually affect the CNS.

CJ Cognitive Skill

Analyze Cues

Reference

Linton & Matteson, 2020, p. 204

Exemplar 19B. Alzheimer Disease (Mental Health Nursing: Older Adult)

Thinking Exercise 19B-1

Answers

Health History	**Nurses' Notes**	Vital Signs	Laboratory Results

11-22-21 Client diagnosed with moderate-stage Alzheimer disease and depression. Alert and oriented × 1. Her partner states that she tends to wander often and tries to go outdoors. She sometimes takes an afternoon nap because she does not sleep well at night. Client has frequent anxiety, especially in unfamiliar places, and sometimes needs assistance with ADLs. Refuses to eat at times. She is able to ambulate without assistive device and recognizes her daughter and granddaughter. ---------------*M. A. Hollister, LVN*

Rationales

The client has moderate or middle-stage Alzheimer disease (AD) and is expected to be disoriented. She wanders to get outside, has difficulty sleeping at night, and is anxious, which places her at high risk for injury. The nurse would want to know that the client needs help at times with ADLs and refuses to eat at times, which can cause impaired nutrition.

CJ Cognitive Skill

Recognize Cues

Reference

Linton & Matteson, 2020, pp. 205–206

Thinking Exercise 19B-2

Answers

Client Finding	Alzheimer Disease	Depression
Partner states that she tends to wander often and tries to go outdoors.	X	
Sometimes takes an afternoon nap because she does not sleep well at night.	X	X
Has frequent anxiety, especially in unfamiliar places.	X	
Sometimes needs assistance with ADLs.	X	X
Refuses to eat at times.	X	X

Rationales

Sleep disturbances, lack of energy necessitating assistance with ADLs, and anorexia commonly occur in clients who are depressed or have Alzheimer disease (AD). The chronic confusion, anxiety, and impaired clinical judgment associated with AD can also affect the client's ability to perform ADLs independently and can cause the client to want to wander.

CJ Cognitive Skill

Analyze Cues

Reference

Linton & Matteson, 2020, pp. 205–206

Thinking Exercise 19B-3

Answers

The nurse identifies the ***priority*** needs of the client, which are to maintain client safety and ensure that basic needs are met.

Rationales

The client who has Alzheimer disease is chronically confused and has impaired judgment. For example, the client at home may leave a stove burner on, causing a fire while cooking. Therefore the client needs to be monitored carefully. In addition, as the disease progresses, the client forgets to bathe, change clothes, or eat.

CJ Cognitive Skill

Prioritize Hypotheses

Reference

Linton & Matteson, 2020, pp. 209–212

Thinking Exercise 19B-4

Answers

Nursing Action	Client Health Problem	Nursing Action for Client Health Problem
1 Validate the client's statements rather than correcting them.	Potential for injury due to wandering	**2** Use an alarm device to notify staff when she tries to leave the unit.
2 Use an alarm device to notify staff when she tries to leave the unit.	Sleep disturbances	**6** Keep the client active during the day, including walking.
3 Ask the client's partner what she likes to eat and drink.	Chronic confusion	**1** Validate the client's statements rather than correct them.
4 Assist the client with ADLs as needed.	Potential for inadequate nutrition	**3** Ask the client's partner what she likes to eat and drink.
5 Reorient the client to reality frequently.		
6 Keep the client active during the day, including walking.		

Rationales

The client is at risk for wandering and needs an alarm system in place to inform the staff of the client's location. Some clients are awake all night and sleep all day. However, the staff would want to keep the client busy and active during the day so that she is tired enough to sleep at night. The client with AD has chronic confusion and cannot be reoriented, especially once she progresses to the middle or moderate stage of the disease. Therefore it is better to avoid arguing and validate the client's feelings or communication. To promote nutrition and prevent dehydration, the nurse would want to ask the client's partner what her food likes, dislikes, and allergies are.

CJ Cognitive Skill

Generate Solutions

Reference

Linton & Matteson, 2020, pp. 209–212

Thinking Exercise 19B-5

Answers

A, C, D, E, G

Rationales

The nurse would first inform the charge nurse about the client's elopement (Choice C). At this time when the client is missing, the nurse would organize a search of the entire unit again and the grounds of the long-term care (LTC) facility (Choices A and E). The nurse would also ask for help to search other units in the LTC facility, while asking staff, visitors, and other clients if they have seen the client (Choices D and G). It is too soon to notify the client's family or guardian or law enforcement. After the client is found (or not), the nurse would document the incident using the facility's variance report. The alarm system can be checked later after the client has been found.

CJ Cognitive Skill

Take Action

Reference

Linton & Matteson, 2020, p. 210

Thinking Exercise 19B-6

Answers

Nurses' Notes	History and Physical	Vital Signs	Laboratory Results

4/20/21 1930 CNA reported to nurse at 1830 that client was missing from her room and the unit. After searching the entire facility inside and outside, client was found folding towels in the laundry room while humming a song. Client stated that she felt very happy and wanted to do laundry. Alert and oriented × 2 (person and place). No apparent injuries. Incontinent of urine with perineal redness. Client had a shower and was assisted to prepare for bedtime. Barrier cream applied to perineum. --*S. M. Littleton, LVN*

Rationales

The client was found to be safe without any apparent injuries. She stated she was very happy and obviously felt comfortable doing laundry. Although she is not oriented × 3, which is normal, she has improved because she was only oriented × 1 earlier. Now she is alert and oriented × 2 to person and place. This change is not unusual for clients who have AD because they often have periods of lucidity and therefore have fluctuating orientations.

CJ Cognitive Skill

Evaluate Outcomes

Reference

Linton & Matteson, 2020, pp. 209–210

Thinking Exercise 19B-7

Answers

D, G

Rationales

The client is in his last stage of Alzheimer disease and has lost his ability or forgotten how to chew and swallow food. The client is not expected to improve and will continue losing weight until he likely dies owing to complications of immobility. It is important for the nurse to discuss this situation with the family or guardian responsible for the client and check his advance directives to determine his end-of-life care requests (Choices D and G). Additional interventions to start an IV or refer the client to another member of the interprofessional health care team would not be appropriate. Most clients have advance directives that prevent aggressive measures, such as insertion of a gastrostomy tube, from being implemented owing to possible complications associated with these procedures.

CJ Cognitive Skill

Take Action

Reference

Linton & Matteson, 2020, pp. 325–327

CHAPTER 20 Elimination

Answers With Rationales for Thinking Exercises

Exemplar 20A. Chronic Kidney Disease (Medical-Surgical Nursing: Middle-Age Adult; Older Adult)

Thinking Exercise 20A-1

Answers

- History of diabetes mellitus type 2 and hypertension for over 20 years
- History of chronic kidney disease managed by diet and diuretic therapy for 6 years
- Reports feeling drowsy and disoriented
- Reports that urinary output greatly decreased over the past few days
- 3+ pitting edema in both ankles and feet
- Vital signs:
  - Temperature = 97.6°F (36.4°C)
  - Heart rate = 86 beats/min and regular
  - Respirations = 20 breaths/min
  - Blood pressure = 168/95 mm Hg
  - Oxygen saturation = 95% (on room air [RA])
- Lab test results:
  - Blood urea nitrogen (BUN) = 72 mg/dL (26.1 mmol/L)
  - Serum creatinine (Cr) = 7.8 mg/dL (689 mmol/L)
  - Potassium = 6.1 mEq/L (6.1 mmol/L)

Rationales

The client has a history of chronic kidney disease (CKD) that has previously been managed by diet and drug therapy. However, today he has several physical and mental changes including a decreased urinary output, 3+ pitting edema in the feet and ankles, and disorientation and drowsiness, a possible decrease in level of consciousness, which could indicate a worsening of his CKD. The client's blood pressure is also higher than the normal or usual range for an adult. The three lab values are above the normal reference ranges, which again indicates that the client's CKD may be worsening as the kidneys are not able to remove waste products from the body.

CJ Cognitive Skill

Recognize Cues

Reference

Linton & Matteson, 2020, pp. 831–833, 837–839

Thinking Exercise 20A-2

Answers

A, E

Rationales

The client likely has increased blood volume as indicated by pitting edema and an elevated blood pressure. This fluid volume excess can cause stress on the client's heart and heart failure (Choice A). The client also has hyperkalemia (increased serum potassium level), which can lead to cardiac dysrhythmias (Choice E). Uremic frost and bone demineralization (loss) can occur in clients who have chronic kidney disease (CKD), but these health problems are not potentially life-threatening. Hypothyroidism, asthma, and stroke are not usually associated with CKD.

CJ Cognitive Skill

Analyze Cues

Reference

Linton & Matteson, 2020, pp. 831–833, 837–839

Thinking Exercise 20A-3

Answers

The nurse recognizes that the ***priority*** needs for this client are to manage his <u>hypervolemia</u>, which can lead to <u>heart failure</u>, and <u>hyperkalemia</u>, which can lead to <u>dysrhythmias</u>.

Rationales

As explained in the Rationales for Thinking Exercise 20A-2, the client is most at risk for two potentially life-threatening complications of CKD. Therefore managing the client's hypervolemia and hyperkalemia are the priority needs for this client.

CJ Cognitive Skill

Prioritize Hypotheses

Reference

Linton & Matteson, 2020, pp. 831–833, 837–839

Thinking Exercise 20A-4

Answers

Nursing Action	Indicated	Contraindicated	Non-Essential
Apply oxygen therapy at 2 L/min.			X
Prepare to assist with central line insertion.	X		
Explain the procedure to the client and his partner.	X		
Administer the prescribed opioid analgesic.		X	
Continue to assess vital signs frequently.	X		
Monitor the client's level of consciousness and orientation frequently.	X		

Rationales

The client does not need oxygen therapy because he does not have any respiratory problems. However, toxins and excess potassium that are usually removed or controlled by the kidneys are increasing in his body and need to be removed quickly by hemodialysis. The nurse would prepare to assist with the insertion of a central line to dialyze the client and explain what is needed to his partner. Because of increased toxins, the client is confused and could experience a decrease in level of consciousness (LOC). The nurse would monitor frequently for these neurologic changes. Opioid analgesics would not be administered because the client has not verbalized that he is in pain. In addition, these drugs are central nervous system depressants, which could cause a decrease in LOC and/or further confusion.

CJ Cognitive Skill

Generate Solutions

Reference

Linton & Matteson, 2020, pp. 833–834

Thinking Exercise 20A-5

Answers

A, B, E, F, H

Rationales

The client may have an infection from the peritoneal dialysis (PD) catheter. Therefore the nurse would take the client's vital signs to determine if he has a fever or tachycardia, common changes associated with infection (Choice A). The nurse would take a culture of the catheter site drainage to send to the lab to identify any infectious agents and perform an abdominal assessment to check for peritonitis (Choices B and E). The nurse would also notify the home health nurse supervisor and the client's primary health care provider about the client's possible infection (Choices F and H).

CJ Cognitive Skill

Take Action

Reference

Linton & Matteson, 2020, pp. 834–836

Thinking Exercise 20A-6

Answers

Client Finding	Is Progressing	Is Not Progressing
Blood pressure = 128/80 mm Hg	X	
Alert and oriented	X	
3+ pitting edema of both ankles and feet		X
Peritoneal dialysis catheter site clean and intact	X	
Serum creatinine = 1.8 mg/dL	X	

Rationales

All of the client's findings have improved, indicating that the client is progressing as a result of having regular dialysis treatments. However, the client still has 3+ pitting edema in his lower extremities.

CJ Cognitive Skill

Evaluate Outcomes

Reference

Linton & Matteson, 2020, pp. 833–838

Thinking Exercise 20A-7

Answers

A, C, D, E

Rationales

The client with severe chronic kidney disease (CKD) has changes in laboratory test results due to major kidney damage. Therefore the client would be anemic owing to decreased renal production of erythropoietin, which is needed to produce red blood cells (Choice A). The client's kidneys would not be able to control the serum level of phosphorus (phosphate), which would cause an elevation (hyperphosphatemia) (Choice D). When serum phosphorus increases, the serum calcium level decreases (hypocalcemia) (Choice C). Severe CKD causes hydrogen ion excess in the body, which decreases the serum pH, making it more acidic. This condition is called metabolic acidosis (Choice E).

CJ Cognitive Skill

Recognize Cues

Reference

Linton & Matteson, 2020, pp. 833–835

Thinking Exercise 20A-8

Answers

Nursing Action	CKD Complication	Nursing Action for Client Complication
1 Restrict fluids based on urinary output.	Hyperkalemia	**6** Administer sodium polystyrene.
2 Administer an aluminum-based antacid.	Anemia	**4** Administer erythropoietin.
3 Provide supplemental oxygen.	Hypervolemia	**1** Restrict fluids based on urinary output.
4 Administer erythropoietin.	Hyperphosphatemia	**2** Administer an aluminum-based antacid.
5 Infuse hypertonic glucose.		
6 Administer sodium polystyrene.		

Rationales

The nurse would give the client sodium polystyrene to remove the excess potassium from the client's body via the GI tract. Giving erythropoietin helps to increase the production of red blood cells, which can improve the client's anemia. Fluid volume excess, or hypervolemia, is managed with fluid restriction or dialysis. Phosphate is a large molecule that cannot be dialyzed. However, it can be bound to aluminum-based antacids and removed via the GI tract.

CJ Cognitive Skill

Take Action

Reference

Linton & Matteson, 2020, pp. 831–838

Exemplar 20B. Intestinal Obstruction (Medical-Surgical Nursing: Older Adult)

Thinking Exercise 20B-1

Answers

Client Finding	Client Finding of Immediate Concern to the Nurse
Severe abdominal pain and distention	X
Vomiting	X
Bilateral fine crackles in lung bases	
Decreased/absent bowel sounds	X
Temperature = 99°F (37.2°C)	
Heart rate = 102 beats/min and regular	X
Blood pressure = 124/66 mm Hg	

Rationales

The client has been vomiting and is likely dehydrated, causing tachycardia. Continued vomiting could worsen dehydration owing to hypovolemia and lead to hypovolemic shock, a life-threatening health problem. Her temperature is only slightly elevated and would not be of immediate concern. The client's bowel sounds are decreased or absent, and she has not been able to have a bowel movement. These changes are causing abdominal pain and distention, which need to be addressed. The nurse expects to hear crackles in the lung bases because the client has a history of COPD. The client's blood pressure is within normal range.

CJ Cognitive Skill

Recognize Cues

Reference

Linton & Matteson, 2020, pp. 849–850

Thinking Exercise 20B-2

Answers

Client Finding	COPD	Intestinal Obstruction
Dyspnea	X	X
Abdominal pain		X
Bilateral fine crackles in lung bases	X	
Abdominal distention		X
Below normal oxygen saturation	X	
Tachycardia	X	X

Rationales

Dyspnea is a common finding in clients who have COPD owing to lack of oxygen diffusion in lung alveoli that have lost elasticity. Dyspnea may also occur in those who have abdominal distention due to intestinal obstruction because of pressure on the diaphragm. Abdominal pain due to distention and decreased or absent bowel sounds occurs in clients who have intestinal obstruction. Other common findings in clients who have COPD are low oxygen saturation and crackles. Tachycardia occurs in clients who have COPD because the heart has to pump more often to compensate for low arterial oxygen. If the client is dehydrated as a result of intestinal obstruction, the body compensates by increasing the heart rate to keep major organs such as the kidneys perfused (oxygenated).

CJ Cognitive Skill

Analyze Cues

Reference

Linton & Matteson, 2020, pp. 849–850

Thinking Exercise 20B-3

Answers

The nurse recognizes that the client's ***priorities*** for care will be to prevent shock and monitor for potential bowel perforation that can result in peritonitis.

Rationales

The client is apparently dehydrated and at risk for hypovolemic shock, a potentially life-threatening complication. As a result of decreased or absent bowel sounds, her bowel is distended, making her also at risk for bowel perforation; this would likely cause peritonitis and probably sepsis, another potentially life-threatening complication.

CJ Cognitive Skill

Prioritize Hypotheses

Reference

Linton & Matteson, 2020, pp. 849–850

Thinking Exercise 20B-4

Answers

Nursing Action	Indicated	Contraindicated	Non-Essential
Insert a nasogastric tube and connect to suction.	X		
Begin IV fluid administration.	X		
Obtain an electrocardiogram (ECG).			X
Apply supplemental oxygen.	X		
Place the client in a flat supine position.		X	

Rationales

At this time the priority for the client's care is to rest the GI tract by decompressing with a nasogastric (NG) tube connected to suction to decrease abdominal distention and pain. IV fluids are needed to treat dehydration resulting from intestinal obstruction, and supplemental oxygen is required to help manage the client's COPD. Positioning the client in a sitting (semi- or high-Fowler) position can improve the ease of breathing because the diaphragm is lowered by gravity and the thoracic space is enlarged. A flat supine position would worsen dyspnea and is contraindicated. An ECG is not necessary at this time.

CJ Cognitive Skill

Generate Solutions

Reference

Linton & Matteson, 2020, pp. 849–850

Thinking Exercise 20B-5

Answers

B, C, D, E, F, G

Rationales

The nurse would keep the client NPO at all times while the NG tube is connected to suction (Choice C). Before irrigating the tube, the nurse would turn off the suction and instill 30 mL of normal saline into the tube. After instillation, the nurse would reconnect the suction (Choices B, E, and F). During this procedure and at all times while the client has an NG tube in place, the nurse would maintain the client's head of the bed to at least a 30-degree elevation to prevent aspiration (Choice G). The nurse would also check that the tube remains in place and is secured with tape or specially designed securement device to prevent tube migration (Choice D). The oxygen does not need to be turned off because the client needs continuous oxygen for COPD.

CJ Cognitive Skill

Take Action

Reference

Williams, 2018, pp. 495–500

Thinking Exercise 20B-6

Answers

Client Finding	Is Progressing	Is Not Progressing
Abdomen soft, round, and nondistended	X	
No report of nausea or vomiting	X	
Respirations = 26 breaths/min and slightly labored		X
Is alert and oriented × 3	X	
Heart rate = 88 beats/min	X	

Rationales

All of the client findings show improvement and resolution of the intestinal obstruction. However, she still has tachypnea as evidenced by her respiratory rate of 26 breaths/min. This finding is likely due to her COPD.

CJ Cognitive Skill

Evaluate Outcomes

Reference

Williams, 2018, pp. 495–500

Thinking Exercise 20B-7

Answers

Action (A) to Take	Potential Condition	Parameter (P) to Monitor
C Maintain sequential compression stockings.	Deep vein thrombosis (DVT)	**3** Leg pain and swelling
G Remind the client to use her incentive spirometer every 1–2 hours.	Atelectasis	**5** Breath sounds
B Keep the surgical dressing clean and dry.	Wound infection	**6** Abdominal incision
A Encourage oral fluids as tolerated.	Acute kidney injury (AKI)	**2** Urinary output
E Introduce fluids to stimulate bowel function.	Paralytic ileus	**1** Bowel sounds

Rationales

After any major surgery, many clients are at risk for DVT and atelectasis. To help prevent these complications, the nurse would maintain the client's elastic and/or sequential compression stockings while the client is in bed. The client's legs should be monitored for signs of swelling, redness, and pain, which could indicate a DVT. The nurse would remind the client to use her incentive spirometer every 1 to 2 hours and deep breathe and cough at least every 2 hours to prevent atelectasis. Clients are also at risk for kidney dysfunction if they are not adequately hydrated. Fluids, in addition to IV fluid therapy, are introduced to help stimulate peristalsis to prevent paralytic ileus and to increase hydration. The nurse would keep the abdominal incision clean and dry and observe for signs of infection, including redness and drainage.

CJ Cognitive Skill

Take Action

Reference

Williams, 2018, pp. 749–755

CHAPTER 21 Metabolism

Answers With Rationales for Thinking Exercises

Exemplar 21A. Hypoglycemia (Medical-Surgical Nursing: Older Adult)

Thinking Exercise 21A-1

Answers

- Drowsy and confused to place and situation
- Reports blurry vision
- Respirations equal and unlabored
- Vital signs: heart rate = 88 beats/min; blood pressure = 98/44 mm Hg; respirations = 14 breaths/min; oxygen saturation = 96% (on room air [RA])
- Skin cool and diaphoretic
- Areas of skin hyperpigmentation present
- Reports join stiffness and pain rated 2/10

Rationales

Several client findings are consistent with the client's history of Addison disease and do not need follow-up. Symptoms of Addison disease include fatigue, weight loss, decreased appetite, GI distress, skin hyperpigmentation, loss of body hair, muscle or joint pain, and sexual dysfunction. Although the client's blood pressure is on the lower end (98/44 mm Hg), the client's heart rate and oxygenation status indicate the client is tolerating the pressure. Client findings that are not normal include acute mental confusion, vision changes, and cool, diaphoretic skin. These findings, especially those reflecting an acute neurologic change, must be followed up by the nurse.

CJ Cognitive Skill

Recognize Cues

Reference

Linton & Matteson, 2020, pp. 990–993

Thinking Exercise 21A-2

Answers

Client Finding	Infection	Hypoglycemia	Stroke
Mental confusion	X	X	X
Blurry vision		X	X
Cool, diaphoretic skin		X	
Drowsiness	X	X	

Rationales

Mental confusion is associated with all three disorders. The client's brain may not be receiving adequate perfusion of oxygenated blood (stroke) or effective supply of glucose (hypoglycemia). Older adults experiencing an infection frequently exhibit confusion and agitation, and this older adult client is at higher risk for sepsis as a result of the recent urinary tract infection. Blurry vision is related to hypoglycemia and stroke. In both situations, vision changes do not result from changes in the eye but instead from a lack of oxygen or glucose to the brain. Rapid onset of cool, pale, moist, and clammy skin is a sign of hypoglycemia. This change in skin is not related to stroke or infection. Drowsiness may be associated with infection, especially when the client experiences a fever or hypoxemia. Clients with hypoglycemia also experience tiredness or lethargy. A client experiencing an acute stroke may experience a decrease in level of consciousness. A client recovering from a stroke may feel fatigue, but drowsiness is not a manifestation of a stroke.

CJ Cognitive Skill

Analyze Cues

Reference

Williams, 2018, pp. 990–993

Thinking Exercise 21A-3

Answers

The client is ***most likely*** experiencing hypoglycemia not associated with diabetes mellitus. The ***priority*** for the nurse is to contact the primary health care provider and report the presence of hypoglycemia symptoms, blood glucose level when symptoms were present, and improvement of symptoms with the increase in blood glucose levels.

Rationales

The diagnosis of hypoglycemia not associated with diabetes mellitus is based on glucose tests as well as three criteria known as the Whipple triad: (1) the presence of symptoms, (2) documentation of low blood glucose when symptoms occur, and (3) improvement of these symptoms when blood glucose rises. The nurse would report symptoms, actions taken, and outcomes, which will assist the primary health care provider in diagnosing the client.

Hypoglycemia not associated with diabetes mellitus can occur with the use of alcohol in chronically malnourished clients or on an empty stomach, and in clients with profound malnutrition, severe liver deficiency, or critical illness, especially with an underlying adrenal insufficiency. Nondiabetes medications can also contribute to hypoglycemia, including beta blockers, quinidine, indomethacin, and trimethoprim/sulfamethoxazole. This client is at risk for hypoglycemia due to adrenal insufficiency (Addison disease) and trimethoprim/sulfamethoxazole prescription for a urinary tract infection.

CJ Cognitive Skill

Prioritize Hypotheses

Reference

Williams, 2018, pp. 990–993

Thinking Exercise 21A-4

Answers

Nursing Action	Indicated	Contraindicated	Non-Essential
Administer 50 g of a carbohydrate.		X	
Consult a registered dietitian nutritionist.	X		
After administering a carbohydrate, recheck blood glucose in 15 minutes.	X		
Teach the client to check capillary blood glucose levels before each meal.			X
Keep the client on bed rest until the hypoglycemic episode resolves.	X		

Rationales

To prevent future hypoglycemia events, the nurse will consult with a registered dietitian nutritionist. Recommended diets for clients without diabetes who experience hypoglycemia differ from a diabetic diet and may consist of complex carbohydrates and increased protein intake. There is no need to teach the client to check capillary blood glucose levels before each meal as this client does not have diabetes mellitus and will not be receiving any insulin. If a hypoglycemia event occurs, the nurse will administer 15 g of a carbohydrate and reassess the client in 15 minutes. Administering more than 15 g is contraindicated as this could cause rebound hyperglycemia. To promote client safety and decrease the risk of falls, the client would be encouraged to remain on bedrest until symptoms of hypoglycemia are resolved.

CJ Cognitive Skill

Generate Solutions

Reference

Williams, 2018, pp. 990–993

Thinking Exercise 21A-5

Answers

Nursing Intervention	Top Three Priority Interventions
Help the client to drink a glass of milk and eat a sandwich.	
Draw blood to assess blood glucose and cortisol levels.	
Administer 50 mL of 50% glucose solution intravenously.	X
Obtain capillary blood glucose level.	X
Position the client in a side-lying position with the neck in a neutral position.	X
Notify the primary health care provider.	

Rationales

Based on the client's recent history, the client is most likely experiencing another episode of hypoglycemia. The nurse will immediately assess the client's capillary blood glucose level at the bedside and administer a source of carbohydrate if the glucose level is low. Because the client is unconscious, the nurse will administer IV glucose instead of oral carbohydrates. The nurse will also place the client in a position that promotes airway patency. Side-lying with a neutral head and neck position is best for an unconscious client. Once the client is safe, the nurse will notify the primary health care provider and draw blood for prescribed diagnostic tests including serum blood glucose and cortisol levels. The nurse will help the client to eat once the client is alert and able to swallow safely.

CJ Cognitive Skill

Take Action

Reference

Williams, 2018, pp. 990–993

Thinking Exercise 21A-6

Answers

A, B, D, G, H

Rationales

The nurse would reinforce teaching focused on recognizing signs of hypoglycemia and actions for prompt treatment. Teaching both the client and the client's family will improve early identification of symptoms (Choice D) and decrease progression to severe hypoglycemia. When the client experiences symptoms of hypoglycemia, the client should ingest 15 g of glucose, which is ½ cup of fruit juice, a full cup of milk (Choice H), or four or five hard candies when beverages are not available (Choice B). The nurse will also reinforce dietary teaching including avoidance of alcohol (Choice G) and ingestion of complex carbohydrates instead of simple sugars (Choice A).

The client does not have an allergy to trimethoprim/sulfamethoxazole. Hypoglycemia is a side effect of this medication; it is not an allergic response. The client is at risk for falls because of neurologic changes secondary to hypoglycemia. Physical therapy cannot assist with this and would not be recommended. Clients with diabetes mellitus are susceptible to injury and poor wound healing. Clients with diabetes are taught to wear appropriate shoes, inspect feet daily, and seek medical care for wounds, blisters, and calluses. This client does not have diabetes and therefore would not need be taught diabetic foot care.

CJ Cognitive Skill

Evaluate Outcomes

Reference

Williams, 2018, pp. 990–993

Thinking Exercise 21A-7

Answers

A, C, D, G

Rationales

Total parenteral nutrition (TPN) is a highly concentrated glucose solution that is administered when the digestive tract cannot be used for feedings. High levels of glucose in the solution cause the pancreas to produce more insulin. When this solution is stopped abruptly, clients typically experience hypoglycemia due to delayed adjustments in the amount of insulin available and being produced. If the TPN bag is completely empty, the nurse will notify the registered nurse immediately for assistance (Choice A) and contact the pharmacy for a new bag of TPN (Choice D). Closely monitoring the client for signs of hypoglycemia (Choice C) and checking the client's capillary blood glucose level (Choice G) will ensure early identification and treatment of hypoglycemia. If the client's blood glucose levels become too low, the nurse will administer a 50% glucose solution intravenously. Oral glucose, such as fruit juice, will not be administered, as the client is receiving TPN and therefore the GI tract may not be available. The nurse will start a 10% dextrose solution until a new bag of TPN is available.

CJ Cognitive Skill

Evaluate Outcomes

Reference

Linton & Matteson, 2020, pp. 709–710, 990–993

Exemplar 21B. Cirrhosis (Medical-Surgical Nursing: Older Adult)

Thinking Exercise 21B-1

Answers

Health History	**Nurses' Notes**	**Vital Signs**	**Laboratory Test Results**

Medical diagnoses

- Spinal disk herniation with diskectomy
- Osteoarthritis
- Hepatic cirrhosis

Social history

- Relationships—widowed, 1 adult child
- Work—retired military
- Alcohol use—prior use = 8–12 beers daily, quit 4 years ago
- Smoking—denies

Medications

- Lactulose 20 g orally three times a day
- Acetaminophen 500 mg orally twice a day
- Propranolol 40 mg orally daily

Rationales

The client's diagnosis of hepatic cirrhosis is relevant to the client's current behavior and appearance. Recognizing that client findings are symptoms of cirrhosis will help the nurse to further analyze if the findings are expected for the disorder or a complication that needs to be addressed. Early signs of cirrhosis are usually subtle and include unexplained fever, fatigue, weight loss, and dull heaviness in the right upper quadrant of the abdomen. Later signs are related to disease progression and include ascites manifesting as a distended large abdomen; jaundice manifesting as yellowish skin; hepatic encephalopathy manifesting as disorientation, agitation, and asterixis (wrist-hand tremors); and hormonal disturbances manifesting as spider angiomas. The client's history of alcohol use is most likely the cause of the cirrhosis and therefore is relevant. The nurse would also recognize medications prescribed for cirrhosis and the client's condition. The client is prescribed lactulose, which eliminates ammonia from the body to decrease symptoms of hepatic encephalopathy, and propranolol, which decreases vascular pressure to prevent complications of portal hypertension.

The client's relationships and work history have no relevance to the client's current behavior or appearance. The client's history of osteoarthritis and spinal disk herniation are also not relevant to the current situation. In addition, the prescribed acetaminophen is most likely taken to manage pain related to these skeletal disorders and is not relevant.

CJ Cognitive Skill

Recognize Cues

Reference

Linton & Matteson, 2020, pp. 770–777

Thinking Exercise 21B-2

Answers

B, C, E, F, H

Rationales

There are multiple complications associated with cirrhosis, but inadequate oxygenation and hemorrhaging are priority complications owing to their life-threatening risks. The nurse will assess for signs of each complication to analyze the client's current situation. Portal hypertension is caused by changes in the liver that obstruct the flow of incoming blood and cause a backup of fluid into the portal system. This backup creates collateral vessels to form in the esophagus, anterior abdominal wall, and rectum. Collateral vessels become distended and engorged with increased pressure and bleed more easily, resulting in GI hemorrhage. Signs of GI bleeding are red or coffee ground emesis (Choice H) and/or black, tarry stools (Choice C). Hemorrhaging also leads to hypotension, tachycardia, tachypnea, pallor, and dizziness or light-headedness (Choice B).

Portal hypertension also leads to the development of ascites, an accumulation of fluid in the peritoneal cavity. As the fluid accumulates, the abdomen presses against the diaphragm, making it more difficult for the client to breathe especially when the client is in semi-Fowler or supine position. The nurse will assess for dyspnea (Choice E), tachycardia, and decreased oxygen saturation (Choice F) to identify respiratory complications secondary to ascites.

CJ Cognitive Skill

Analyze Cues

Reference

Linton & Matteson, 2020, pp. 770–777

Thinking Exercise 21B-3

Answers

The client is ***most likely*** experiencing several complications of cirrhosis. The nurse is most concerned about the client's <u>vital signs</u> and the possibility of <u>GI bleeding</u>.

Rationales

Although all of the client's findings must be addressed, the vital signs indicate a potentially life-threatening condition that the nurse must prioritize. The client's vital signs indicate tachycardia and a borderline low blood pressure. These findings with the client's report of light-headedness indicate that the client is most likely hypovolemic. Based on the client's medical history, the nurse will conclude that GI bleeding is the most likely cause of vital sign changes. The nurse will assess for additional signs of bleeding and initiate treatment to increase fluid volume by contacting the primary health care provider.

CJ Cognitive Skill

Prioritize Hypotheses

Reference

Linton & Matteson, 2020, pp. 770–777

Thinking Exercise 21B-4

Answers

Nursing Action	Indicated	Contraindicated	Non-Essential
Administer the prescribed lactulose.	X		
Assist the client when ambulating to the bathroom.	X		
Provide the client with a meal high in calories, carbohydrates, and vitamins.		X	
Have client lie in a supine position.		X	
Refer the client to Alcoholics Anonymous.			X

Rationales

Although the client is prescribed lactulose, the client's current neurologic assessment indicates he most likely has not been taking the prescription, which decreases ammonia-producing bacteria in the intestines through fecal excretion. Some clients attempt to avoid the discomfort of severe diarrhea by not taking the lactulose when feeling well. However, ammonia levels can increase quickly and decrease the client's ability to effectively reason and make decisions. The nurse would administer the prescribed lactulose dose and then assist the client to the bathroom as needed. The client's vital signs and report of light-headedness increase the client's risk for injury when ambulating. The nurse will need to assist the client to promote safety and decrease potential injury.

The nurse will also help the client to sit in an upright position, which promotes lung expansion by using gravity to lower the distended abdomen. Lying in a supine position would be contraindicated, especially with the client's report of nocturnal dyspnea. A diet high in calories, carbohydrates, and vitamins is usually prescribed to clients who have hepatic cirrhosis. The nurse is concerned that the client may be bleeding internally, and therefore the nurse would not provide a meal at this time. Treatments for GI bleeding include procedures that will require the client to be NPO. Although the client may benefit from participation in a support group such as Alcoholics Anonymous, the client is acutely ill and neurologically impaired. This referral is not relevant at this time, and the client indicated that he quit drinking alcohol 4 years ago.

CJ Cognitive Skill

Generate Solutions

Reference

Linton & Matteson, 2020, pp. 770–777

Thinking Exercise 21B-5

Answers

Responses by the Nurse	Daughter's Questions	Appropriate Response by the Nurse for Each Question
1 "Liver disease can cause fluid to leak into the abdominal cavity, causing it to expand."	"What is causing my father to bleed?"	**7** "GI bleeding occurs when vessels in the esophagus, stomach, or intestines tear. Liver failure causes these vessels to bleed more easily."
2 "Bleeding episodes may be treated with a blood transfusion as well as medications to lower pressure in the liver and improve clotting."	"Why did he faint on the toilet?"	**6** "Syncope is a temporary loss of consciousness due to insufficient blood to the brain. The intestinal bleeding has caused a decrease in blood volume."
3 "Alcoholic beverages are full of calories and sugar, which can lead to weight gain."	"Will he need blood transfusions?"	**2** "Bleeding episodes may be treated with a blood transfusion as well as medications to lower pressure in the liver and improve clotting."
4 "Poor nutrition leads to an ineffective clotting process called thrombocytopenia. This occurs in clients with cirrhosis and promotes GI bleeding."	"My father has always been skinny. Why has he gained so much weight in his belly?"	**1** "Liver disease can cause fluid to leak into the abdominal cavity, causing it to expand."
5 "Blood transfusions may be needed if surgical interventions are not successful."		
6 "Syncope is a temporary loss of consciousness due to insufficient blood to the brain. The intestinal bleeding has caused a decrease in blood volume."		
7 "GI bleeding occurs when vessels in the esophagus, stomach, or intestines tear. Liver failure causes these vessels to bleed more easily."		

Rationales

Clients with cirrhosis are at high risk for hemorrhage due to impaired coagulation and fragile varices. Vessels in the esophagus, stomach, and intestines are distended and fragile owing to portal hypertension and may be triggered to bleed by irritants or increased intra-abdominal pressure. Thrombocytopenia, a low platelet count, is a hematologic disorder associated with cirrhosis, but it is not caused by poor nutrition and does not promote GI bleeding. Hemorrhage increases the client's risk for syncopal events due to deceased blood volume and oxygen-carrying capacity.

Treatment of GI bleeding usually includes IV octreotide, which constricts blood vessels and lowers pressure in the hepatic circulation, as well as blood transfusions, vitamin K, and proton pump inhibitors. In emergency situations surgical procedures may be performed to shunt blood from engorged varices to other veins. Sclerotherapy may also be used to inject a solution that causes varices to harden and close. The use of blood products is based on laboratory results and client findings, not a result of ineffective surgical procedures. The client's weight gain is most likely associated with fluid and sodium retention due to excess aldosterone, and fluid shifting from intravascular space (blood vessels) to interstitial space (third space). Although alcohol use contributed to the development of hepatic cirrhosis, calories from alcohol did not cause the client's ascites or weight gain.

CJ Cognitive Skill

Take Action

Reference

Linton & Matteson, 2020, pp. 770–777

Thinking Exercise 21B-6

Answers

Statements by the Client or His Daughter	Effective	Ineffective	Unrelated
"We will consult the doctor before starting any herbal treatments."	X		
"I will eat a low-protein diet."		X	
"I will monitor my father for any signs of confusion or fatigue."	X		
"We will contact the community resources you provided."	X		
"I will sleep in my recliner because I'm most comfortable there."			X

Rationales

Many medications and herbal treatments are metabolized by the liver, and some are toxic to the liver. The client will be taught to take only medications, including herbal therapies, that are approved by the primary health care provider. The client and his daughter will be taught to notify the primary health care provider regarding increased fluid retention, black tarry stools, bloody vomitus, increased fatigue, and/or confusion. The nurse will provide information about community resources to assist the client and his daughter. These resources may include the American Liver Foundation and home health nursing services.

The client will be taught to eat a balanced diet and follow nutritional guidance provided by the registered dietitian nutritionist (RDN). Protein restrictions, previously prescribed to prevent the accumulation of ammonia, are no longer recommended. The RDN will most likely recommend normal or increased protein to prevent malnutrition. The client may sleep wherever he is comfortable. There are no restrictions on where or how he sleeps.

CJ Cognitive Skill

Evaluate Outcomes

Reference

Linton & Matteson, 2020, pp. 770–777

Thinking Exercise 21B-7

Answers

A, B, D, F, H

Rationales

Ongoing assessments are essential for the nurse to monitor for signs and symptoms of cirrhosis complications including bleeding, ascites, encephalopathy, and renal failure. The nurse will monitor daily weights (Choice A), intake and output, and abdominal girth (Choice F). Good nutrition is essential for regeneration of liver tissue, but clients with cirrhosis have complex nutritional needs as well as difficulty managing fluid and electrolyte imbalances. The nurse will request a consultation with a registered dietitian nutritionist to help manage the client's nutritional needs (Choice D).

Cholestyramine is administered to increase the excretion of bile salts. Bile salts, which are normally processed by the liver, can build up when the liver is not functioning properly. An accumulation of bile salts can lead to salt deposits under the skin, which create intense pruritus. Nursing activities focused on relieving itching of pruritus include gentle bathing with mild soap and tepid water, thorough rinsing, and application of moisturizing lotions (Choice H). Diuretics are administered to treat ascites through the reabsorption and elimination of abdominal cavity fluid. To prevent complications, the nurse will monitor daily weights (Choice A), intake and output, and serum potassium levels. The nurse will also assess for signs of hypokalemia including heart palpitations (Choice B), muscle cramps, and weakness or fatigue.

CJ Cognitive Skill

Take Action

Reference

Linton & Matteson, 2020, pp. 770–777

CHAPTER 22 Coordinated Care *(Medical-Surgical Nursing: Older Adult)*

Answers With Rationales for Thinking Exercises

Thinking Exercise 22-1

Answers

A, B, E, F, G

Rationales

The assistive personnel (AP) are certified nursing assistants who have been educated to record intake and output, feed residents, take vital signs, and perform passive range-of-motion exercises (Choices A, B, E, and F). In addition, AP can use an oral catheter to suction excessive secretions that accumulate in the mouth (Choice G).

CJ Cognitive Skill

Take Action

Reference

Williams, 2018, Chapter 10

Thinking Exercise 22-2

Answers

C, D, F, H

Rationales

The client's stroke caused him to have right-sided weakness and ADL dependence. Therefore he needs physical therapy to help him with mobility skills and eventually ambulation, and occupational therapy to help him learn how to be independent in ADLs (Choices C and F). Because he has difficulty swallowing, he needs to be seen by the speech-language pathologist (SLP) to determine the extent of his dysphagia and what type or consistency of food he can safely have. In addition, the SLP can also assist him with communication (Choice D). The registered dietitian nutritionist would plan the client's diet based on his swallowing assessment (Choice H).

CJ Cognitive Skill

Take Action

Reference

Linton & Matteson, 2020, pp. 402–408

Thinking Exercise 22-3

Answers

As a result of the nurse's conversation with the client, the nurse recognizes that the informed consent was not adequate. Therefore the nurse contacts the surgeon to ensure that the client understands the surgical procedure prior to having his amputation.

Rationales

The client gave consent for the surgery but apparently did not understand the surgical procedure. As a result, the nurse is obligated to contact the surgeon to ensure the client is well informed.

CJ Cognitive Skill

Analyze Cues

Reference

Linton & Matteson, 2020, p. 272

Thinking Exercise 22-4

Answers

The day nurse organizes and prioritizes care by planning to assess Resident 1 and Resident 3 ***first*** to ensure safety.

Rationales

Residents 1 and 3 have had experiences that could have caused injury either at the time of the experience or within the 24 to 48 hours after the experience. For example, Resident 1 experienced a fall, which could cause a cerebral hematoma or other injury that might manifest itself well after the fall. Resident 3 wandered out of the building and could have fallen, causing a delayed injury. Therefore the nurse would check on these residents as the first priority.

CJ Cognitive Skill

Prioritize Hypotheses

Reference

Linton & Matteson, 2020, pp. 195–198, 205–206, 383–385, 402–408

Thinking Exercise 22-5

Answers

Nursing Action	Resident	Appropriate Nursing Action for Resident
1 Perform a finger stick blood glucose (FSBG).	Resident 1	**3** Assess the client's level of consciousness for change from baseline.
2 Determine the client's mental status and compare with baseline.	Resident 2	**6** Confirm that the client will begin physical and occupational therapy today.
3 Assess the client's level of consciousness for change from baseline.	Resident 3	**2** Determine the client's mental status and compare with baseline.
4 Perform a skin assessment for integrity.	Resident 4	**4** Perform a skin assessment for integrity.
5 Monitor the client's blood pressure every 4 hours today.	Resident 5	**7** Perform a neurologic assessment for new symptoms.
6 Confirm that the client will begin physical and occupational therapy today.		
7 Perform a neurologic assessment for new symptoms.		

Rationales

Resident 1 experienced a fall last night and should be followed up by means of neurologic assessments for the next few days, especially the level of consciousness (LOC). The first indication of neurologic decline is a change in LOC. Resident 2 was admitted for rehabilitation services, and therefore the nurse would check that these therapies begin as soon as possible. Resident 3 has moderate-stage Alzheimer disease, which means that her mental/cognitive status will likely fluctuate and she may have periods of lucidity. Resident 4's pressure injury is likely due to her impaired nutritional state, and she is at risk for additional tissue breakdown. Therefore the nurse would perform a skin assessment to monitor for further tissue integrity problems. Resident 5 was admitted after a transient ischemic attack (TIA) last evening. Although the client has a history of hypertension, the nurse's priority is frequent monitoring for new neurologic symptoms indicating another TIA or a stroke.

CJ Cognitive Skill

Generate Solutions

Reference

Linton & Matteson, 2020, pp. 195–198, 205–206, 383–385, 402–408

Thinking Exercise 22-6

Answers

Potential Client Discharge Activity	Appropriate for the Nurse to Perform	Not Appropriate for the Nurse to Perform
Assist in completing the agency transfer form.	X	
Reinforce discharge health teaching.	X	
Obtain informed consent.		X
Perform medication reconciliation.	X	
Check on client transportation to the rehabilitation facility.	X	
Notify the client's family or designee about the planned transfer.	X	

Rationales

All of these activities are important for the nurse to implement for a successful transfer to another health care agency, except that there is no indication for informed consent to be obtained. Informed consent is not part of the nurse's role at any time.

CJ Cognitive Skill

Generate Solutions

Reference

Linton & Matteson, 2020, pp. 859–862

Thinking Exercise 22-7

Answers

B, C, D, E

Rationales

The nurse would recognize that the client may be experiencing fluid overload from the transfusion and would stop the transfusion immediately (Choice E). Because the client is having respiratory distress, the nurse would prepare to administer supplemental oxygen and report the findings to the RN to transfer the client's care in this potential emergency (Choices B and D). The nurse would also document the client's findings and actions taken to care for the client at this time (Choice C).

CJ Cognitive Skill

Take Action

Reference

Linton & Matteson, 2020, p. 539

Thinking Exercise 22-8

Answers

B, F, G, H

Rationales

The charge nurse is responsible for a large 48-bed nursing unit and has to make the decisions about how best to ensure that the residents' needs are met. The LPN is a new graduate who has been designated as a medication nurse. However, the LPN would not be physically able to administer multiple medications to all 48 residents but could perhaps give them to 30 or so residents. The charge nurse could also help with the medication pass. Both nurses would want to supervise the CNA staff (Choice B). If there is time, the charge nurse might assign the new LPN to monitor the tube feedings, suction the resident's old, well-established tracheostomy, and maintain oxygen therapy as ordered (Choices F, G, and H).

CJ Cognitive Skill

Generate Solutions

Reference

Williams, 2018, Chapter 10

CHAPTER 23 **Pharmacology** *(Medical-Surgical Nursing: Older Adult)*

Answers With Rationales for Thinking Exercises

Thinking Exercise 23-1

Answers

A, C

Rationales

The client has a low blood pressure (systolic less than 100 mm Hg), and her heart rate is at the lower end of the normal heart rate range. Therefore the nurse would hold amlodipine and losartan because they are given for hypertension. One of the side effects of both drugs is hypotension. Given that the client is already hypotensive, the nurse would not want to give medication that would worsen this problem.

CJ Cognitive Skill

Take Action

Reference

McCuistion et al., 2021, pp. 492, 524–526

Thinking Exercise 23-2

Answers

The nurse recognizes ***priority*** health teaching needs, including reinforcing the need for the client to have laboratory testing to monitor <u>thyroid-stimulating hormone</u> levels due to being on levothyroxine and <u>electrolyte</u> levels due to being on HCTZ.

Rationales

Clients receiving levothyroxine must take this medication as lifelong treatment for hypothyroidism. The client needs to have frequent monitoring of thyroid-stimulating hormone (TSH) levels so that the dosing of her medication can be adjusted as needed. An elevated TSH level indicates that there is a need to stimulate the thyroid gland to release more thyroxine into the bloodstream. In this case the dose of levothyroxine would need to be increased because the client still has an underactive thyroid gland. Conversely, a below-normal TSH level indicates that there is more than adequate serum thyroxine and the dose of levothyroxine may need to be decreased. HCTZ is a diuretic that can cause sodium and potassium depletion. Therefore these electrolyte levels need to be monitored.

CJ Cognitive Skill

Prioritize Hypotheses

Reference

McCuistion et al., 2021, pp. 503, 613

Thinking Exercise 23-3

Answers

A, B, E, F, G, H

Rationales

The nurse would teach the client the need to take all medication doses because two of the drugs are antibiotics to treat the infection (Choice A). However, many antibiotics can cause GI distress, especially nausea and diarrhea, which can cause dehydration in a client over 65 years of age (Choice B). Pantoprazole is a proton pump inhibitor that can cause loss of magnesium and bone loss. Therefore the client should have a baseline serum magnesium and bone density for comparison after the drug regimen is discontinued (Choices E and F). Pantoprazole also decreases gastric pH, which can predispose older adults to pneumonia (Choice G). Alcohol can cause a severe interaction with metronidazole, including possible vomiting, severe headache, and seizures. The nurse would teach the importance of avoiding alcohol while the client is taking this drug (Choice H).

CJ Cognitive Skill

Take Action

Reference

McCuistion et al., 2021, pp. 568–569

Thinking Exercise 23-4

Answers

B, C, D, E, F

Rationales

Most drugs given to clients for management of rheumatoid arthritis affect the immune response and can cause infection. Therefore the nurse teaches the client to avoid crowds and people who have infection (Choice B and D). Hydroxychloroquine is an antimalarial drug that helps decrease joint inflammation, but it can cause retinal damage. Therefore the nurse reminds the client to have frequent eye examinations (Choice C). MTX can cause bone marrow suppression and damage to the liver, lungs, and kidneys. Therefore the client needs to follow up with all laboratory testing to monitor for these changes (Choice E). MTX is taken weekly and should be taken on the same day and time each week to maintain serum drug levels (Choice F).

CJ Cognitive Skill

Take Action

Reference

McCuistion et al., 2021, pp. 359, 601

Thinking Exercise 23-5

Answers

Client Finding	Effective	Ineffective	Unrelated
States she is feeling stronger today	X		
Temperature = 97.2°F (36.2°C)	X		
States that she has no more "night sweats"	X		
Has a productive cough		X	
Reports frequent indigestion after meals			X
Reports having no chest discomfort	X		

Rationales

The client condition has improved, but she still has a productive cough. Her report of indigestion is not related to the management of pneumonia.

CJ Cognitive Skill

Evaluate Outcomes

Reference

McCuistion et al., 2021, pp. 324–325

Thinking Exercise 23-6

Answers

Based on the client's morning FSBG value, the nurse would give <u>22</u> units of NPH insulin and <u>3</u> units of regular insulin at 7:30 a.m. (0730). Because of the peak action of NPH insulin, the nurse would monitor the client for hypoglycemia beginning at <u>11:30 a.m. (1130)</u>.

Rationales

The client has an order for NPH insulin 22 units to be given every morning before breakfast. Based on his current FSBG value of 198 mg/dL, the nurse would also administer 3 units of regular insulin according to the prescribed sliding scale. The peak action of NPH insulin is 4 to 8 hours, so the nurse would begin to monitor for a significant drop in blood sugar at 11:30 a.m. If the client eats an adequate breakfast, his blood sugar should not become too low as a result of the additional regular insulin dose.

CJ Cognitive Skill

Analyze Cues

Reference

McCuistion et al., 2021, pp. 623–627

Thinking Exercise 23-7

Answers

A. Client's Drugs	B. Drug Class	C. Correct Drug for Drug Class
1 Fluoxetine	Antiepileptic drug	**2** Gabapentin
2 Gabapentin	Cardiac glycoside	**4** Digoxin
3 Baclofen	Dopaminergic drug	**5** Carbidopa/levodopa
4 Digoxin	Nonsteroidal anti-inflammatory drug	**6** Celecoxib
5 Carbidopa/levodopa	Antispasmodic drug	**3** Baclofen
6 Celecoxib	Antidepressant drug	**1** Fluoxetine

CJ Cognitive Skill

Take Action

Reference

McCuistion et al., 2021, pp. 222–223, 230–231, 246–247, 267, 279–281, 485–486

References

Ignatavicius, D. D., Workman, M. L., Rebar, C. R., & Heimgartner, N. M. (2021). *Medical-surgical nursing: Concepts for interprofessional collaborative care* (10th ed.). St. Louis: Elsevier.

Leifer, G. (2019). *Introduction to maternity and pediatric nursing.* (8th ed.). St. Louis: Elsevier.

Linton, A. D. & Matteson, M. A. (2020). *Medical-surgical nursing.* (7th ed.). St. Louis: Elsevier.

McCuistion, L .E., DiMaggio, K. V., Winton, M. B., & Yeager, J. J. (2021). *Pharmacology: A patient-centered nursing process approach.* (10th ed.). St. Louis: Elsevier.

Morrison-Valfre, M. (2017). *Foundations of mental health care.* (6th ed.). St. Louis: Elsevier.

Williams, P. A. (2018). *deWit's Fundamental concepts and skills for nursing.* (5th ed.). St. Louis: Elsevier.